The Mechanics of Sports Injuries

Sports Injuries

An Osteopathic Approach

The Mechanics of Sports Injuries

An Osteopathic Approach

Cynthia Tucker
DO, MRO

Illustrated by T. K. Deoora
DO(Hons), MRO

OXFORD

Blackwell Scientific Publications

LONDON EDINBURGH BOSTON
MELBOURNE PARIS BERLIN VIENNA

Blackwell Scientific Publications
Editorial offices:
Osney Mead, Oxford OX2 0EL
25 John Street, London WC1N 2BL
23 Ainslie Place, Edinburgh EH3 6AJ
3 Cambridge Center, Suite 208
  Cambridge, Massachusetts 02142,
USA
54 University Street, Carlton
  Victoria 3053, Australia

First published 1990

Set by Setrite Typesetters Ltd
Printed and bound in Great Britain by
Cambridge University Press,
Cambridge

DISTRIBUTORS

Marston Book Services Ltd
PO Box 87
Oxford OX2 0DT
(*Orders*: Tel: 0865 791155
        Fax: 0865 791927
        Telex: 837515)

USA
  Year Book Medical Publishers
  200 North LaSalle Street
  Chicago, Illinois 60601
  (*Orders*: Tel: (312) 726−9733)

Canada
  The C.V. Mosby Company
  5240 Finch Avenue East
  Scarborough, Ontario
  (*Orders*: Tel: (416) 298−1588)

Australia
  Blackwell Scientific Publications
  (Australia) Pty Ltd
  54 University Street
  Carlton, Victoria 3053
  (*Orders*: Tel: (03) 347−0300)

British Library
Cataloguing in Publication Data
Tucker, Cynthia
  The mechanics of sports injuries.
  1. Sports & games. Injuries. Therapy
  I. Title
  617'.1027

ISBN 0−632−02583−2

Contents

Foreword by Sebastian Coe and Peter Coe   vii

Preface   ix

Acknowledgements   xi

1 Osteopathy   1

2 General Health   12

3 Why Do Injuries Occur?   24

4 Classification of the Different Types of Injury   32

5 Tissue Injuries   46

6 The Shoulder Girdle   76

7 The Elbow   101

8 The Wrist and the Hand   118

9 The Hip and the Thigh   137

10 The Knee Joint   157

11 The Lower Leg   185

12 The Ankle   207

13 The Foot   221

14 The Head and the Neck   244

15 The Thorax, Ribs and Diaphragm   277

16 The Lumbar Area and Abdomen   301

17 The Pelvis, Sacrum and Coccyx   321

18 Various Sports and their Commonly Related Injuries   340

19 Psychological Problems of Sport   380

20 In Attendance at a Sporting Event   386

Index   391

Foreword

by Sebastian Coe and Peter Coe

Sport at the highest level is extremely demanding. It requires tremendous application in both intensity and duration. Getting to the top is hard, staying there is even harder. The intensity is the quality of the training and the duration is your competitive life in the sport. Yet these two elements are simultaneously your essentials and your enemy.

In distance running, the statistics show that the average age at which the top ten male milers achieved their best performances was 27.8 years, with women achieving their best at 25.8 years. Thus a coach should have as his prime objective the maintenance of his young charges who may be only 12 or 14 years of age and must have no serious injuries for as long as 15 years if they are to achieve their full potential.

If they intend to stay at the top for another five years then it should not need pointing out (although unhappily it does) that the coach and the athlete should develop a very thorough maintenance programme, the best of which is a preventive one.

We work in a sport which demands thousands of hours training, most of which is running. But if running is defined as very long repetitions of a rather narrow range of movements with an awful lot of impact stress, then we are also defining a programme with a high risk of overuse injuries. Structures are easily damaged by combined stresses such as bending and torsion or with repeated applications of impact stress, something we expect to do in running and frequently without much thought.

The sedentary person with an acute injury might limp around on it until it gets better and perhaps get away with it. An athlete in hard training will not, he will only aggravate the injury. Frequently athletes will return again and again to the poor physiotherapist for relief. Not being a magician he cannot cure them until the fundamental cause is removed. If any active person continues exercising they will be obliged to favour the injury to relieve the pain, but all that they will be doing will be structural damage leading to a chronic condition. It can be a very long process indeed to repair such damage.

Structural changes are not easy to spot with an untrained eye. Many youngsters have developed a tilted pelvis which has remained undetected, but the ensuing pain when training has manifested itself. Similarly it needs only a slight misalignment of the spine to limit activity and to give rise to much lower back pain. Those in endurance events need to take as much care as those in contact sports if they want to avoid the services of the orthopaedic surgeon.

We first came to osteopathy to remedy a back problem that, quite frankly, should not have been allowed to develop. (Black mark to the coach.) Not surprisingly, it is now an essential part of our maintenance programme.

Good osteopathy is not only receiving treatment. An osteopath will also give you good advice on avoiding the condition for which you are being treated and can often detect the signs of impending trouble. Good coaches and athletes should have the arrows of osteopathy and massage in their quiver of medical backup − it can lessen the need for far more drastic treatment later. We know, we have been together in sport for 20 years, 14 of them at the top, and we freely acknowledge the invaluable help that we have received from the author in the art and science of osteopathy.

Sebastian Coe
Peter Coe

Preface

Sport should be enjoyed at all levels but true enjoyment can only be experienced by thoroughly fit athletes. Their bodies need to be capable of physical activity without suffering stress or damage. The body's efficiency can be lowered psychologically, dietetically, chemically, by infection, or mechanically. Emphasis in this book is on the mechanical and structural problems which can affect the efficiency of the human machine.

Throughout the text I use the word 'athlete' to cover all sports-persons, not only those involved in track and field events. I also use the pronoun 'he' to include members of both sexes.

The largest body system is the musculoskeletal. All others respond to its demands. For example, the heart rate and respiratory rate increase greatly during exercise. A disorder in one body system can affect another, but it is the sport-related musculo-skeletal problems seen in clinical practice which are dealt with in this book.

A body which is working efficiently is responsive to physical stress. Generally if it can cope with the physical stress of sport it can also withstand those stresses of day-to-day living.

Before any injury can be treated it has to be diagnosed correctly and the cause found. Each athlete must have a thorough examination and the injury related to the whole body and never isolated from it, as well as being related to the specific sport. This ensures that any predisposing factors are noted, such as a difference in leg lengths giving rise to a lateral spinal distortion (scoliosis). Body types vary, some being less suitable to particular sports than others. Noting these points is helpful when considering the athlete as a whole.

Although injuries are described separately, it is important to remember that they frequently occur in multiples, one problem complicating another and one region being stressed as a result of a problem elsewhere.

An injured athlete is often told 'to give up sport'. This can cause considerable psychological damage. Once there is an improvement in the physical condition the psychological change can be dramatic. Athletes are keen to 'get fit' again; their recovery is often swift and they will cooperate more than most patients. The danger lies in athletes being overkeen to return to sport; they are often reluctant to give their bodies enough time to recover completely. As a practitioner one has to be very strict on this point as good work must never be undone for the sake of a few more days rest. It helps to overestimate the recovery time when first giving the athlete a prognosis, so he will be delighted when he returns to sport sooner than he had anticipated!

There are, of course, limitations to all forms of treatment and osteopathy is no exception. Yes, some athletes will need to be referred to other practitioners − possibly for surgery. I have included guidelines on the need for referral where relevant.

My intention is to share with my colleagues the valuable experience which I have gained in the treatment of athletic injuries. These have occurred in athletes at international, club and fun levels many of whom had been advised to 'give up' but were able to continue sport.

Acknowledgements

My sincere thanks to all those who have given me encouragement and practical help, in alphabetical order. Martin Barlow, Alfred Chan, Margaret Emmans, Alan Gayfer, David Haslam, Chris Horrod, Ros Lake, Ethel Mason, Denise Parnell, Jonathan Smith and to my colleagues who are all registered osteopaths, Gloria John, Ian Collinge, Vaughan Cooper, Ros Foster, Gerry Gajad-harsingh, Andrew Harwich, Fiona Hendry, Denise Markovic, Elizabeth Rhattigan, Paul Stamp and to my future colleagues, Ruth Coventry, Simon Curtis and Kevin McGhee.

Without their help I would have been unable to produce this book. My special thanks go to my colleague Tajinder Deoora who has been responsible for the illustrations.

Chapter 1   Osteopathy

1.1   Definition

Osteopathy is a system of manual skills which are used both in diagnosis and treatment. It lays much emphasis on the structural framework of the body, especially in the way it functions.

Osteopaths contend that much of the disability and pain which people suffer stems from abnormalities in the function of the body framework (the musculoskeletal system), rather than from various disease processes which are collectively known as pathologies. The musculoskeletal system is the largest system in the body and enables us to move about. The visceral system provides nourishment to it and removes waste products as well as enabling damage to be repaired. The third system of the body is the nervous system which keeps the other two systems informed of each other's needs and condition. In health, all three systems work in perfect harmony and the body is said to be in 'good health'. This is total body health.

1.2   Basic principles

Osteopaths are concerned with the integrity of the musculoskeletal system and the mechanical disorders which frequently occur within it. Mechanical problems can result from disturbances such as incorrect posture, old injuries, athletic strains, occupational stresses, wear and tear, mental stress, malnutrition, vascular insufficiency, any condition which reduces the mechanical integrity of the musculoskeletal system. Osteopaths also believe that such stresses can have a widespread effect elsewhere in the body through the nervous system in a reflex way. Treatment is aimed at the musculoskeletal system but the effect can also be elsewhere. A common complaint is pain in the leg but the root of this problem may be in the spine where treatment is needed and the leg symptoms thus relieved.

Alternatively pain in the leg may be due to a local problem and this in turn may be related to trouble elsewhere, so differential diagnosis is vitally important when assessing any condition. Why are so many clinical conditions recurrent? The answer may be due to a repeated strain or to some predisposing factor which must be recognised and dealt with if present.

Inherent healing ability of the body

Osteopathy was founded in America in 1874 by Dr Andrew Taylor Still who was a doctor in a small frontier town in the mid-west. He realised that one of the principles of osteopathy was that 'structure governs function' which is as true today as it was then. This means that if the body is working correctly mechanically, there will be minimal stress on the musculoskeletal system and muscles and joints will be subject to minimal tension. The second principle which Still realised is that the body has the power to heal itself. This ability will depend on the mechanical integrity of the moving and supporting structures.

A common complaint is pain in the hamstrings which probably started while running. On questioning the patient carefully, it develops that there is a history of a previous low back problem which may have led to an area of faulty mechanics in the lumbar spine or pelvis where there may be loss of normal mobility in one or more joints. The additional stress on the hamstrings as a result of this mechanical fault may not only have led to the immediate strain but will impede healing and lay the patient open to further trouble. For healing to occur as perfectly as possible the previous injury must be dealt with, and then the body's in-built healing ability can be fully released.

Structure governs function − function governs comfort

Pain is the complaint which causes more patients to seek advice than anything else. In the absence of pathology it is usually due to faulty function, certainly as far as the musculo-skeletal system is concerned. Scoliosis and excessive anteroposterior curves are often seen in practice but the patient may have no symptoms if these apparent abnormalities are functioning well. If, however, the patient strains his spine he may well suffer pain, but the symptoms are as a result of the strain and not necessarily due to the underlying deformity. The practitioner has to decide whether or not the strain was predisposed by the deformity as this could have an adverse effect on the function of the spine. Just as function governs comfort, so dysfunction governs discomfort.

Osteopathic treatment is structured to the individual requirements of the patient and is designed to improve the function of the parts of the musculoskeletal system so that the inherent healing ability of the body can conduct itself unimpeded by structural faults. However, osteopathy is not a panacea for all ills and has certain limitations. There are also times when alternative therapies are preferable.

1.5

Osteopathic training

The General Council and Register of Osteopaths was set up in 1936 on the recommendation of the Minister of Health. Membership is open to graduates of the several schools of osteopathy which are recognised by the GCRO. The level of training has to conform to the high standards required for professional registration – 'MRO'. The training course is four years full-time. Entrance requirements are the same as those needed to enter colleges of further education elsewhere, viz, usually three A levels. The subjects needed are the sciences and/or mathematics with variations for mature students. Tables 1.1 and 1.2 show the components of the course and assessment schedules typical of one of the recognised schools.

Osteopathic concepts are not at variance with medical teaching. Many of the medical subjects are taught by registered medical practitioners while the osteopathic subjects are taught by registered osteopaths.

The early part of the course covers the basic sciences and is designed to prepare the students for clinical work in the outpatients' clinics which are attached to the various schools. There is great emphasis on anatomy, especially surface anatomy and much time is spent on the osteopathic examination of the patient as a whole and of individual joint and associated soft tissue integrity.

Technique classes are held at all levels of the course starting with basic handling and advancing to more complicated treatment techniques. Great emphasis is placed on safety throughout. Gradually the osteopathic student develops a 'tissue sense' and can assess the condition of various different parts of the body by careful palpation.

The clinical course is the longest part of the training and more than 1500 hours are spent in the training school clinics by the students before graduation. There are general and specialised clinics and students gain experience in all of these, which deal with both adults and children. Senior students are supervised by clinical tutors as they treat patients themselves, the tutors providing assistance where needed. Throughout the clinical course the students are assessed on their osteopathic skills and their developing professionalism.

By the end of the gruelling four year course the young graduate is capable of dealing with the problems he will face in practice. He will be able to carry out a complete examination, give a diagnosis and suggest suitable treatment, osteopathic or any other which he feels will accelerate the recovery of the patient. He will be able to give a prognosis and any advice on supports, exercises or diet, etc.

Table 1.1   The components of the osteopathy course of one of the recognised schools.

Topic	Year One			Year Two			Year Three			Year Four		
	1	2	3	4	5	6	7	8	9	10	11	12
Anatomy − regional; Myology; Osteology; Arthrology	█	█	█	█								
Embryology	█	█	█									
Physiology	█	█	█	█								
Quantitative methods		█	█									
History of osteopathy	█											
Introduction to technique and diagnosis	█	█	█									
Technique				█	█	█	█	█	█	█	█	█
Applied technique				█	█	█	█	█	█	█	█	█
Osteopathic diagnosis					█	█	█	█	█			
Osteopathic principles					█	█	█					
Applied anatomy physiology and pathology of osteopathic practice					█	█	█	█	█			
Pathology Gastro-intestinal disorders; orthopaedics and rheumatology; neurology; clinical emergencies; nutrition and dietetics; cardiovascular and respiratory diseases; ear, nose and throat; dermatology; obstetrics; gynaecology; urinary tract diseases; endocrinology.					█	█	█	█	█			
Clinical osteopathy					█	█	█	█	█	█	█	█
Clinical methods					█	█	█	█	█			
Medical statistics							█					
Clinical psychology					█	█						
Radiodiagnosis					█						█	
Business studies											█	
Osteopathic care of children								█				
Applied psychology												█

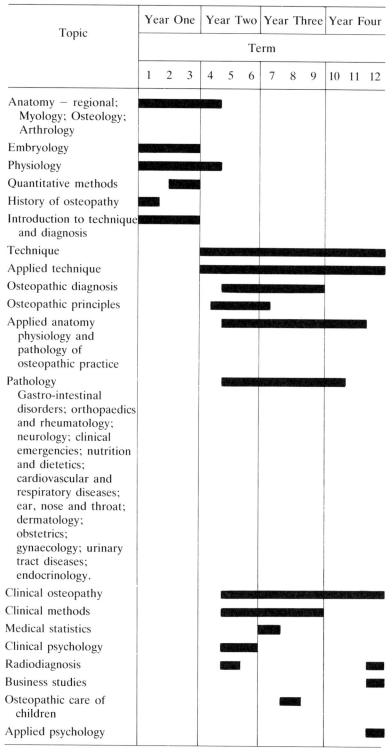

Adapted from The British School of Osteopathy Syllabus

Table 1.2 The assessment schedule of the osteopathy course of one of the recognised schools.

Topic	Year One			Year Two			Year Three			Year Four		
	1	2	3	4	5	6	7	8	9	10	11	12
Anatomy − regional; Myology; Osteology; Arthrology	■	■	■	▶								
Embryology	■	■	■	▶								
Physiology	■	■	■	▶								
Quantitative methods	■	■	■	▶								
History of osteopathy												
Introduction to technique and diagnosis												
Technique	■	■	■	■	■	■	■	▶	■	■	■	▶
Applied technique												
Osteopathic diagnosis	■	■	■	■	■	■	■	■	▶			
Osteopathic principles	■	■	■	■	■	■	▶					
Applied anatomy physiology and pathology of osteopathic practice	■	■	■	■	■	■	■	■	■	■	■	▶
Pathology Gastro-intestinal disorders; orthopaedics and rheumatology; neurology; clinical emergencies; nutrition and dietetics; cardiovascular and respiratory diseases; ear, nose and throat; dermatology; obstetrics; gynaecology; urinary tract diseases; endocrinology.	■	■	■	■	■	■	■	■	■	■	▶	
Clinical osteopathy	■	■	■	■	■	■	■	■	■	■	■	▶
Clinical methods												
Medical statistics	■	■	■	■	■	■	■	▶				
Clinical psychology												
Radiodiagnosis	■	■	■	■	■	■	■	■	■	■	■	▶
Business studies												
Osteopathic care of children												
Applied psychology												

Adapted from The British School of Osteopathy Syllabus

1.6   **The osteopathic dimension**

Osteopathic skill can be acquired only by years of diligent practice based on thorough training. A sophisticated palpatory sense is developed by repetitive practice and involves precision timing, localisation, a sense of tissue tension and accuracy together with speed when applying a specific force through a joint. The speed or 'high velocity' as it is more usually called, must also be given at low amplitude to avoid injury to the joint concerned. All this is very specialised and is the osteopath's armoury. The examination of any one joint consists of a unique method of mobility testing. Each joint has an accepted range of movement in any one direction. Experience will guide the osteopath as to whether this is reduced or excessive. The joint is tested in all its ranges both actively and passively. Any deviation from normal can thus be detected. At the same time the condition of the surrounding soft tissues will be examined. Any distinction between normal and abnormal soft tissue tone may be slight but a well developed sense of palpation will reveal this difference to the osteopath if it is present. These abnormalities of tissues will alter the function of that tissue and this is reassessed after treatment has been given when there should be a palpable change and associated improvement.

Any abnormality within the musculoskeletal system has to be related to the function of that system as a whole and never isolated from it. An injury in the foot will result in some abnormality of gait. This in turn can affect the weight distribution of the body and can lead to problems elsewhere. Even a painful arm can result in it being carried awkwardly, resulting in increased tension in the muscles of the shoulder girdle and neck. Osteopaths will always examine the patient as a whole and consider the immediate symptoms as part of the complete body, never isolating them from the whole person.

1.7   **Osteopathic examination**

Osteopaths begin examination of the patient the moment they see him for the first time, probably as the patient walks into the treatment room. How is the patient weight bearing? Does he seem to be symmetrical right and left? They note the physical build, sex and age and general tension of the patient. Is this tension due to apprehension? Does the patient appear to be in pain? If so, is it extreme?

After taking the personal details, name, address, age, occupation, leisure activities, marital state, number of children, height and weight, the practitioner will need to know why the patient has come for advice, the history of the complaint and duration and any variations which have occurred. Is the patient aware of the causes of such variations? Is the pain localised or does it radiate? What are the aggravating and relieving factors? What treatment or advice has the patient already received? What were the effects of this? In this way the osteopath will build up a picture of the patient as a whole and of the specific clinical condition with which he presents.

There is emphasis on the general health of the patient: does the remainder of the body function normally? Has the patient been subjected to excessive stress recently? Has there been previous trouble in the area and if so was it similar to the present problem? Is there a history of previous injury or accident which may have caused tissue damage? What treatment did the patient receive for this? A thorough history will guide the osteopath to the probable cause of the patient's symptoms but the diagnosis will follow the clinical examination.

Initially the patient will be asked to stand up and the osteopath will look at him from the rear, side and front, noting any obvious abnormalities. Is the patient carrying his weight evenly? Are there excessive or reduced curves in the spine? Is there a scoliosis present; if so does there appear to be a leg length discrepancy? Are the shoulders level? Is the head held straight? Are there any areas where the muscle development seems excessive or reduced? This examination is carried out with the patient wearing one layer of underclothes. Any skin discolouration is noted.

Next the patient is asked to carry out active movements. Assuming there is a low back problem, the patient is asked to bend forward, backwards, sideways to right and left and to rotate to both right and left. The range of movement is noted and the quality of that movement as well as the quantity. Any pain is noted and at what point that pain comes on and/or subsides. The examination so far is purely one of observation by the practitioner. The tone of various muscles is noted and at this point the osteopath will probably feel this, noting any differences for example between the right and left hamstring muscles. He may want to check for any wasting which appears to be present. He may even use a tape measure to detect the difference in the muscle bulk of the two limbs while the patient is weight bearing. If there is involvement of an extremity joint any obvious differences between that and the one on the unaffected side of the body is noted. Active movements of this joint may be carried out in the standing position, e.g. of the shoulder joint. In the sitting position active movements may be assessed, it is easier to examine the neck this way. Any alteration in weight bearing is noted in the sitting position as the 'base' of the body now becomes the pelvis whereas it was the feet when the patient stood. This examination is especially important if the patient has a sedentary occupation as this is the position he most frequents. Throughout, the osteopath notes how the body tissues react to the particular movement the patient is carrying out and the general comfort of the patient.

Passive examination of the joints follows. Usually the patient is lying down. In the lumbar area, flexion, extension, side-bending to right and left are examined with the patient side-lying and rotation with the patient sitting up. The quality of the movement at each spinal level as well as the quantity of movement is noted. The state of the surrounding soft tissues is palpated and any areas of unusual tone or local oedema is felt and noted. Should there be any referral of symptoms, this is also noted, be they caused by gentle pressure or by any passive movement. All other joints of the body are examined along routine orthopaedic lines but emphasis is always placed on the condition of the surrounding soft tissues which are palpated with great care. The palpatory sense of the osteopath is highly refined after years of experience.

Should there be need for further clinical examination, for example of the central nervous system, cardiovascular system, blood or urine tests or X-rays, these will be carried out along established clinical lines.

The purpose of an examination is to reach a diagnosis and then to decide the best treatment for the patient. By the end of this examination the osteopath should be able to give a diagnosis, outline a treatment plan and give the patient a prognosis, both short-and long-term.

| 1.8 | **Head zones** |

From each spinal level nerves pass to specific parts of the body with only minor variations of pattern. Osteopathy aims to restore normal mobility to joints and to relieve abnormal tension in the surrounding tissues. The effect of this is twofold: firstly the local discomfort is relieved and the body is able to adapt once more to it's environment, and secondly the possibility of referred symptoms via the nervous system is lessened. We have already discussed the effect of a mechanical disturbance within the spine and the way it can cause nerve irritation. Figures 1.1 and 1.2 show the spinal levels associated with the various areas of the body.

Osteopaths believe that there is a reflex pathway both from the spine to the various organs and in reverse. A great deal of work has been carried out in the USA at the Texas College of Osteopathic Medicine especially by Professor Irwin Korr, showing this to be true. He has also shown that interference of the nerve pathway can lead to dysfunction of organs. If this is true and the pathway runs both ways then it must be possible to improve disturbed organ function by restoring normal spinal mechanics. We are back to the truism that structure governs function, which can be local or distant in its effect.

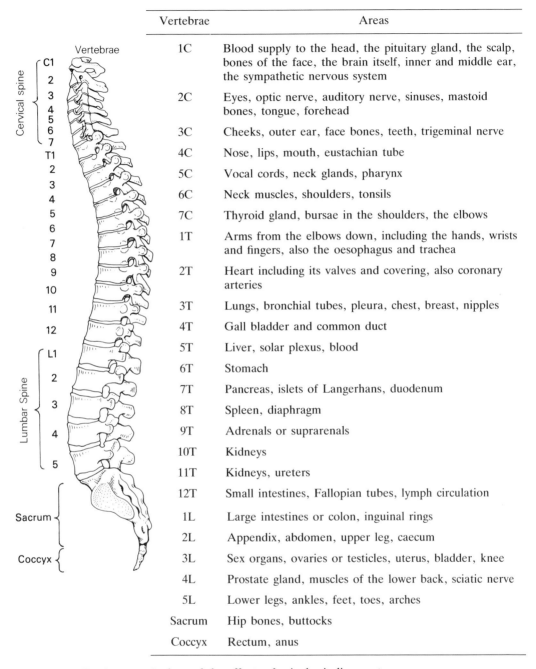

Vertebrae	Areas
1C	Blood supply to the head, the pituitary gland, the scalp, bones of the face, the brain itself, inner and middle ear, the sympathetic nervous system
2C	Eyes, optic nerve, auditory nerve, sinuses, mastoid bones, tongue, forehead
3C	Cheeks, outer ear, face bones, teeth, trigeminal nerve
4C	Nose, lips, mouth, eustachian tube
5C	Vocal cords, neck glands, pharynx
6C	Neck muscles, shoulders, tonsils
7C	Thyroid gland, bursae in the shoulders, the elbows
1T	Arms from the elbows down, including the hands, wrists and fingers, also the oesophagus and trachea
2T	Heart including its valves and covering, also coronary arteries
3T	Lungs, bronchial tubes, pleura, chest, breast, nipples
4T	Gall bladder and common duct
5T	Liver, solar plexus, blood
6T	Stomach
7T	Pancreas, islets of Langerhans, duodenum
8T	Spleen, diaphragm
9T	Adrenals or suprarenals
10T	Kidneys
11T	Kidneys, ureters
12T	Small intestines, Fallopian tubes, lymph circulation
1L	Large intestines or colon, inguinal rings
2L	Appendix, abdomen, upper leg, caecum
3L	Sex organs, ovaries or testicles, uterus, bladder, knee
4L	Prostate gland, muscles of the lower back, sciatic nerve
5L	Lower legs, ankles, feet, toes, arches
Sacrum	Hip bones, buttocks
Coccyx	Rectum, anus

Fig. 1.1   Head zones. A chart of the effects of spinal misalignments.

1.9   **Pathology**

Pathologies are not often seen in athletes. They must be suspected if a trivial injury gives rise to extreme symptoms, or if the patient appears to be generally unwell. Any possibility of bone or joint pathology must have further investigation immediately.

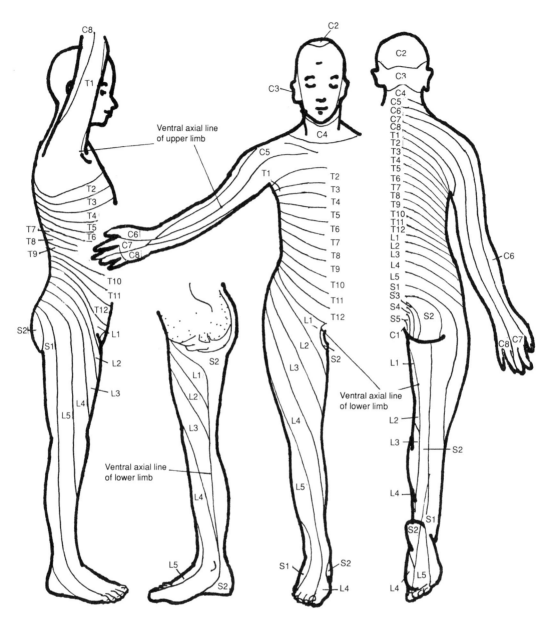

Fig. 1.2   Dermatomes of the body.
(From *Grants Atlas of Anatomy* by James Anderson.)

Fracture

Pathological fractures are of two types: in apparently normal bone they are stress fractures while others occur in abnormal bone.

Stress fractures are considered to be the result of repeated compression of bone — as in the pars interarticularis of L5 in fast bowlers — or extreme muscular action. The common sites are the pars interarticularis, pubic rami, shaft of the tibia, shaft of the fibula, patella, calcaneum, metatarsals (especially 2nd) and the shaft of the humerus (especially in adolescents taking part in throwing sports). There is often a history of strenuous exercise. Pain is felt at the site of fracture with possible redness and swelling. Pain will be exaggerated if the bone is subjected to passive bending and X-rays usually show the lesion.

Pathological fractures occur in otherwise abnormal bone. The stresses of exercise may precipitate such an injury and may be the first sign of an underlying disease of the bone. Although the likelihood is small, the possibility must always be considered of conditions such as Paget's disease, post-traumatic disuse, cyst, osteomalacia, osteoporosis, osteomyelitis, secondary deposits, hyperparathyroidism or tumours of either bone or cartilage. Also, osteochondritis which is comparatively common and may or may not be relevant to the clinical condition.

Pathological fractures are discussed further in section 5.6.

Chapter 2 General Health

2.1 Definition

An athlete can be said to have good general health when he can carry out his normal daily routine free from discomfort or mental or physical stress. He is then mentally and physically fit.

The normal daily routine of the athlete will include more physical activity than that of the sedentary worker but it has been shown that the latter performs his daily work more efficiently when he too partakes of physical exercise. There was a report in the *Sunday Times* on 20 September 1987 about a school near Glasgow where violence had broken out among the children at primary school level. A regime of graduated physical exercise was introduced on a daily basis and the 'daily PE helped them perform better in the classroom.' The report continues to say that mathematics showed the 'most noted improvement, especially among children aged 11 and 12.' There were also significant improvements in the pupils' attitudes towards their school, and violence decreased markedly.

The normal daily routine in factories in the Far East includes physical exercise classes and the management claim that work performance is improved thereby.

These two situations suggest that physical fitness and mental fitness may be related. There seems to be a correlation between mental stability and the 'letting off' of excess physical energy as any parent knows. It is reasonable to assume that some form of sporting activity will be beneficial to everyone provided certain guidelines are followed, and it is becoming evident that an awareness of the need for such exercise is more common now than it was a few years ago.

2.2 Physical fitness

This is the individual's physical development related to his daily activity. Sedentary workers need less muscular development than full-time athletes who are on an intensive training schedule. But sedentary workers by keeping 'fit' will enjoy a better sense of wellbeing, both physical and mental.

The human body is designed to maintain a state of good general health and has inherent healing powers, but this ability to remain 'fit' can be interfered with in several ways. The essential components of fitness are a good balanced diet, adequate rest, graduated muscular exercise, minimal physical and psychological stress and the absence of toxic substances namely drugs and invasive infections.

There is a common misconception that one can partake of sport to 'get fit' whereas it is essential to be fit to partake of sport safely. Injuries occur when the body is not fit enough for the sport or the technique is incorrect. The only other injuries which can be seen in practice are those of an extrinsic nature, for example in body contact sports, or perhaps falling off a horse or bicycle. These are often the worst type of injury. From the osteopathic viewpoint, good general health is normal and it is essential to remove the factors which interfere with this normal state. In a perfect situation if all such factors could be removed, the general health of the athlete would be superb and the effect of training and coaching, maximal. However, this is seldom seen in reality but training along established lines will always improve performance, such improvement depending on the particular individual.

There is one other important point and that is the suitability of the individual to the specific sport. There are several different body types which are inherent and often familial. For instance, the slightly built, asthenic build is unlikely to achieve great success in the endurance sports such as distance swimming, but is more suited to gymnastics.

In order to improve the physical fitness of any individual it is essential that there is a regulated programme of muscular exercise and also the mental determination on the part of the individual to carry out such a programme over a period of time. The rewards can then be great.

There has always been a great deal of controversy especially between athletes who follow different sports themselves as to which sport produces the fittest competitor, or alternatively which sport demands most from the competitor. In *The Times* on 30 May 1986 there was an article on the work of Dr Craig Sharp who tested up to 100 practitioners of each sport for six different attributes and a table adapted from his findings is shown in Fig. 2.1.

Strength was tested by pulling and pushing on various machines. Muscle endurance was tested by some demanding task, flat out, until the build up of lactic acid made the athlete collapse. Then the recovery rate was measured as the test was repeated. Muscle speed involved the time it took an athlete to reach peak power. Cardio-respiratory fitness tested aerobic fitness; obviously sprinters who perform entirely anaerobically had a low score. The flexibility tests involved various ranges of body movement, some of which sound quite horrifying! The percentage of body fat for male athletes was about 10% and 22% for females.

Training can improve the characteristics of the athlete's body which are required by his particular sport, but sport produces more than just physical fitness as Dr Sharp points out.

SPORT	Score out of ten						
	Cardio-respiratory fitness	Muscle speed	Strength	Local muscle endurance	Flexibility	Low body fat	TOTAL
Olympic gymnastics	6	9	9	10	10	9	53
Stage dance	8	8	7	8	10	10	51
Karate	6	9	9	8	9	6	47
Swimming: 1,500 m	7	6	7	9	8	7	44
Slalom canoeing	8	7	7	9	6	7	44
Squash rackets	9	7	5	8	6	9	44
Cycle-cross	9	7	8	8	5	7	44
Basketball	9	8	5	7	5	8	42
Sprint canoeing	6	6	8	10	5	7	42
Rowing: single and pair sculls	8	7	7	9	5	6	42
Windsurfing	6	5	8	10	7	6	42
White-water canoe	7	7	6	9	6	6	41
Shinty	8	7	6	7	6	7	41
Sprint cyclist	8	10	6	7	1	8	40
Rowing: fours, eights	7	6	8	9	4	6	40
Football: 1st division	6	7	7	8	5	7	40
Hurling	7	7	6	7	6	7	40
Road cyclist	10	6	4	9	1	8	40
Rugby: back	7	8	5	6	5	7	38
Netball	8	7	5	6	5	7	38
Badminton	7	7	4	6	6	7	37
Athletics: sprinting	4	10	8	5	4	6	37
Lacrosse	6	7	5	7	5	7	37
Athletics: middle distance	8	7	4	7	2	8	36
Hockey	6	8	4	6	5	7	36
Volleyball	7	7	5	6	5	6	36
Speed-skating	7	7	6	6	4	6	36
Cross-country skiing	10	2	4	9	2	9	36
Tennis	5	5	6	7	5	7	35
Athletics: distance	9	4	2	9	1	10	35
Table tennis	5	7	4	7	5	6	34
Rugby: forward	6	5	10	5	4	4	34
Long distance swimming	7	2	7	10	3	1	30

Fig. 2.1 The attributes of different sports.

Adapted from *The Times* spectrum section 30 May 1986

2.3   **Diet**

There has always been a great deal of controversy about what constitutes a good balanced diet and what is ideal for the maintenance of good health. However, there are several points which are universally held to be accurate.

The *daily calorific intake* should be sufficient to maintain the optimum body weight. Meals should be taken at regular intervals but prior to strenuous exercise, a meal should not be taken within three hours of starting time. This is because exercise increases the peripheral circulation thus reducing the blood supply to the gastro-intestinal tract so digestion is less efficient. Conversely, after a large meal the peripheral circulation is reduced and muscular activity is less efficient. During exercise, body salts and water should be taken to maintain the required level especially in hot weather when perspiration is at its greatest. Many proprietary drinks are available and are especially useful in endurance sports when the loss of fluid can be considerable.

The body requires a balanced intake of carbohydrate, protein and fat together with water, vitamins and minerals, Malnutrition can result if any of these is deficient. There are several books on this subject and I recommend the advice given in Robert Haas' book, *Eat to Win*. Such advice has proved useful to many athletes, particularly professional tennis players.

The importance of a high *fibre* diet has been recognised recently. Foods which contain fibre are the natural foods such as fruit, vegetables and whole grains. Fresh fruit and vegetables should constitute a large part of the athlete's daily intake of food, as cooked and processed foods are more difficult to digest and assimilate in the body and generally contain a lower proportion of essential vitamins and minerals than do fresh foods.

There is also a great deal of controversy about the need for *protein* to be in the form of animal products but it is now believed that red meats are not the best protein available. Nuts and pulses provide protein in a more easily assimilated form. Time was when wrestlers used to eat two pounds or more of meat per day, but the fashion has changed. Fish is a pure source of first class protein and is also a valuable source of iodine and is easily digested and assimilated.

So, to sum up, an ideal diet should contain as much fresh food as possible including nuts, and fish is preferable to red meats. My own feeling is that the diet should be supplemented with vitamins and minerals especially during the winter when it is not always easy to obtain really fresh foods. Those which are available have travelled from far away places and they are often past their optimum condition.

Foods to avoid are: highly processed foods, highly refined foods such as white flour and sugar, excessive alcohol, overcooked foods. Foods to include are: fresh fruit and vegetables, fish, nuts and pulses, whole grains, unrefined sugar.

Meals should always be taken at regular intervals and in a relaxed frame of mind and never rushed. One should never overeat. Drinking with meals is not to be encouraged and the intake of liquid should be sufficient to assuage thirst only. It should be taken between meals; water or fresh fruit juices are the best sources of liquid rather than stimulants such as coffee or alcohol.

Physical factors

There are obvious variations in body type which are inherent and cannot be altered which are defined in the Sheldon classification (see Fig. 2.2). The endomorphic type is short of stature and rather 'square' of shape. He is ideal for such sports as long distance swimming as he has reserves of subcutaneous fat and will conserve his body heat well, but he is poorly suited to most other sports. The *ectomorph* is long and lanky and will find sports such as basket ball ideal to his build. The *muscleman* appears to be triangular in shape and is best fitted for the power events such as weight lifting. Should this type attempt a sport such as high jump he may well find he is subject to more frequent injury than the ectomorph. There are, of course wide variations to be found within this classification.

Occupational factors also have to be considered. The person who is bound to the office desk for eight hours or more per day will get little or no exercise whereas the musical conductor has many hours of regulated albeit gentle exercise during his working life. The former will need to devote more of his time on daily fitness exercise than the latter. To improve the general condition of the body any exercise has to work the muscles and the cardiac and respiratory systems progressively, a little harder than usual. This leads to progressive increase in strength and efficiency of these muscles. The fact that some occupations already work the muscles and heart and respiratory systems while others do so to a lesser degree will have a direct bearing on any fitness program devised for a particular individual. No two people are exactly alike.

Similarly the pastimes of an individual must be taken into consideration. The person who owns a dog will of necessity have to walk daily whereas the person who is interested in oil painting will spend his spare time being physically less active. The housewife receives a fair amount of exercise as does the amateur gardener and it is of great importance to assess the lifestyle of each individual. At the other extreme is the disabled person but he, too, is capable of enjoying sport provided he is prepared for it.

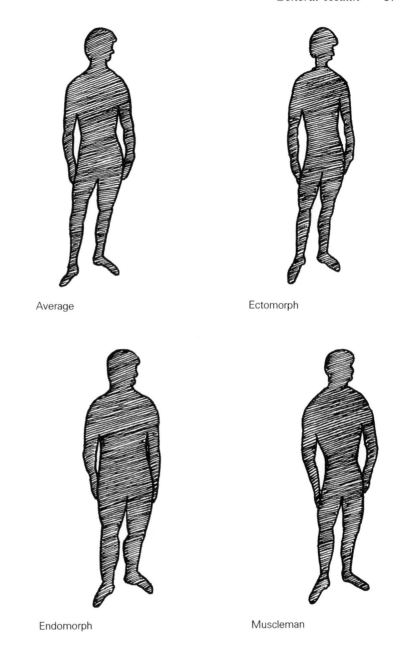

Average

Ectomorph

Endomorph

Muscleman

Fig. 2.2 Types of physique

The age of the athlete will also have a bearing on his general health. The basic difference between a young and old person is the elasticity of his tissues. Extreme elasticity is seen in a small child as he lies in his pram eating both feet at once! Sadly this is lost progressively as we grow older but again the rate varies considerably from one person to another. Less elastic tissues are more easily strained and need to be more thoroughly warmed up before strenuously used in sport.

There are fundamental differences between men and women both anatomically and physiologically. These differences give a great advantage to men in all sports which involve strength endurance and power. However great a player Steffi Graf is, she would find it impossible to compete against Ivan Lendl on equal terms, but in a sport such as show jumping where technique is of prime importance, men and women can compete equally.

The heavier male skeleton is less likely to suffer from stress fracture but would find the floor exercises of the gymnast more difficult to perform. The female pelvis is built wider than the male so there is a greater slope to the female thigh which makes the likelihood of dislocation of the patella greater in the female (see Figs 2.3 and 2.4).

Graduated muscular exercise

The purpose of exercise is threefold, namely to increase stamina, strength and suppleness.

Stamina or *muscular endurance* is the ability to continue an activity for many hours without feeling fatigued. It is essential in all endurance sports and is required in everyday activities to prevent tiredness at work and enable the athlete to enjoy leisure hours. There are two ways to develop stamina − the first is to do an exercise which you can repeat only once or twice, for example a push up, and gradually increase strength to repeat up to say twenty times. The alternative and better way is to reduce the initial load and repeat at that level until progression can be made to a harder level. The easiest level of the push up is done against a wall with the hands at shoulder level, followed later by the hands at a lower level (at waist height) then lower still (at hip height) and progressing to knee level and finally floor level.

There is much written about this type of exercise and suggested reading is the outline programme for marines. These exercises are safe provided all precautions are noted and followed carefully. The advantage of this regime is that it can be self-regulated and done without much equipment. The programme is designed for both men and women up to middle age. Any distress should be checked out by a doctor.

All these exercises depend on the principle of progressive overload. Such conditioning helps to prevent sprains, strains and stress fractures. Joints and ligaments become more capable of absorbing shock and withstanding stress. In addition, the cardiovascular system develops more capillaries thereby improving peripheral circulation and increasing aerobic energy.

Although endurance is advantageous generally, *strength* is required in many sports. This is the measure of the power of a muscle or muscle group when exerting maximal force, as in weight

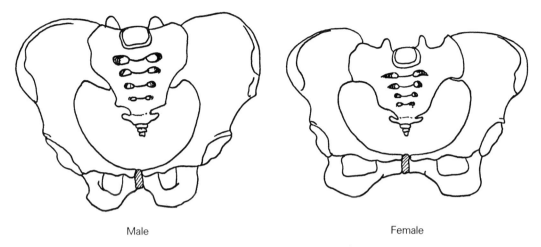

Male   Female

Fig. 2.3   Male and female pelvis, anterior aspect.

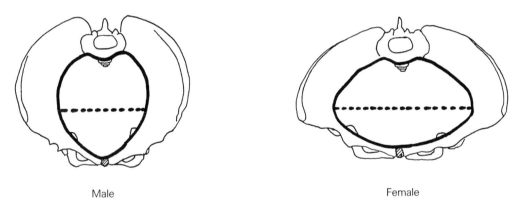

Male   Female

Fig. 2.4   Male and female pelvis, transverse diameter of the pelvic inlet.

lifting. Strength is increased by lifting a weight no more than once or twice and then repeating, after a period of rest and recuperation until that weight can be lifted eventually up to eight times. At that point the weight can be increased and the process repeated. The advantages of great strength are limited in everyday life but certain sports require it. The athlete should train under an experienced coach to develop strength safely.

The third purpose of exercise is to develop *suppleness* and it is this which is of most significance to the osteopath. There is an optimum range of movement in all joints of the body and loss of this mobility is often seen as a contributory factor in injury. The causes of joint immobility are many, including soft tissue shortening or 'tightness' and facet locking at the joint surface. These conditions are seen in spinal joints most frequently but also occur in peripheral joints. The problems may be due to old injury where the recovery has been incomplete or to occupational and postural problems. All these must be carefully analysed by the osteopath when examining the patient, and related to the patient's daily life and his sport in particular. Only years of experience in the clinical field will make this task easier.

Assuming that the joints of the body are functioning correctly the soft tissues will need constant attention and the best way to improve their flexibility is to carry out repeated stretching exercises. Again much is written on this subject but I would recommend any book on the subject which is based on the principles of Hatha Yoga.

Any lack of natural suppleness will display as stiffness in the body which can be seen in many people and is often considered 'normal' in older people. This is not necessarily true and regular stretching will overcome the problem but it must be done carefully and progressively. Many yoga teachers are fully qualified and their help can be invaluable.

Stiffness will also develop to avoid or alleviate pain. Any underlying joint problem will be accompanied by muscular guarding which acts as a protection, reducing movement and thus reducing pain, so again the integrity of joint physiology is of prime importance.

Emotional problems can also cause muscular stiffness. Stress will often produce tightness of the upper thoracic muscles especially across the shoulder area and if suspected, the presence of stress must be recognised by both osteopath and patient if it is to be relieved.

Stretching is a way of becoming aware of the comfort of the body. Every stretch leads to increased awareness which is a process of self-analysis and a safeguard against injury, and the fear of injury is lessened thereby.

Some sports will increase one or more of these three aims of exercise. Swimming – hard swimming, that is, will increase all three.

Some dangers of exercise

At times, athletes present with injuries which have occurred following some relatively minor trauma. Careful history taking will reveal a long history of often repeated exercises which strain ligaments, stretch nerves and possibly pressurise blood vessels. Undue load may be placed on vertebrae, intervertebral discs, meniscii and cartilage, to name but some of the tissues which can be damaged.

The guidelines of safety are that stretching should never cause pain and should be carried out gently and repetitively – hence my suggestion that yoga is a safe discipline, because pain is not caused.

Ideally, stretching should be carried out while the athlete is not weight bearing as his muscles are in use when he is in the upright position more than when he is non-weight bearing.

Extra care is needed when doing the following exercises: toe touching puts great strain on the ligaments of the low back, beyond which the muscles cannot give support. Hurdler's stretch can over-stretch the pubic symphysis and medial ligaments of the knee joint. Deep knee bends and squats can stress the meniscii of the knee. The ballet bar stretch can irritate the sciatic nerve. The yoga plough can damage the cervical vertebrae; this particular exercise should only be carried out by those who are advanced in yoga. Sit ups must always be done with safety in mind, or the posterior ligaments of the spine can be stretched too much.

Circuit training has helped athletes to exercise groups of muscles with but a few repetitions, returning to the circuit for further repetitions, encouraging strength without overstrain. This system will increase the effectiveness and reduce the risk of injury. (See Chapter 18, Weights.)

Table 2.1, based on a table *Looking After Yourself* published by the Health Education Council shows how three aspects of exercise vary with different sports.

2.7　　**Mental factors**

Considering the patient as a whole, he is 'body, mind and soul'. His general health can be affected adversely by mental factors – problems which have to be considered. Perfect general health includes the ability of the patient to cope with stress in his everyday life as well as when he is competing at sport. The response to stress such as that at the start of a race has the effect of increasing the adrenaline level in the blood, which in turn can be beneficial at such a time. However, long-term stress has a detrimental effect and the body is less able to perform well under such conditions. The effect can be seen in musculature which can become tense; the fibres are not able to relax as they should after exercise and when in this state, are more liable to injury. The special systems of the body can also be affected – digestion may be impaired, the heart and circulation may be less than optimally efficient and the endocrine glands may be affected as well. Any or all of these deficiencies tend to be cumulative in their effect so the body efficiency lessens progressively. To overcome these stress problems a regulated system of yoga as a daily routine is ideal and there are many books written on the subject.

An example of extreme stress is the feeling of being 'scared stiff'

Table 2.1 The varying effects of different sports on stamina, suppleness and strength.

Sport	Stamina	Suppleness	Strength
Badminton	**	***	**
Canoeing	***	**	***
Climbing stairs	***	*	**
Cricket	*	**	*
Cycling (hard)	****	**	***
Dancing: ballroom	*	***	*
disco	***	****	*
Digging (garden)	***	**	****
Football	***	***	***
Golf	*	**	*
Gymnastics	**	****	***
Hill walking	***	*	***
Housework (moderate)	*	**	*
Jogging	****	**	**
Judo	**	****	**
Mowing lawn by hand	**	*	***
Rowing	****	**	****
Sailing	*	**	**
Squash	***	***	**
Swimming (hard)	****	****	****
Tennis	**	***	**
Walking (briskly)	**	*	*
Weightlifting	*	*	****
Yoga	*	****	*

*	No real effect
**	Beneficial effect
***	Very good effect
****	Excellent effect

From: *Looking After Yourself* by The Health Education Council.

when it is impossible to move at all. Most people are subjected to a lesser form of stress during their daily lives and it is wise to overcome the effects of this daily condition by routine stretching and relaxation. The added discipline of regulated deep breathing is also most beneficial and is included in yoga.

Steve Davis was asked recently what makes a champion; his reply was a natural ability, constant practice, dedication and temperament. It is interesting that two out of four necessary requirements, in his opinion, can be classified as mental factors. Many an athlete knows that winning depends on 'what lies between the ears'.

2.8

Rest

A full-time athlete needs about eight hours rest daily but there are individual variations. During intensive training the metabolic rate of the athlete is high and periods of physiological rest are essential as these times allow mental and muscular relaxation to occur. Muscles which do not have sufficient rest will accumulate the chemical by-products of muscular activity which will impede further muscular efficiency and may lead to an increased likelihood of injury. Sleep is the body's natural period of recuperation.

During intensive periods of physical exercise short periods of rest are also beneficial as they minimise tissue overuse and will increase the body's general efficiency.

Rest following injury is of prime importance as most damaged tissues will benefit from rest at least for a short time. In these cases, rest has to be carefully balanced with whatever body activity is needed to keep the athlete generally fit without causing further damage to the injury suffered. It is important to maintain general fitness if at all possible. Rest in cases of injury may be complete i.e. bed rest, or it may be of only part of the body, for example by strapping, bandage or plaster-of-Paris cast. In general, rest is advised initially as it certainly helps tissues to heal but it is wise to get the athlete mobile again as quickly as possible in most cases. The exception may be in cases of tissue overuse which has lead to injury.

Training programmes as laid down by coaches are precise and most are scientific and excellent. Many coaches insist on a day free from training at regular intervals, usually once a week thus providing physiological rest. This is also the case the day before a competitive event and it is important that the guidelines laid down by the coach are adhered to at all times. These rest days protect the athlete from overtraining which can lead to an increase in the likelihood of injury. The need for tissues to have rest days is well recognised in athletic training programmes.

Chapter 3   Why Do Injuries Occur?

General

It has been estimated that of the cases which attend accident, emergency and casualty units in the UK, 10% are due to sports injury. In addition, 10% of sports injuries will result in loss of work as well as sport by the patient. It therefore becomes obvious that sports injuries are not insignificant to the nation's economy and have to be taken seriously by practitioners and athletes alike.

Most of the injuries which occur are of a minor nature, namely strains, sprains, abrasions and contusions and these should not prevent return to normal sport as recovery should be good. There are, however, injuries of a more serious nature such as fractures, concussion and trauma to internal organs where incorrect diagnosis and treatment can lead to chronic disability. The long-term prognosis will in all cases depend on correct diagnosis and treatment which includes full rehabilitation before sport is resumed.

There are codes of safety which are laid down and regulated by the governing bodies of the various sports. In many cases these rules are enforced by the referee or umpire. The referee has to make sure that the game is conducted in such a way that the safety of every participant is ensured so that injury is unlikely to result. Where there is no such person present it is the responsibility of the athlete to observe the rules for his own safety and for the safety of everyone else concerned.

In short, if the athlete is fit for the sport and the rules are observed and the technique is correct, injury should not occur.

3.2   **The individual**

Age

The incidence of injury will vary with the age of the athlete. Young persons may suffer from *greenstick fractures* or *epiphysitis* both of which are unknown in adult bone. The former is usually as a result of direct injury and the latter of overuse. Where there is overuse of a muscle in a growing athlete an irritation of the insertion commonly results, such as in the insertion of the patellar tendon into the tibial tubercle − Osgood Schlatter's Disease. *Osteochondritis* is another condition frequently found in adolescents especially in the spine and is thought by some practitioners to be a result of overstress of the vertebral column. If a child complains of pain it should always be taken seriously especially if it is worse following sport and appears to be skeletal in origin.

During adolescence the muscle power increases and there is a greater likelihood of *stress fractures* occurring as well as muscle tears. Young adults often have more enthusiasm than is good for them and may become too competitive with sports such as weight training. They can overdevelop musculature which stresses their bone structure and back problems are often seen in this age group. It seems that the bones are not yet strong enough to withstand the muscular stresses to which they are subjected. Adolescent bone is often not strong enough to withstand repeated compression such as in rugby. The intervertebral discs may become inflamed and cause erosion of the vertebral bodies which consequentially become biconcave, but this is not seen so much these days as the rules of the game have been modified.

Once the musculoskeletal system has reached full maturity the athlete may be subjected to a severe training programme, so *overuse injuries* are more frequently seen. With a progressive increase of achievement in sport, these injuries are likely to be even more common in the future. At this age, the enthusiastic amateur will have less time available for training yet he will still wish to compete and his chance of injury will increase accordingly. There is also more risk from body contact sports once full maturity is reached.

Middle age brings different injuries again as the athlete finds it more difficult to maintain his fitness level and his tissues are beginning to lose elasticity. Early *degenerative changes* will start to appear and tendons and ligaments are more subject to trauma. The full-time athlete will need to spend even more of his time stretching his body to lessen his chance of injury and his recovery time will be progressively longer as he advances in age.

Older people are less likely to partake of strenuous sport or that which involves body contact. Degenerative changes will be present and the body less adaptable to sports which require sudden bursts of energy such as squash. Soft tissue injuries become common and complete tears are more often seen, such as *ruptures* of the tendo Achilles or even the long head of the biceps in the upper arm. The advantage which these older athletes have is an increase in skill and experience which may well protect them from injury. However, they are more likely to partake of the endurance sports such as marathon running and in such events may collapse, literally. Other less strenuous sports such as golf may lead to rotational strains, especially in the lumbar spine where elasticity is reduced and degenerative changes are present. Recovery also takes longer but these people are less impatient in their adversity and will more readily accept the fact that tissue repair takes time.

Sex

The female skeleton is usually lighter than the male and the male musculature is usually heavier than the female. These two factors give men positive advantages over women in most sports as strength and endurance will be greater in men. There is a greater chance of muscular and tendinous injury in men due to the additional pull on the bone. As women tend to have greater flexibility there is an increased chance of ligamentous injuries and a corresponding incidence of hypermobile joints. The lighter bone structure of women also leads to an increased tendency to stress fracture especially in the foot.

Men are more likely to be subjected to body contact sports where direct injury is a risk such as American football or rugby whereas women may overstretch tissues in sports such as gymnastics especially in the floor events. The increased likelihood of patellar dislocation in women due to the greater angle of the femur has already been mentioned in section 2.4.

The sexual skeletal differences develop with puberty. Up to the age of about 10, girls tend to be taller and heavier than boys and can compete with them as there is little or no difference in strength between the sexes. However, there is a peak rate of growth which occurs earlier in girls than boys. At about the same time oestrogens in girls cause an increase in body fat and in its distribution, whereas androgens in boys cause an increase in muscle bulk and a reduction of body fat. At this point in their development, boys gain the advantage over girls in strength and tend to partake in strength and endurance type sports. From then on, there are few events where the sexes can compete equally and the pattern of injuries will vary accordingly. (See also section 2.4.)

Body type

See section 2.4 where reference has already been made to the different body types. The *average* frame can partake of a variety of different sports depending on sufficient training. Those which involve extreme flexibility such as gymnastics will be found to be difficult as will those which require extreme strength (weightlifting) or extreme endurance, but this type of frame can safely partake in all the average sports.

The *endomorphic* type is best suited to long distance swimming events where the additional body fat which is usually present will protect him from cold. He will never be extremely fleet of foot but events such as equestrian sports may well suit his type (though not as a jockey where he will be too heavy).

The *ectomorphic* type is often described as the bean pole and will excel at events such as high jump, volley ball and basket ball –

i.e. any event where he elevates himself off the ground. He will have great 'spring'.

The *muscleman* type will find weightlifting and other power sports suitable to his body, but any sport which involves flexibility will be difficult for him. If the sport is unsuitable for the individual, the risk of injury is increased. The forces which are applied to the musculoskeletal system by unsuitable sports will produce excessive stresses which the body may be unable to withstand.

Psychology

What makes an athlete want to compete? When I asked this question of an athlete I was told that it produced a tremendous sense of satisfaction and achievement. The feeling which results from pushing himself beyond what he ever thought was possible has increased his belief in himself. To better one's own personal best is thrilling and exciting and may well lead to an increased strength of personality as well as physical achievement. Many athletes enjoy the competitiveness of sport and every serious sportsman will strive to win in his event; second best is never good enough! In addition, sport is a great equaliser in what is otherwise, often a very unequal world. The energy outlet is physically and mentally satisfying, giving a feeling of enormous personal satisfaction.

There are also the social aspects together with the companionship and the development of team spirit, especially in the various team sports. Maybe these factors assist athletes in adapting to the harrowing problems of living and working in close proximity with others.

Injury, however, leads to psychological problems. The competitive athlete is extremely frustrated as he is no longer able to partake of his chosen sport. In general, these are the most 'impatient patients' we see in practice! They believe that their problem is worse than it really is, often due to fear and ignorance. This frustration only starts to be relieved when a practitioner gives a definite diagnosis and prognosis. The athlete needs to be told when he will be able to resume his sport; in the meantime it is useful to give him some alternative to do, preferably as part of his treatment.

For example, a patient with a hamstring injury can safely be encouraged to swim using a float between his legs at least in the early stages of recovery. It may not be his chosen sport but at least swimming provides physical activity and will help to maintain his general fitness.

Athletes like to talk about their sport and to know that the practitioner understands it. To explain the injury to the athlete and relate the injury to his sport is most important as this will help to establish full co-operation between patient and practitioner which is essential if the best possible result is to be achieved.

An athlete will seldom consult a practitioner unless he has been personally recommended, usually by another athlete who may have had a similar condition. He needs to have faith and full trust in the practitioner probably more so than the average non-athletic patient. The professional sees his future at stake – a serious matter, and he will do his utmost to ensure it. This is apparent in that the professional is more liable to know when he is safe to resume training. The amateur will tend to go back to training too soon, thus risking recurrence of injury. Virginia Wade was asked recently to what she attributed her long career in professional tennis; she replied that she had always given her injuries sufficient time to recover. What a wise lady! The resumption of normal training may take some time and has to be gradual. Here, co-operation between practitioner, athlete and his coach is ideal as all three should work together. Reassurance as to when training can start again is vital to the athlete; even if he is not receiving treatment at this time he will need to be in contact with the practitioner if only by telephone. As so many have said to me 'it is nice to know that you are there!'

To be able to gain the confidence of the athlete, the practitioner has to have confidence in himself and this only comes with experience. It is so much easier to treat a condition when one has treated similar cases before. Most widely experienced practitioners have gained invaluable knowledge by working at the grass roots level often without remuneration. I would advise all young graduates to gain as much experience as possible by attending as many events as they can in many different sports. The knowledge gleaned is cumulative and will lead to a wider understanding of sports injuries and a greater confidence in how best to deal with them.

3.3		**Tissue fitness**

Tissues need to be fit to withstand the forces applied to them when an athlete is performing, without breaking down under the stress of the sport.

Let us consider *muscles* first. Skeletal muscle (see Fig. 3.1) consists of a number of individual fibres each of which is surrounded by a membrane – the sarcolemma. Each fibre is an individual cell. Within the cell are numerous myofibrils which are capable of causing the muscle to contract. Each myofibril consists of two small elements of protein, the larger being myosin and the smaller actin. It is thought that there is an instantaneous union of myosin and actin whereby they pass over the myosin tightly, following nerve stimulation which comes from the brain. This causes shortening of the myofibril. The energy required for this to take place is provided by adenosine triphosphate (ATP). ATP is present in the muscle in small quantities only, approximately enough to cause

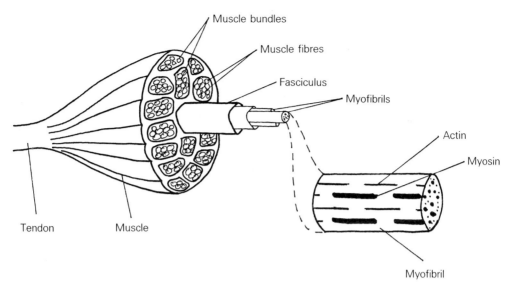

Muscle bundles

Muscle fibres

Fasciculus

Myofibrils

Actin

Myosin

Tendon   Muscle

Myofibril

Fig. 3.1   Skeletal muscle.

contraction for half a second so it has to be replenished swiftly. Creatin phosphate is also found within the muscle and can be converted into ATP but the result of this is to cause contraction for another five seconds only. The next process which occurs is conversion of glycogen into ATP, the glycogen also being stored within the muscle. This process is known as anaerobic glycolysis. This will provide energy for muscular contraction for a further forty-five seconds. All these processes are anaerobic as no oxygen is needed for them to be carried out. When glycogen is broken down to form ATP anaerobically, lactic acid is formed as a by product. This causes an increased acidity which prevents further muscular contraction and the acid must be eliminated swiftly by the blood stream. It is this chemical reaction within muscle which prevents any runner, however well trained, from sprinting flat out for more than 400 metres without seizing up.

Aerobic glycolysis now takes place. In the presence of oxygen more of the muscle's store of glycogen is converted into ATP and further contraction can occur. Within each myofibril are several thousand mitochondria which produce the enzymes required to break down oxygen and glycogen into more ATP so that muscle contraction may continue. To ensure the increased supply of oxygen the athlete will need to breathe faster and deeper. One of the easy ways to assess increased fitness is to see how much longer it takes to get out of breath when running at the same pace.

Even deep respiration during strenuous exercise supplies only part of the oxygen required for the recovery phase if the exercise lasts for more than a minute. The athlete goes into oxygen debt and his respiration rate is increased for a time following exercise. During light exercise no oxygen debt is incurred.

For oxygen to reach the mitochondria a plentiful supply of blood is needed via the capillaries. The heart has to beat efficiently. The resting heart rate of an untrained person is about 72 beats per minute. If during exercise his heart rate increases to 180 beats per minute he has increased his cardiac output by two and a half times, in theory. A trained athlete may have a resting heart rate of 40 beats per minute so when his rate increases to 180 beats per minute he has an increase of four and a half times, theoretically. Some of this increase will benefit the capillaries of the heart muscle itself but most will improve the oxygen supply to the skeletal muscles and improve the efficiency of removal of by-products of muscular contraction.

Oxygen is taken into the body through the trachea to the lungs where it passes into the blood stream. The lungs consist of millions of alveoli where the gaseous exchanges occur (oxygen in and carbon dioxide out). The range of chest movement during inspiration reduces the pressure within the chest thus forcing air in: this range depends on free movement of the diaphragm and ribs and the integrity of action of the intercostal and abdominal muscles.

The effects of training will improve the lung capacity, increase cardiac output, increase peripheral circulation as there is an increase in the number of capillaries within the muscles, and increase the number of mitochondria within the myofibrils. All this will help the athlete run faster and for a longer period.

Tendons and ligaments are elastic tissues and have an optimum length for efficiency. Injury of a ligament will often result in lengthening of the structure (which may lead to instability of a joint). Tendons may shorten if insufficient exercise is taken. They respond to rhythmic stretching exercises as do tendon sheaths where present and are less likely to be injured when regularly stretched. There are several good books on stretching techniques.

Warming up properly and warming down after physical exercise will reduce the risk of *injury* enormously. Professional athletes are fully aware of the need, but sadly amateurs are not prepared to spend time on this invaluable discipline. There is no doubt that warming up reduces the likelihood of pulled muscles and helps to allay anxiety before an event. It should consist of comfortable free running or jogging until the whole body feels warm or is possibly gently perspiring. This takes at least ten minutes or longer in cold weather. Stretching then follows and every part of the body which will be used during the sporting activity needs to be progressively stretched. Following the event it is essential to run or jog gently at a decreasing pace and if any muscles feel sore, a warm shower is advisable.

Recurrent injuries are seen all too often. They are frequently due to insufficient recovery time. The moral is, if in doubt as to whether you should compete or not, *don't* unless advised by a professional person that you are fit to do so.

3.4   **Prevention**

To sum up, many injuries are preventable.

(1) Make sure that you are fit for the event.
(2) Observe the rules of the sport.
(3) Accept that you have a responsibility to others and to yourself.
(4) Always warm up and warm down adequately.
(5) Always wear correct clothing.

Footwear

Socks should be of the correct size and made of a pure natural fibre usually pure cotton. This will absorb perspiration and two pairs may be necessary. Shoes should fit properly. They should be designed for the particular sport and always be in good repair. Worn out shoes will be distorted in shape and will not support the foot correctly. Because the feet are normally covered up they are often neglected. First and foremost they should be kept clean. Nails should be kept short and round taking the shape of the toe and never protruding beyond the end of it. Any sore area on the foot should be attended to properly. Advice from a State Registered Chiropodist especially with regard to callouses, athletes foot or verucae can save the athlete a great deal of trouble in the long run.

Clothing

This should be correctly fitting and comfortable to wear. If it hampers movement there is an additional risk to the wearer or if it is too loose he may have to fiddle with it during his sport. Natural fibres are usually preferable to man-made ones as cooling of the body by evaporation of perspiration is not impeded. Any garment made of man-made fibre should be of an open weave especially in any sport involving high energy expenditure.

Protective clothing is required in many sports. It must never put other players at risk like the shoulder pads used by rugby football players, which have now been banned. All such clothing should be made of materials which can be cleaned easily and maintain the protective properties.

Finally, all athletes need common sense! Some are downright dangerous to both themselves and to others, often carried away by their enthusiasm and excitement and oblivious of the risks they are taking which are possibly contrary to the rules and regulations of their sport.

Chapter 4   Classification of the Different Types of Injury

4.1   Primary injury

This type of injury is directly related to a sporting activity. It is obvious and the history will often reveal the cause and time when the injury was sustained, especially in acute cases. Primary injuries can be subdivided into intrinsic and extrinsic injuries.

Intrinsic injuries are caused by some force which has been generated within the patient's own body, or can be said to be 'self-inflicted'. Extrinsic injuries on the other hand are caused by some force which was generated outside the patient's body and to which he was unfortunately subjected. The latter injuries are generally more severe as an extrinsic force is likely to be greater than an intrinsic one. Such extrinsic injuries can be considered as 'accidents' and are identical with other accidental injuries which may have no bearing whatever on sporting activities. The only difference may be in the way such an injury is treated because of the need for the athlete to continue his sporting career. His tissue response and speed of recovery may also be better than that of the non-athlete.

Intrinsic injury is a result of a breakdown of technique under stress especially when the athlete is trying extra hard and makes a sudden lunge or sharp movement. His co-ordination breaks down while he is making that particular movement. So many intrinsic injuries occur spontaneously. There are, however, intrinsic injuries which are of a chronic nature and which build up over a period of time, such as the spin bowler's finger in cricket. Many such chronic injuries come about from repeated stresses which are not given sufficient time to recover when they first occur. There is an increase of fluid within the tissues following exertion which is normally absorbed after a short period of rest. If this period is not long enough for fluid absorption to be complete and the exertion is repeated too soon, a build up of fluid occurs. Initially there is a localised swelling, an increase in fluid pressure and damage to the surrounding tissues may result in fibrotic change or scarring.

Acute intrinsic injuries include ligament strains – the common sprained joint, muscle tears, tears of the musculotendinous junction, fascial sheath tears, tendon tears, dislocations for example of the first tarsometatarsal joint or even fractures (stress fractures). The soft tissue tears are the most frequently seen injuries.

Chronic intrinsic injuries include repeated minor tears of muscle or ligament, but the one most frequently seen is *tendonitis* especially of the tendo Achilles at the heel. The end result of repeated trauma to this tendon may well be rupture which seems to be more common if the tendon has been infiltrated with hydrocortisone in the past. *Bursitis* also tends to be a result of chronic intrinsic injury where there is a resultant thickening of the wall of the bursal sac due to excessive friction on the bursa during joint movement. Interference of the blood supply will also lead to a chronic intrinsic injury and is seen typically in the anterior compartment syndrome. The anterior (front) and lateral (outside) muscles lie within a tight sheath of fascia. If this sheath becomes tighter still, there is interference of the blood supply to those muscles (ischaemia) and pain is felt which becomes progressively worse as the muscles are used. Generally speaking, deep soft tissues are only sensitive to pain caused by ischaemia which is a reduction of blood supply. This may be pressure on the vessels directly or as a result of a build up of fluid within the fibres thus reducing local circulation. Either way the effect on tissues is the same. The clinical picture of these chronic intrinsic injuries will be a history of repeated minor traumata and palpable changes within the tissue concerned.

By contrast, the *extrinsic injury* is seldom chronic and often severe. The force applied to the athlete may be great, especially where a high velocity is involved such as in motor racing. The equipment used in the sport may cause injury, for example when a player is struck by a squash racket. The confines of the court increase the chance of such an injury. Body contact sports carry the risk of being struck by another competitor and the force will be greater if the sport includes moving at speed. Lastly some sports have an element of risk of being struck by chance, for example, during rock climbing or skiing but these injuries are comparatively rare. The type of injury seen will include fractures, dislocations, lacerations and probably severe bruising. First aid treatment is often needed and as the injuries are frequently severe the recuperative period is often long. Shock may be an added complication.

4.2

Secondary injury

Secondary injuries result from primary injuries but affect other structures — i.e. they are complications. They may be obvious, for example, the shortening of a leg following fracture leading to a scoliosis for which the athlete cannot compensate, with resultant low back pain. They may be less obvious, for example, knee pain resulting from a chronic ankle injury often in the opposite leg. As a rule it is essential to examine the patient *as a whole* and not just the area of which he is complaining in order to build up a true clinical picture.

Treatment of these injuries will involve attention to the primary injury even if it is no longer giving symptoms. The patient must be helped to accommodate for the primary injury, for example, by modifying his balance and posture. For instance, a heel lift may help take some of the stress off a scoliosis secondary to a leg fracture. Each case needs complete body assessment.

A retraining programme may be necessary especially if there is muscular weakness from the primary injury or even a change of sporting activity may have to be considered.

<table>
<tr><td>4.3</td><td></td></tr>
</table>

Predisposition to injury

The various body types and their suitability or otherwise to various sports has already been discussed. Unsuitability of body to sport will increase the risk of injury and should always be pointed out, if relevant, to the athlete.

Congenital abnormalities may be present and predispose the athlete to injury – i.e. that particular injury might well not occur if the abnormality were not present. *Congenitally shortened muscles* will lead to abnormal mechanics. Those commonly affected are the hamstrings (posterior thigh) and the gastrocnemius (posterior calf). These may well tear when put on stretch if already shortened. Tendons may be shortened congenitally, the commonest one being the Achilles tendon at the heel. Some cases are so severe that surgical lengthening is necessary. Shortened tendons, too, are more likely to tear when put on stretch.

Congenitally lax ligaments occur in approximately 5% of the population and there is joint hypermobility as a result. This does not necessarily lead to instability, for acrobats need this flexibility to perform. However, the incidence of recurrent dislocation of the shoulder joint and of the patella is increased where lax ligaments are present. (These are not extreme cases as seen in certain clinical conditions such as Marfan's syndrome.)

Congenital Pes Planus is not rare. Secondary to this is the increased pronation of the foot which places mechanical stress on the body, especially the knee and ankle joints and can make weight bearing sports difficult. Such people may well perform better in sports where running or jumping are not required – e.g. swimming.

Congenital abnormalities are also seen in bone. The tibia is normally curved forward but this curve may be excessive in some people. When activities such as jumping or running are undertaken, the curve is accentuated as the weight is placed on the limb. Is it possible that this could be a contributory factor in the development of *shin splints*? This very common condition is pain along the anterior margin of the bone and X-rays suggest tiny stress fractures are present. The periosteum is also painful and oedematous (swollen), probably where it has been stretched due to the underlying swelling in the bone. There is a great deal of argument about shin splints but I postulate that this increased curve of the tibia may well be relevant in some cases. An *os trigonium*, present in 7% of the population may become inflamed and painful in excess springing − e.g. jumping (see Fig. 4.1).

A difference in the length of the two legs is commonly seen and is considered to be of clinical importance if the difference exceeds 0.3 cm and symptoms are present. Many greater differences are seen in clinical practice, however, which do not appear to cause problems. The effect of a leg length difference is the development of a *scoliosis* which is usually convex in the lumbar area on the side of the short leg and concave in the thoracic area on that same side (see Fig. 4.2). This can lead to problems especially in sports which require the use of some implement in one hand. Some of these curvatures certainly seem to have a family pattern and I wonder if they may be transmitted genetically.

Cervical ribs are not rare. They can cause trouble in some sports especially those which involve a great deal of arm elevation such as rock climbing or badminton (see Fig. 4.3).

A congenital fault in the *pars interarticularis* in a lumbar vertebra will increase the chance of a *spondylolisthesis* developing later, especially in sports which demand extension of that area of the spine, such as diving or fast bowling at cricket. The fault is often not found until a spondylolisthesis develops (see Fig. 4.4).

Anomalies of bone structure are fairly often seen. The *acetabulum* in the pelvis may be shallow leading to reduced movement of the hip joint on one or both sides (see Fig. 4.5). It can often be suspected but only finally diagnosed at surgery as the labrum is cartilagenous and will not show up on an X-ray.

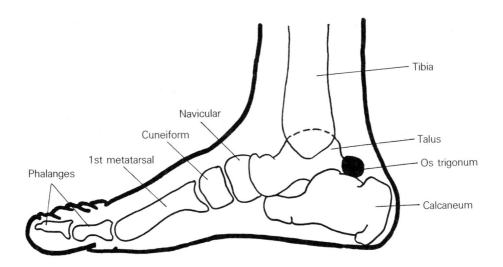

Fig. 4.1   Os trigonum, medial aspect of the foot.

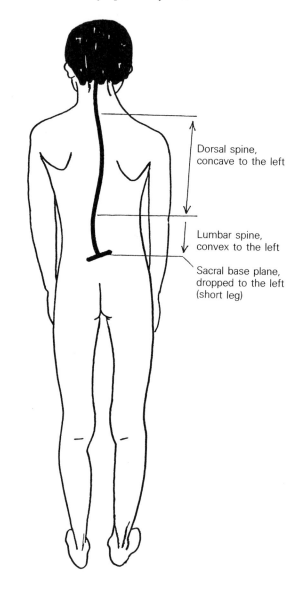

Dorsal spine,
concave to the left

Lumbar spine,
convex to the left

Sacral base plane,
dropped to the left
(short leg)

Fig. 4.2 Spinal
scoliosis. Lateral
curvatures resulting
from a short leg (left).

Anomalies are fairly common at the *lumbosacral joint*. The two
most often seen are some alteration of the plane of the facets of
that joint (see Fig. 4.6) or possible *sacralisation* (see Fig. 4.7).
Sometimes there are six instead of five lumbar vertebrae (see
Fig. 4.8) or there is incomplete union of the sacral vertebrae (see
Fig. 4.9). All these conditions will lead to altered mechanics at that
level, increasing the possibility of joint strains. Again these abnormalities are seldom discovered until the patient develops pain.
Occasionally there is fusion of two or more vertebrae which leads
to a reduction of movement at that level, thus placing additional
stress on the surrounding joints where strains may well develop.

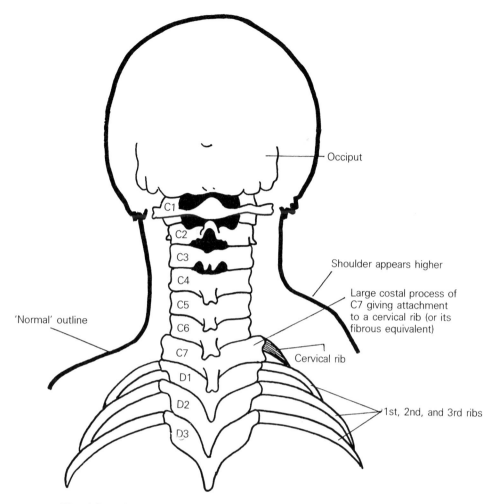

Fig. 4.3   Posterior aspect of cervical spine with right cervical rib.

The fused area itself will not produce symptoms as stress cannot be placed there by movement.

There are certain familial tendencies seen in practice. Certain spinal curves, hallux valgus (bunion) and the tendency to develop varicose veins may all increase the likelihood of injury during sporting activities.

Abnormalities which are acquired are invariably irreversible but the effect of such a condition may well be reduced clinically. The fact that the disabled are capable of competing in sport bears this out: many are first class athletes in particular events. There may have been a fault in the development of the individual often for no apparent reason, i.e. where the aetiology is unknown.

Cases of *reduced spinal curvature* in the A–P plane (i.e. those which curve from the front to the back of the body) will reduce the

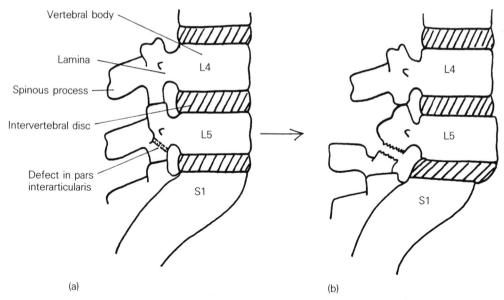

Vertebral body

Lamina

Spinous process

Intervertebral disc

Defect in pars
interarticularis

L4

L5

S1

L4

L5

S1

(a)

(b)

Fig. 4.4   (a) Congenital fault across the pars interarticularis (but no shift of the vertebral body); (b) development of a spondylolisthesis. The body of L5 has shifted forward and the pars interarticularis defect has widened.

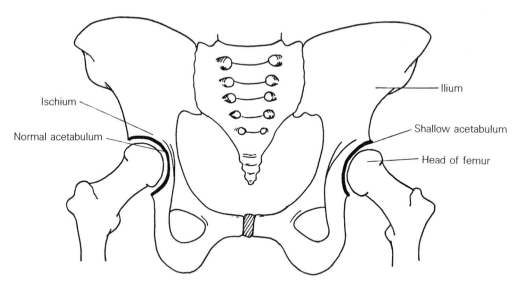

Ischium

Normal acetabulum

Ilium

Shallow acetabulum

Head of femur

Fig. 4.5   Normal and shallow acetabula, anterior aspect of pelvis.

mechanical efficiency of the spinal joints and render them more likely to strain. Conversely those curves may be excessive − the typical *kypholordotic curve* where there will be shortening of soft tissues on the concavity of the curve and lengthening on the convexity leading to soft tissue contraction and stretching respectively.

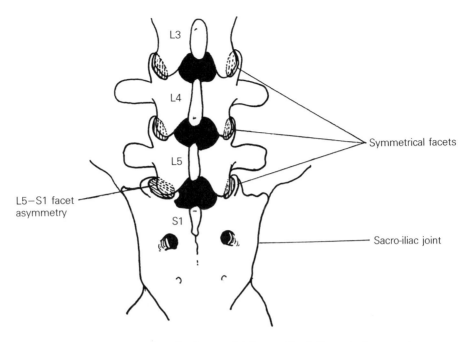

Fig. 4.6   Anomalous lumbosacral joint on the left, posterior aspect.

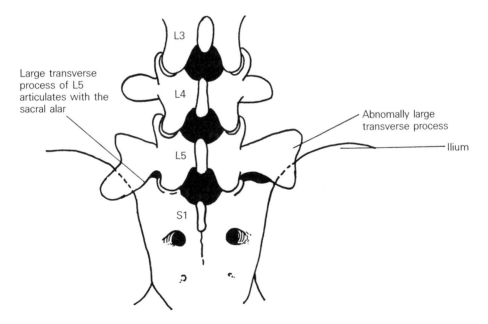

Fig. 4.7   Sacralisation of the lumbosacral joint.

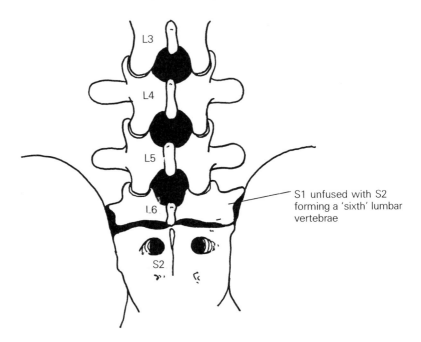

Fig. 4.8
Lumbarisation
of S1.

S1 unfused with S2
forming a 'sixth' lumbar
vertebrae

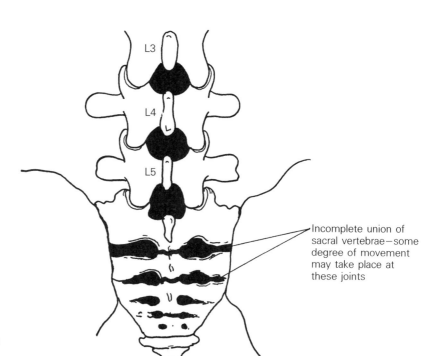

Fig. 4.9 Incomplete
union of sacral
vertebrae.

Incomplete union of
sacral vertebrae—some
degree of movement
may take place at
these joints

Here too, the centre of gravity line of the body will not pass through the weight bearing parts of the vertebrae and excessive wear may result (see Fig. 4.10).

There are cases of *scoliosis*, too, which have developed for no apparent reason; in these cases asymmetrical movement occurs (see previous discussion and Fig. 4.11).

There are two conditions found in the knee usually for no apparent reason. *Genu valgum* (or knock-knees) may lead to additional weight bearing stresses being placed on the medial (inner) aspect of the joint. Osteoarthritis is likely to develop here later in life but symptoms of ligamentous origin may well develop earlier, especially if the knee is subjected to a great deal of weight bearing stress. The ligaments on the medial (inner) side of the joint will be progressively stretched. *Genu varum* (bow legs) leads to additional weight bearing stress being placed on the lateral (outside) part of the joint where symptoms of ligamentous stretch and/or osteoarthritis have an increased chance of developing (see Fig. 4.12).

Abnormality may result from accident. The typical example is a fractured bone where it may be shorter than before or it may be

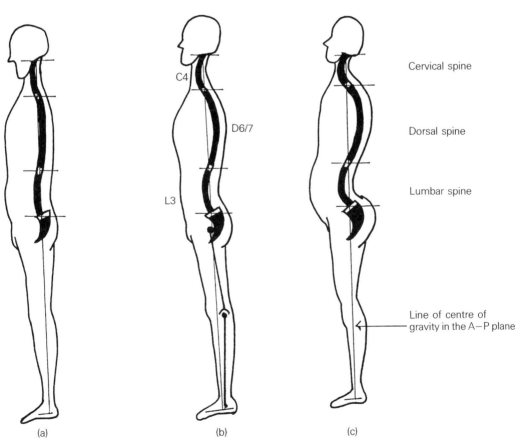

(a)   (b)   (c)

Fig. 4.10   A−P curves of the spine. (a) Reduced; (b) normal; (c) increased.

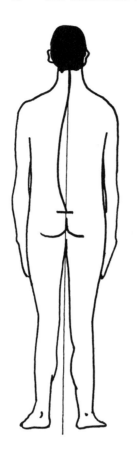

Fig. 4.11 Two types of scoliosis (lateral curvatures).

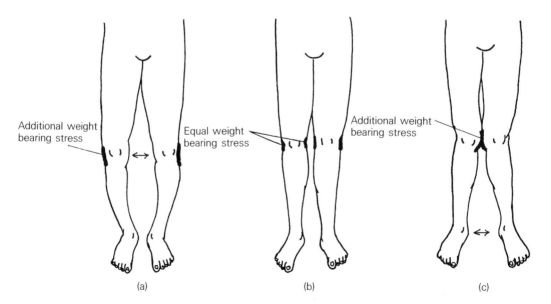

Additional weight bearing stress

Equal weight bearing stress

Additional weight bearing stress

(a)   (b)   (c)

Fig. 4.12   (a) Genu varum; (b) normal; (c) genu valgum.

distorted in shape. A shortened long bone in a leg may lead to a *scoliotic spine*. The clavicle (collar bone) is frequently misshapen and shortened following fracture. This may lead to the shoulder joint being held anteriorly (forward) with resultant strain on certain muscles during activities such as throwing. Fractures can also cause injury to other surrounding tissues, the function of which may never completely recover, particularly blood vessels and nerves.

Repeated stresses also produce their effect. If bone is subjected to repeated pressure it may well develop an *exostosis* (outgrowth). An exostosis can be obstructive and is often sensitive to further pressure. The back of the heel is a typical site for an exostosis to appear, caused by shoe pressure over a period of time (see Fig. 4.13). Repeated compression to the spine may lead to distortion of the shape of the vertebral bodies (see Fig. 4.14). This used to be seen in young rugby players who had been in the scrum too often and may be seen in adults still as a result of such compression in their youth. The young intervertebral discs become swollen and enlarged and actually erode the young, soft bone so that the vertebral body becomes biconcave instead of nearly square (see Fig. 4.15).

Certain inflammatory conditions can lead to permanent changes within the skeleton. *Epiphysitis* and *osteochondritis* are typical examples. If the epiphysis (growing point) becomes inflamed there is a proliferation of bone at that site. Osteochondritis has a similar effect and leads to wedging of the vertebral bodies in the spine. The net result of this is an increased *kyphosis* (see section 5.9). This condition is very common indeed and Dr Alan Stoddard considers it to be a contributory factor in 60% of adults who

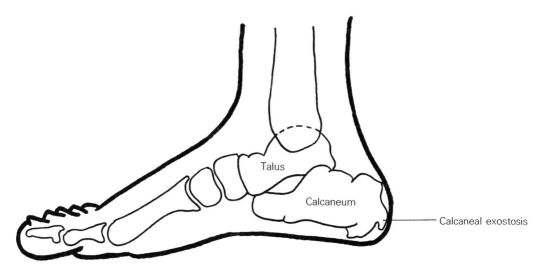

Fig. 4.13   Calcaneal exostosis.

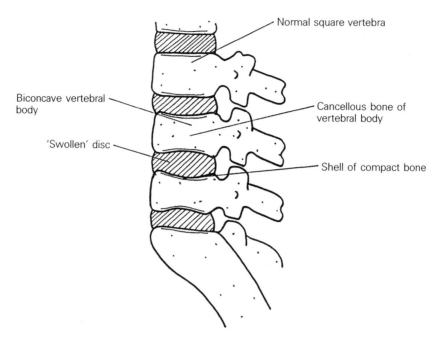

Fig. 4.14   Compression of vertebral body in the adolescent.

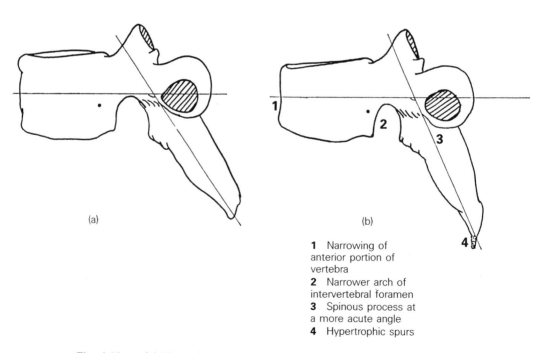

(a)   (b)

1 Narrowing of
anterior portion of
vertebra
2 Narrower arch of
intervertebral foramen
3 Spinous process at
a more acute angle
4 Hypertrophic spurs

Fig. 4.15   (a) Normal dorsal vertebra; (b) distorted vertebra due to repeated
compression.

complain of low back pain. It is often overlooked in childhood when it is in the active phase but the effects are all too often seen in adults. Both osteochondritis and epiphysitis are self-limiting conditions and are still dismissed as 'growing pains' in young people. However, if detected in the active phase the child should be limited in physical activities to minimise the resultant deformity both from a cosmetic and skeletal efficiency aspect.

The musculoskeletal system can be affected by infectious disease and deficiency conditions. *Poliomyelitis* attacks the anterior (motor) cells of the spinal cord leading to possible paralysis of an area of the body from which it never recovers. The effect of conditions such as *rickets* is still sometimes seen in clinical practice with the resultant deformities.

Any of these predisposing factors can lead to mechanical faults, disturbance of coordination or poor body balance. Posture in the upright position requires perfect coordination in joints, muscles and other soft tissues and is largely controlled by nervous reflexes. Muscular activity is needed to maintain the upright posture as well as to propel the body along and move it about, and any interference in this delicate balance, from whatever cause, will render the athlete more susceptible to injury during his sporting career. It is essential, therefore, that all aspects of imperfect body mechanics are detected and their effects fully considered when assessing the true extent and complexity of all sporting injuries.

It is important to remember that other conditions may present as apparent sporting injuries. Pathologies of bone, joint or muscle may be present although thankfully they are rare, while such conditions as multiple sclerosis may render the patient more liable to injury during sport. A clue to the need for further investigation may be severe symptoms from a comparatively minor injury or the patient giving a somewhat unusual symptom picture. Such cases should never be dismissed without full examination.

Chapter 5   Tissue Injuries

5.1   **Skin**

The three layers of the skin are shown in Fig. 5.1. It acts as a tough outer protection to the body and having a good blood supply, normally heals well following injury. The thickness of the epidermis varies; it is thickest on the soles of the feet where it receives a great deal of pressure.

A *bruise* is caused by a blow on the surface of the body which does not actually break the surface of the skin. Bleeding occurs in the underlying tissues accompanied by pain and swelling. Treatment consists of the application of an ice pack firmly secured to minimise the bleeding. If the skin is not broken, tincture of arnica is a useful treatment. Arnica can also be given by mouth and should be continued for five days.

The complication of a bruise is *scarring* in the underlying tissues, leading to reduced elasticity. This seldom needs treatment but will respond to ultrasound if necessary. The area should be moved during the healing period to minimise the amount of scar tissue formed.

A *burn* is damage to the skin usually as a result of heat, but a friction burn or an ice burn may also occur. If the skin is exposed to excessive strong sunlight, sunburn may result. This is preventable

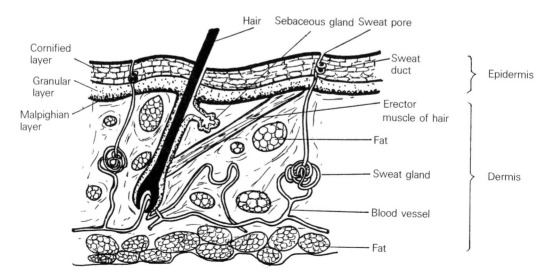

Fig. 5.1   Cross section through the skin.

by protecting the skin during exposure and should not occur to the point where it needs treatment. A burn caused by heat is seldom seen as a sport injury. A friction burn, however, is relatively common, usually caused by a player falling and sliding on a rough surface. It is often accompanied by a *graze*. These burns should be treated by cooling the skin surface as quickly as possible, by applying ice or plunging the area into cold water.

An ice burn is likely in sports where the athlete is exposed to very cold conditions and the area should be warmed gently but never heated. Sometimes an ice burn is caused by overenthusiasm in the application of ice packs. It can be prevented if the skin is given protection by smearing oil on before the ice pack is applied – a natural precaution to take. Severe burns need specialist treatment and the patient should be sent to a casualty unit as quickly as possible.

Burns are classified according to the depth of tissue damaged (see Fig. 5.2). A first degree burn affects the epidermis, a second degree affects the dermis while a third degree burn affects the subcutaneous layer. All third degree burns need specialist treatment as do all burns which cover an area of skin greater than approximately 2.5 sq. cm. Small first degree burns should be exposed to the air; no adhesive dressing should ever be applied as it will tend to remove the damaged epidermis and cause an open wound, thus risking infection.

A *blister* is caused by repeated friction. The epidermis is lifted away from the dermis and fluid collects in the resultant space (see Fig. 5.3). A blister is very painful as the nerve endings become

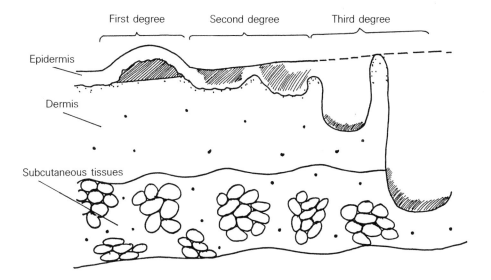

Fig. 5.2   Skin, degrees of burns.

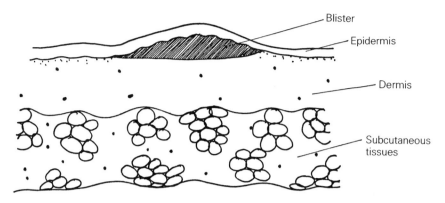

Fig. 5.3   Blister formation.

exposed when they are no longer protected by the adherent epidermis. Should the skin be subjected to continuous friction over a period of time, the epidermis will thicken and a callous will form. These are most often seen on the soles of the feet, or the palms of the hands in athletes such as tennis players where the racket causes friction. Callouses tend to crack due to the epidermis becoming less elastic. They should be treated by an expert, such as a chiropodist and may soften somewhat with the application of lanolin. Blisters are treated by removing the fluid with a sterilised needle and then covering the area with a clean dressing. The epidermis should never be cut away.

A *graze* is usually caused by a fall where the epidermis is removed by friction. They are very painful as the underlying nerve endings are exposed. Quite severe bleeding may occur. The area should be cleaned with a disinfectant and covered with a clean dressing. Healing usually occurs quickly and specialist treatment is only necessary when a large area of epidermis has been removed, possible as a result of a motorbike accident.

A *laceration* involves damage to both epidermis and dermis and the subcutaneous tissue is exposed. If the wound is long it may need stitching or at least the sides should be held together with 'butterfly' dressings. If the wound is of the puncture type such as that caused by a dart or arrow, there may be damage to underlying tissues and specialist treatment is required. A simple wound will heal adequately if kept clean and covered. Infection may be a complication of a laceration and specialist treatment is then needed. Some scars adhere to the underlying tissue especially in boxers who are injured over the eye. Some people produce hypertrophic scar tissue which is not only unsightly but has a tendency to crack open. Some scars which form after a graze has been infected may be raised above the level of the surrounding skin. All three of these conditions need to be treated by a specialist. The other complication of a laceration is the possibility of tetanus or lockjaw. All athletes should keep their immunity up by regular booster injections.

Occasionally an athlete is subjected to a *crush injury*. This will cause bleeding which may escape if the skin is broken. Severe crush injuries need specialist treatment especially where a wide area of the body is injured but mild cases will recover on their own and should be treated as bruises.

5.2   Muscles, tendons and fascial sheaths

A *skeletal muscle* is composed of many individual fibres which are capable of contracting and shortening. A motor unit is a small group of these fibres around which the blood vessels which supply the muscle, run together with the nerves. The whole muscle is surrounded by a sheath of connective tissue known as the fascial sheath. The muscle is fleshy and has a good blood supply. A *tendon* is composed of thick collagen fibre with a poor blood supply (see Fig. 5.4). It is designed to connect muscle to bone and tapers from the point where it joins the muscle – the musculo-tendinous junction – to the point where it is attached to the bone. Surrounding the tendon is the paratenon, a membrane which provides nourishment to the fibres of the tendon. In addition, a

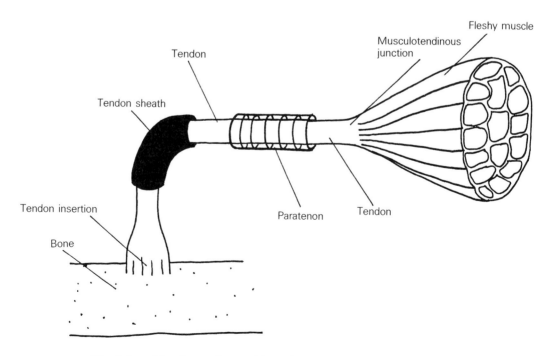

Fig. 5.4   Muscle, tendon and bone junction.

tendon may be surrounded by a '*tendon sheath*' which is thick walled and is protective in sites where the tendon would be liable to injury, for example where the tendon runs round an angled bone. The mechanism by which muscle contracts is explained in section 3.3.

Muscle and fascial sheath injuries

A muscle can *tear* from an intrinsic or extrinsic force. The effect will be the same and will include damage to blood vessels. A complete tear will result in some loss of function but a partial tear or 'pull' will not impair function. In each case bleeding will occur within the muscle and pain will be felt on contraction.

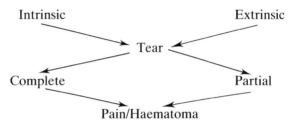

The local injury will be obvious and the history clear. Pain is felt at the site of injury which is increased on contraction or on passive stretch and there is local swelling and tenderness. With an intrinsic tear a sharp pain is felt suddenly and the patient may say he thought he had been hit.

Treatment in the early stage is designed to reduce the internal haemorrhage – i.e. ICE which stands for Ice, Compression and Elevation. Two days later gradual active exercise is started and ultrasound or short wave diathermy are useful to accelerate repair. A complete tear does not significantly impair the function of the muscle and surgical repair is seldom needed. There is often a strange contour to the muscle thereafter; the commonest site for this is in the front of the thigh, especially in the rectus femoris (see Fig. 5.5). Complications of muscle injury are not seen as often these days as they used to be as treatment has improved greatly. Infection and cyst formation are rare and both require expert treatment. Scarring, however, is inevitable and results in shortening of the muscle made worse by the fact that pain is exacerbated by stretching during the repair phase. Subsequent injury is therefore more likely to occur and this is why recurrent muscle tears are all too common. The most important part of treatment of muscle tears has to be progressive mobilisation and stretching, if the muscle is to avoid further damage in subsequent sporting activities.

Calcium deposits may develop within the muscle following a tear especially where the injury was caused by a direct blow, and will produce considerable disability, a condition known as *myositis*

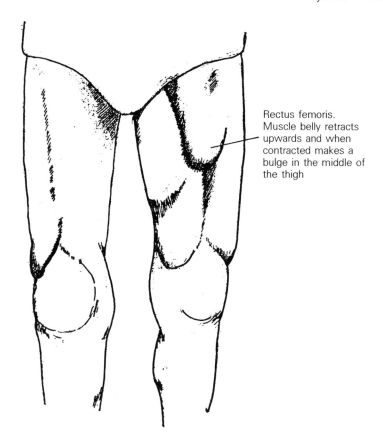

Rectus femoris.
Muscle belly retracts
upwards and when
contracted makes a
bulge in the middle of
the thigh

Fig. 5.5 Rupture of
the left rectus femoris
at the lower
musculotendinous
junction.

ossificans (see Fig. 5.6). A hard mass will be palpable within the
muscle at the site of injury and X-rays will show the deposit.
Progressive mobilisation of the muscle will increase the deposit
and is contraindicated if this condition is suspected. Short wave
diathermy is thought to be helpful but surgical treatment may be
necessary once the active stage has passed if there is too much
disability.

Muscle *stiffness* following unaccustomed activity is common. It
can be prevented by sufficient preparation for the sport and relieved
by heat following such activity. Rubifacients are also helpful but
adequate preparation, warm up and warm down should be carried
out. Muscle bruising may occur without a tear and is treated as a
skin bruise. Calcium deposits may be a later complication of this
injury. Occasionally bleeding may occur within the muscle and
track down the limb as the blood flows between the tissue planes
forming a vivid discolouration at a site well away from the original
injury. Recovery is swift and treatment is as for a muscle bruise.

The fascial sheath may *rupture*, usually at the musculotendinous
junction when its normal pressure on the muscle fibres will be
reduced rendering contraction of that muscle difficult if not impossible. (See Fig. 5.7 for normal synovial sheath). The patient

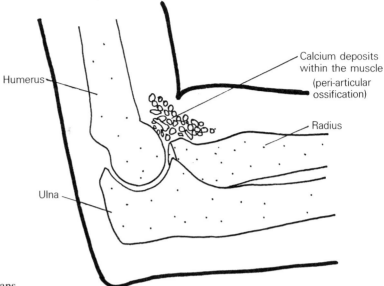

Fig. 5.6 Myositis ossificans.

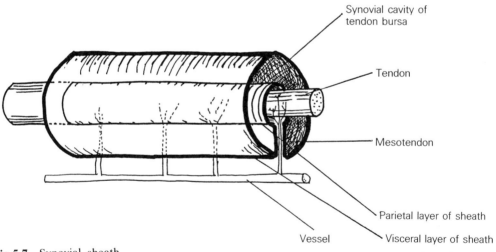

Fig.5.7 Synovial sheath.

complains of pain in the area which is worse when the muscle is used. There is often bruising present and a localised tender swelling which becomes larger as the muscle is contracted. Small lesions of the fascial sheath will repair but large tears may need surgical intervention. Recurrence of this injury is not common.

In some parts of the body there are fascial sheaths just under the skin which are subjected to the stresses of powerful neighbouring muscles causing them to become painful at their attachments. The common sites are the plantar aponeurosis in the sole of the foot and the fascial sheath on the lateral aspect of the thigh. Examination reveals an area of tenderness which is often widespread, with slight warmth and increased tension. Treatment to relax the hypertonic fibres by gentle stretching, passively, will relieve symptoms.

Fibrotic changes occur in some athletes usually in the muscles at the back of the shoulder girdles. It is a serious condition and frequently progressive. The patient will complain of pain, tenderness and stiffness which is aggravated by use and only marginally relieved by rest. There is a history of similar previous attacks which get progressively more severe and last longer. Heat and deep massage to the affected muscles is beneficial followed by progressive stretching to the area. Examination reveals an increased tension in the muscle and there is marked tenderness within the fleshy parts.

Muscle spasm is frequently seen in practice and is associated with joint injury. The muscles around the injured joint tighten up probably to form a type of natural splint and reduce the chance of further injury to the joint. Although the muscle will respond to soft tissue massage type treatment the condition will recur if the joint problem is not treated satisfactorily so that the spasm is no longer necessary for joint protection. The condition is most frequently seen in the spine where joint strains are very common. The muscles will be sensitive to palpation and there will be some abnormal mobility of the underlying joint with possible pain on one or more active movement. Muscle spasm is not the same as the shortening which occurs following a muscle tear.

The osteopathic approach to muscle injuries will include examination of all of the joints which are acted on by the injured muscle as there is likely to be a resultant mechanical fault somewhere. For example, if a hamstring muscle has been injured, the knee, hip and/or pelvic joints may be functioning imperfectly, the knee joint includes the superior tibiofibular joint. The hamstrings arise partly from the pelvis and are attached as low down as the tibia and the fibula. Similarly, an osteopath considers that a mechanical fault in any one or more of those joints can predispose the athlete to such an injury. If the joint mechanics are at all impaired there will be an undue stress placed on the muscle which may well give way under it; so the prevention of muscle injuries generally, will depend on perfect body mechanics, or as near perfect as it is possible to achieve for that individual.

Even then the rules of warming up and down must be carefully observed. When sport is resumed and especially in cold weather, it is wise to suggest that the athlete rubs the old injury well with some rubifacient to promote the circulation and to continue doing this until he has not the slightest twinge on full activity.

Skeletal muscle may suffer from *cramp*, which is a generalised form of spasm. It is very painful and the spasm cannot be controlled voluntarily. Cramp occurs when the muscle goes into oxygen debt and normal contraction is no longer possible.

There are two distinct types of cramp − runners cramp and swimmers cramp. In the former, the muscles of the legs go into oxygen debt when they are subjected to extended running which causes muscle fatigue. If the circulation is not very good, runners cramp is more likely to occur. Swimmers cramp is a similar condition where oxygen debt is the principal cause. However, swimmers are more likely to suffer from cramp after a meal when extra blood is required by the digestive system to digest food. There is then less for the peripheral circulation. In addition, the water may be cold so the peripheral circulation will be diminished, and while swimming the breathing is intermittent and breath is taken at longer intervals than when running. The muscles of the legs and also of the abdominal wall are those most frequently affected. Stomach cramps will generally bend an athlete in half with pain while leg cramp can lock the leg with great force and pain.

Treatment is designed to increase the blood flow by stimulating the circulation and thus reducing the oxygen debt. Fresh blood can be encouraged to the area affected, by friction and deep squeezing of the area together with deep breathing to increase the oxygen supply to the body.

5.4   **Tendon and tendon sheath injuries**

The word 'tendon' derives from the Latin meaning 'stretch' which is a misnomer as tendons are bundles of thick, fibrous, collagen fibres which are inelastic and their inelasticity progresses with age. For this reason tendons are more likely to be injured in older athletes as distinct from muscles which are often injured in the young. Tendons may be long and slender or short and compact. All are surrounded by a 'paratenon' and some by a 'tendon sheath' too. Injury is usually intrinsic in origin, from some abnormal sudden movement or from progressive stress, rarely from direct extrinsic origin. A tendon tear may be partial or complete.

Tendinitis is inflammation of the tendon where there is no tendon sheath and is associated with shortening of the related muscle in most cases, which will result in an extra pull along the tendon. The common sites are the patellar tendon, often caused by stress from jumping, the biceps tendon in the upper arm, often following rupture of the ligament which holds the tendon in the bicipital groove, and the Achilles tendon, from progressive overuse or possibly from friction − e.g. shoe pressure. The condition responds well to deep friction and stretching of the associated muscle fibres. Any fault in the mechanical integrity of the surrounding joints must be rectified. A period of relative rest followed by progressive use is needed and full use should only be started again when there is no remaining discomfort.

Rupture most usually occurs from progressive overuse and weakening. The patient will complain of sudden sharp pain and may think he has been shot or kicked. The common sites are the Achilles tendon (see section 11.3) and the long head of the biceps in the arm (see Fig. 5.8).

Displacement may occur and the common sites are the biceps in the arm and the peronei on the lateral aspect of the ankle (see Figs. 5.9 and 5.10). The biceps tendon displaces from within the bicipital groove after damage to the transverse humeral ligament which normally retains it there. The peroneal muscles normally lie, in their tendinous form, posterior to the lateral malleolus at the ankle. If displaced, the tendons may lie obliquely across the fibula, near its lower end. In cases of displacement, surgical repair is needed or the efficiency of the muscle will be permanently impaired.

Avulsion of a tendon may occur from a sudden excessive movement and if present, needs surgical repair.

Ossification within a tendon can be seen for about 2−3 cm from its attachment to bone. Minor stress fractures at the point of

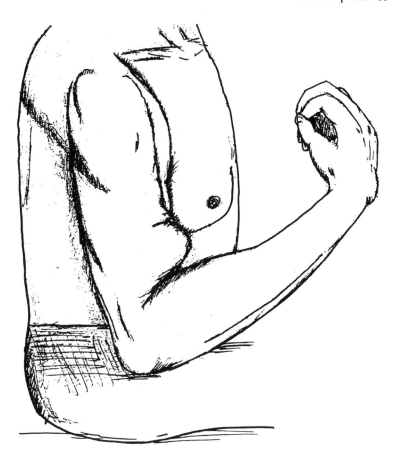

Fig. 5.8 Appearance of rupture of the long head of biceps.

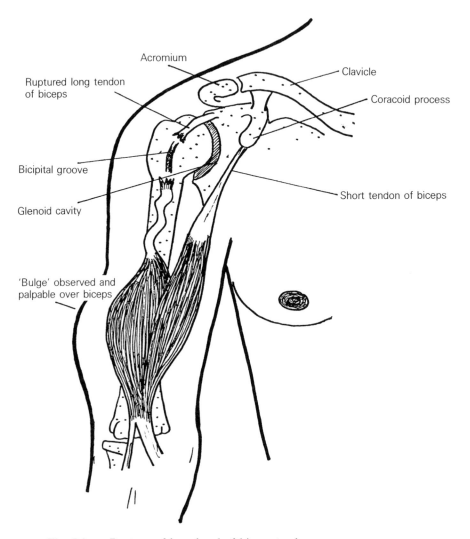

Fig. 5.9   Rupture of long head of biceps tendon.

attachment of a tendon to a bone probably due to excessive pull, can sometimes lead to this condition but it is seldom of clinical importance and gives no symptoms.

Damage may occur to the peritenon around the tendon. It is usually caused by excessive use or unaccustomed activity, after which the pain and disability are quick to appear. There is a palpable swelling around the tendon but it will subside in most cases with rest (possibly including strapping) and any anti-inflammatory treatment. Stretching to the relevant muscle fibres is also helpful. If the condition does not resolve or becomes recurrent with activity, surgery to remove adhesions present may be necessary.

Localised thickening of the tendon sheath may occur usually for no apparent reason although it can be caused by active rheumatic

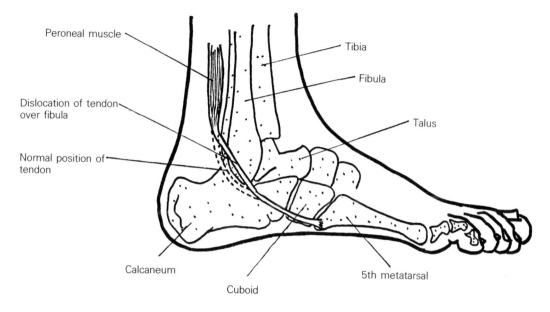

Peroneal muscle

Dislocation of tendon over fibula

Normal position of tendon

Tibia

Fibula

Talus

Calcaneum

Cuboid

5th metatarsal

Fig. 5.10   Dislocation of peroneal tendon, lateral aspect.

disease such as gout or rheumatoid arthritis. The condition is only of importance if symptoms result, when it is necessary to reduce any local inflammation and improve local mechanics.

Tenosynovitis is a condition where there is an increase of the synovial fluid which normally acts as a lubricant between the tendon and its sheath. It is usually caused by acute overuse but can be due to a blow. In the acute phase, local swelling can be seen and pain is felt due to an associated inflammation of the tendon. Crepitus may be palpable over the area. Rest is essential at this stage with, possibly, splinting or strapping too. If the condition becomes chronic, adhesions may occur between the tendon and its sheath and impairment of function of the muscle together with pain on use, will result. Friction may reduce the adhesions or infiltration may be necessary or even surgery in the most persistent cases.

Occasionally the pull of the tendon on the bone to which it is attached is so strong that a fragment of bone may become detached as in the Mallet finger suffered, for example, by cricketers fielding in the slips (see Fig. 5.11). This is an extremely painful injury and requires splinting for the fracture to heal.

Complications of tendon injury are rare but the associated muscle will need careful rehabilitation after the tendon lesion has healed.

5.5   **Musculotendinous injury**

Anywhere where one tissue blends with another is potentially a weak place in the body and this is the case at all musculotendinous

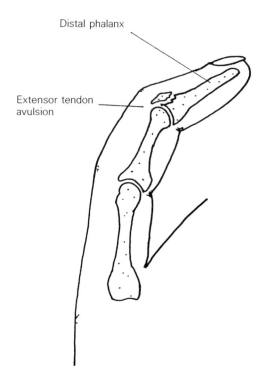

Distal phalanx

Extensor tendon avulsion

Fig. 5.11 Mallet finger. Avulsion of a fragment of the distal phalanx.

junctions. So it is essential to know these sites when treating sporting injuries. If the injury is more muscular than tendinous, treatment as for muscle injuries will produce excellent results, namely soft tissue and stretching techniques to the muscular component. However, surgery may be necessary in some cases where there is more of a tendinous involvement although conservative treatment should always be tried first. Tears may be partial or complete and are invariably intrinsic in origin. Repetitive minor traumata may well result in pain and disability over a period of time.

5.6

Bone injury

A *fracture* is the condition where there is a break in the continuity of a bone or where it is separated into two or more parts (see Fig. 5.12). Most fractures occur as a result of some extrinsic force often applied across the bone. It would probably be able to withstand an equal force if applied along the length of the bone. The history will often lead to suspicion of fracture. There is often considerable damage to the surrounding soft tissues with swelling, loss of function and disability, possible deformity and possible grating at the site of the break. If the force applied was not excessive there may have been some underlying weakness of the bone structure from

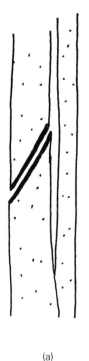 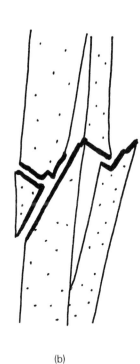

Fig. 5.12 (a) Oblique fracture; (b) comminuted fracture.

(a)   (b)

some pre-existing disease. Such a condition should be suspected in cases of fracture with comparatively small forces.

X-rays will reveal most fractures but some are not apparent until callous formation is present. This starts one to four weeks following the fracture and is usually complete by six weeks. Any suspicion of fracture must always be referred for further investigation.

Stress fractures are relatively common and are due to excessive loads especially where there has been a change in the training programme. The onset is usually insidious rather than sudden and such a fracture causes pain which is exacerbated following exercise and also at night. The pain is localised and there may be localised swelling. In the early stages, X-rays are invariably normal in appearance but will show the fracture in the later stages. A common site is in one of the metatarsals where there is usually an area of localised erithema (redness) on the under surface of the foot below the fracture. Treatment is rest, possibly with some mechanical support to relieve the pain, and sport must not be resumed until the patient is completely symptom-free. Recovery is usually quite swift.

Pathological fractures are occasionally seen in athletes and are due to some underlying bone disease. The possibility of such a fracture should be considered if there is excessive bone damage from a relatively minor injury. Further investigation is essential.

Other sinister conditions may present as sports injuries and should be considered when there is a complaint of intractable bone pain. These conditions are usually not relieved by various factors as one might expect, for example the pain will be the same throughout the twenty-four hours.

An *exostosis* is a bony outgrowth and is invariably caused by a blow or a series of repeated frictional irritations, for example on the posterior aspect of the calcaneum from persistently ill-fitting shoes, or in hockey players where there has been a history of blows on the shins from hockey sticks. These seldom give any symptoms once the initial bruising has elapsed. However any 'lump' on any bone which is getting bigger must be taken seriously and must be investigated further. Exostoses may be widespread and intra-articular, for example on the anterior aspect of the ankle joint in footballers.

5.7

Epiphyseal conditions

Epiphysitis is an inflammatory condition of the epiphysis (growing area) of a bone. It may be localised or generalised. It is thought to be due to excessive pressure applied to the growing skeleton and often results from parental pressure on a youngster. Pain is felt at the epiphyseal line which is exacerbated during and after exercise, and later there will be disability and loss of movement in the neighbouring joint. The usual sites are in the long bones of the lower extremities. Treatment must be to rest the areas and only return slowly and progressively to active sport when the symptoms have subsided. General osteopathic treatment to the surrounding joints especially of an articulatory type is helpful but must be gentle and of short duration, as the inflammatory changes must not be exacerbated by treatment. The 'slipped epiphysis' is a much more serious condition and occurs in the upper femoral epiphysis (see Fig. 5.13). This condition resembles a pathological fracture and is thought to be due to an underlying abnormality. X-rays confirm the diagnosis but specialist treatment is essential. The condition is commoner in boys than girls, the age for boys is usually about 15 whereas girls suffer at about 12 years of age. The youngster will complain of pain which is worse on any weight bearing activity. On clinical examination there is loss of internal rotation and abduction to some degree, but all active and passive movements may be somewhat limited. This condition may present as the result of a sporting activity but is not commonly seen in osteopathic practice.

5.8

Accessory bone

In 7% of the population there is a small accessory bone present, posterior to the ankle joint (see Fig. 4.1). Normally it is of no

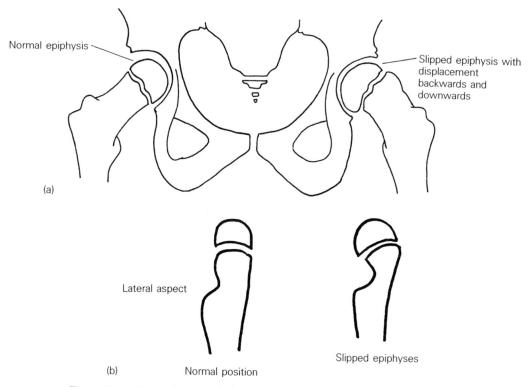

Normal epiphysis

Slipped epiphysis with displacement backwards and downwards

(a)

Lateral aspect

(b) Normal position

Slipped epiphyses

Fig. 5.13 Slipped epiphysis (coxa vara). (a) Anterior-posterior aspect; (b) lateral aspect.

consequence whatever, but in some sports, for example jumping, it may be compressed and become inflamed. Pain will be felt deep to the tendo Achilles and a tender spot may be palpable there. The symptoms will be aggravated by any excessive compression of the inflamed bone. Treatment will be to reduce the inflammation and reduce the compression stress on the bone. Occasionally, if the symptoms persist and really handicap the athlete, excision may be necessary.

In the sole of the foot there are several sesamoid bones – the exact distribution varies from one person to another. Under the big toe, embedded in the insertion of the flexor hallucis brevis muscle, two of these are always present (see Fig. 5.14). The larger is on the medial aspect of the toe and is sometimes double, in which case an X-ray of the bone may be mistaken for a fracture which is not the case. On forced dorsiflexion of the first metatarsophalangeal joint, the sesamoid may be subjected to trauma if the athlete comes down from a height, for example in tennis, especially on hard court surfaces. The injury is often repetitive and there is a resultant inflammation set up in the bone. Pain will be felt, aggravated by running or jumping and there will be a localised

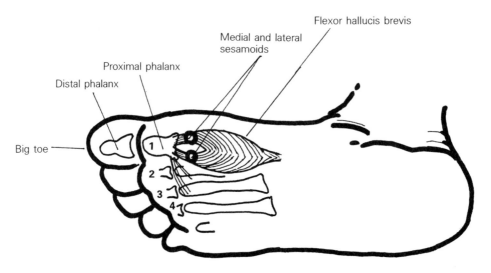

Flexor hallucis brevis

Medial and lateral
sesamoids

Proximal phalanx

Distal phalanx

Big toe

Fig. 5.14   Sesamoid bones of hallux.

tender area with possible swelling felt on palpation. Treatment is
designed to take some of the weight off the irritated bone, for
example by strips of chiropody felt on either side of the sesamoid.
Rest from jumping and/or running may be necessary and possibly
a thicker soled shoe to minimise the chance of recurrent trouble.
Excision is seldom required.

5.9

Avascular necrosis of bone

Bone tissue may die as a result of infection or if there is interference
of the blood supply.

Although rarely seen in athletes, infection such as *osteomyelitis*
or *tuberculosis* could present as an athletic injury. In such a case,
the patient would not be in good general health and might have a
raised body temperature. Enlargement of the adjacent lymph nodes
would be likely. He would probably complain of pain in one joint
of insidious onset, although it might have started following physical
activity. Clinical examination would reveal limitation of movement
in all ranges of the affected joint together with pain at the extreme
of all movements. There might well be some guarding felt at the
extreme of all passive movements. These findings should guide the
osteopath to seek further investigation for the patient.

The blood supply to a bone may be cut off following fracture or
dislocation of a joint. Fracture of the scaphoid, talus and femoral
head and dislocation of the ankle leading to necrosis of the talus,
wrist dislocation leading to necrosis of the lunate and dislocation of
the hip joint leading to necrosis of the head of the femur may
occur. In all these cases there would be a history of fracture and/or
dislocation.

There will also be stiffness in the joint and local tenderness may be present. X-rays will show increased bone density and possible bone deformity. Specialist treatment is needed in such a case. Excessive alcohol intake (of more than 75 g daily) or extensive treatment by corticosteriods can also lead to bone necrosis. The history should reveal the latter but the former might well be denied by the patient! The hip, knee or even the shoulder are the most likely sites.

Necrosis of the head of the femur, Perthe's Disease, may present as an apparent sporting injury. The patient will be a child usually four to eight years of age; it is commoner in boys and may occur bilaterally. The only symptoms are an ache and slight limp. On clinical examination, the joint is found to be limited in all ranges of movement with discomfort at the extremes of movement. Abduction in flexion is most clearly limited. Orthopaedic treatment is necessary. As the process continues, the head of the femur flattens and becomes 'mushroom shaped' (see Fig. 5.15). This predisposes to degenerative change later in life but the active process is self-limiting, so the less severe cases are revealed when degenerative changes occur rather earlier in life than might be suspected. Such cases may well present as sporting injuries where the degenerative joint may have been subjected to stress from physical activity.

Osteochondritis is seen very often in practice. Crushing osteochondritis presents in the spine (especially the thoracic), the navicular, metatarsal, lunate and capitulum. Increased bone density and bone deformity are characteristic. In the active stage, which will be in youngsters who are experiencing a 'growth spurt' or an increase in physical activity, rest is essential to minimise the deformity. Osteopathic treatment to improve the mechanics of the affected areas will relieve pain and may help reduce deformity as it is likely that the blood supply will improve with such treatment. The long-term effects of the disease will reduce certain movements

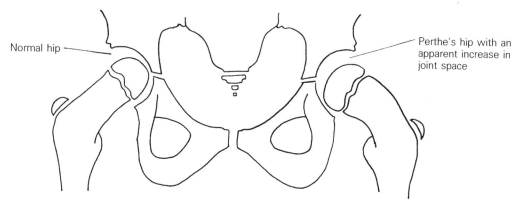

Normal hip

Perthe's hip with an apparent increase in joint space

Fig. 5.15   Perthe's disease.

and osteopathic treatment, designed to normalise such movement
as far as possible, will help to reduce any disability.

Splitting osteochondritis (see Fig. 5.16) usually occurs in young
men. It is thought to be due to repeated minor traumata causing
small fractures at certain sites; the fragment of bone becomes
necrotic. The sites are the lateral surface of the medial condyle in
the knee, the anteromedial tip of the talus in the ankle, the
superomedial part of the femoral head, the capitulum of the
humerus and the first metatarsal head. Healing may occur in some
children but it may take up to two years. The detached fragment
may be asymptomatic but if it becomes displaced it may give rise
to irritation and possibly have to be removed later in life.

Pulling osteochondritis (see Fig. 5.17) is a condition where the
pull of a strong tendon on the growing area of a bone leads to
detachment. The common sites are the tibial tubercle and the
calcaneal apophysis. Pain is felt especially on physical activity and
if severe immobilisation is necessary. Only occasionally is surgery
needed, if there is total detachment.

5.10   **Joints and ligaments**

A joint is where two or more bony surfaces meet and a specific
range of movement occurs. Most joints are of the synovial type

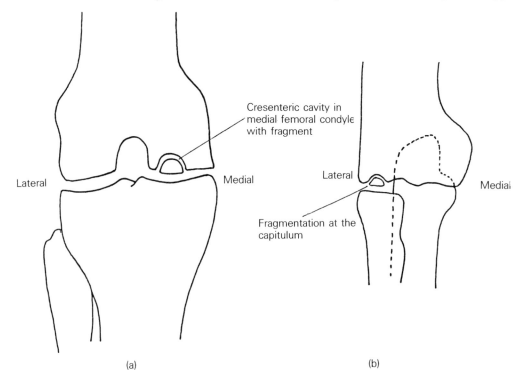

Cresenteric cavity in
medial femoral condyle
with fragment

Lateral   Medial   Lateral   Mediai

Fragmentation at the
capitulum

(a)   (b)

Fig. 5.16   Splitting osteochondritis (dissecans). (a) The knee; (b) the elbow.

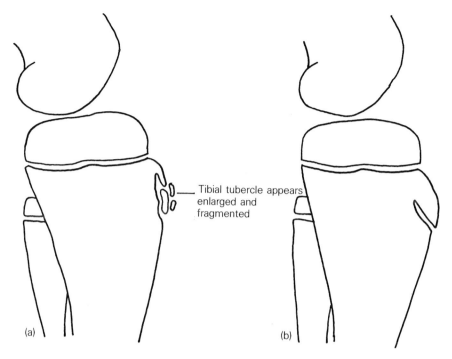

Tibial tubercle appears enlarged and fragmented

(a)

(b)

Fig. 5.17   (a) Pulling osteochondritis of the tibial tubercle (apophysitis); (b) normal tibial tubercle.

(see Fig. 5.18); the opposing bone ends are covered with articular cartilage and the whole joint is surrounded by a capsule which is lined with synovial membrane except where weight bearing occurs. The synovial membrane secretes synovial fluid which is a lubricant of the joint. The capsule is reinforced by ligaments which strengthen areas which are subject to particular strain during movement of the joint. Some joints have additional ligaments within the joint which are designed to strengthen the joint still further, for example the cruciate ligaments in the knee (see Fig. 5.19) and the ligamentum teres in the hip. Average active movement in any joint is that which occurs during normal everyday activity. Maximal active movement is greater in all ranges and occurs with full muscular pull on the joint. Passive movement is greater still and occurs when any outside force is applied to the joint which is not great enough to damage the joint. If the joint is forced beyond it's passive range of movement, damage will result. At that point the ligaments are placed under stress which is too great for them to withstand.

5.11   **Ligament injuries**

In normal function a joint is stable; it does not wobble around and is capable of moving through it's normal range of movement which

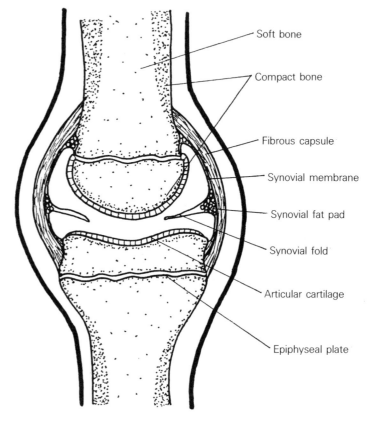

Fig. 5.18 A section through a synovial joint.

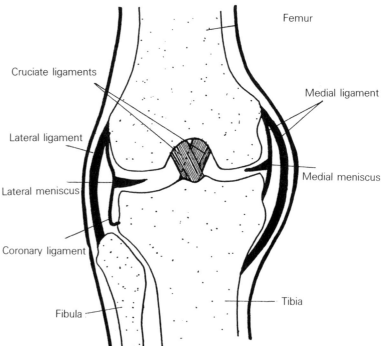

Fig. 5.19 Cruciate (anterior and posterior) ligaments of the knee.

is produced by muscular action. If, however, the joint is subjected to some force either intrinsic or more commonly extrinsic, which forces it beyond it's passive range of movement, the ligaments on one side of the joint and the capsule there, are stretched. A minor stretch will result in a minor tear of ligamentous fibres but the force can be great enough to cause a complete tear (see Fig. 5.20). This condition is known as a *joint sprain*. It is characterised by a history of injury, pain is felt especially when movement stretches the damaged ligament, and swelling may occur due to involvement of the synovial membrane. Active movement will then be limited as will passive movement and one passive movement in particular will cause more pain than the others. Minor tears are best treated initially by rest and swelling can be minimised by elevation of the limb and the application of ice packs. Strapping to support the injured fibres while they heal will minimise lasting stretching of the fibres. Chronic overstretch of a ligament results in instability of a joint in at least one range of movement and is difficult to treat and predisposes to degeneration.

During the repair period, joint activity is encouraged without weight bearing until weight bearing is no longer painful − i.e. only uncomfortable. Once the fibres have healed, any mechanical fault which remains in the joint must be treated to ensure a full recovery. If the force is greater than the ligaments can withstand, dislocation or subluxation of the joint will occur. Here the alignment of the joint

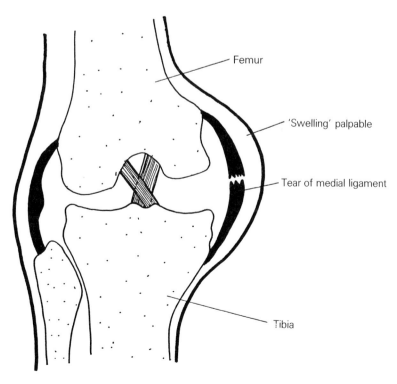

Fig. 5.20 Medial collateral ligament tear of the right knee.

Femur

'Swelling' palpable

Tear of medial ligament

Tibia

surfaces is completely upset. Dislocation is most likely to occur in joints which are anatomically unstable, such as the sternoclavicular joint and the shoulder. Reduction of the dislocation should never be attempted as there is always the possibility of some other damage, for example a fracture. Reduction of dislocations is definitely a specialist's task. Once the tissues have healed, any remaining fault in the joint can safely be treated by osteopathic means.

Chronic ligamentous stretch leads to instability of a joint and there is hypermobility of movement in one or more ranges. If the joint affected is not under voluntary muscular control, for example the sternoclavicular joint, the sacro-iliac joint or the symphisis pubis, the condition is often virtually untreatable except by some mechanical support. If the pain caused by such a condition is great, infiltration into the supporting ligaments followed by restriction of movement is required. If however, the joint has muscles around it which act upon it, treatment is aimed at strengthening them to help support the chronically strained ligament.

| 5.12 | **Synovial membrane and capsule injury** |

This is similar to injury to a ligament, but is more widespread as the whole capsule is affected. As the synovial membrane is irritated, there will be considerable joint effusion. The initial injury may have been sufficiently severe to have caused dislocation; in fact many capsule injuries are as a result of dislocation. Provided the joint is not left unstable, these injuries respond well to ice, pressure and possible elevation initially, followed by a programme of muscular re-education. Any fault which may remain in the joint should be treated by osteopathic means. The capsule of the shoulder joint is an exception to the above rule. Following trauma it has a nasty habit of tightening progressively, the well known 'frozen shoulder'. Articulatory techniques designed to methodically stretch the shortened fibres will finally result in full movement but recuperation is often long and arduous.

In some injuries swelling may occur immediately and so rapidly that it is almost visible. This is invariably due to haemorrhage within the joint. Of itself this is not necessarily important, but if there is continuous bleeding or if a thrombus forms a serious situation could result. So all immediate swelling should be referred for expert advice. This condition is known as *haemarthrosis*.

| 5.13 | **Intra-articular injury** |

Structures within a joint may be injured, usually by some extrinsic force. A *loose body* may result for example, if a snippet of cartilage becomes detached due to some force (see Fig. 5.21). There is a history of injury and the symptoms occur in sudden attacks possibly

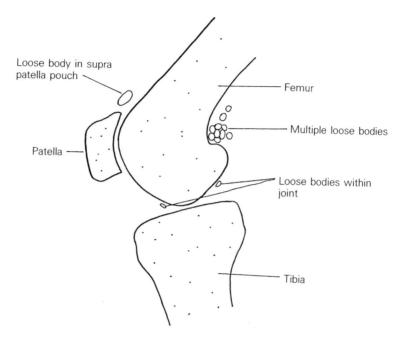

Loose body in supra patella pouch

Femur

Multiple loose bodies

Patella

Loose bodies within joint

Tibia

Fig. 5.21 Multiple loose bodies at the knee.

associated with a certain movement. Often it is difficult to reproduce the symptoms on examination. X-rays will reveal a loose body only if it is radio opaque. The joint may lock and the patient may have found how to shake it free. Such cases require surgical treatment as the joint will never function normally until the fragment is removed.

The cruciate ligaments in the knee may be *stretched* or even *torn*. This is a common football injury often caused by one player falling on another striking him from behind as he falls to the ground. On examination there will be excess movement in the A−P plane − i.e. when the tibia is shifted forward and backward on the femur with the knee flexed at 90°. Some of the less severe cases recover but it takes a long time. Muscular strengthening is essential to both the quadriceps and the hamstrings and surgery may be necessary in severe cases.

Any joint in the body can suffer from a *facet lock*. This is a condition where there is loss of mobility of the joint in one or more of it's movements within the normal range of the joint. Such a condition can be caused by some abnormal intrinsic muscle pull or from some extrinsic force. In the early stage there will be muscle spasm around the whole joint and some degree of inflammation and pain. There will be loss of normal movement in at least one range, both actively and passively. Meticulous osteopathic examination of the joint will reveal the condition, and specific osteopathic techniques need to be used to right the mechanical fault. In a chronic stage there will be the same mobility loss but the initial muscle spasm will have subsided and the joint will be less inflamed. This condition is frequently found in a series of joints, especially in the spine.

5.14

Mobility injury

Stiffness is a common complaint of athletes and usually follows injury to a joint, probably because the surrounding muscles went into protective spasm at the time of injury. It follows therefore that any stiffness condition may be due to a muscular rather than a true joint condition and every joint should be examined and the surrounding muscles checked for tightness. This is especially common around the knee — for example there may be limitation of extension due to a hamstring condition which can resemble locking. All stiff joints need to be handled carefully and the cause of the stiffness diagnosed before treatment is started.

Hypermobility has already been dealt with in section 5.11.

5.15

Bursal injury

A bursa is an enclosed sac which secretes a lubricant and is placed at a site in the body where there would be friction on some structure, for example where a tendon passes over a bony area or under the skin at points where there is likely to be pressure — e.g. in front of the patella. If injured, the bursa may swell and become painful and possibly obstructive. The usual cause of bursitis is pressure which may be from a single blow or from a series of recurrent traumata. The area will be swollen and possibly painful to touch while the history will usually make one suspect the condition. The common sites are around the knee, on the point of the elbow, deep to the tendo Achilles (see Fig. 5.22), in the subdeltoid space in the shoulder and under the insertion of gluteus medius into the greater trochanter (see Fig. 5.23). Treatment with ice packs in the early stages with rest is usually effective, but the condition may become chronic and if obstructive, aspiration or even excision of the bursa may be necessary.

5.16

Blood vessel injury

Blood vessels are usually injured when the skin is broken. If an artery is damaged the blood will exude in a pulsating fashion but will be steady if the injury is to a vein. In all cases the most important thing is to stop the bleeding by the application of a pressure pad over the wound and the area should be elevated above the level of the heart. In severe cases of arterial bleeding from a limb, pressure may be applied to either the brachial or

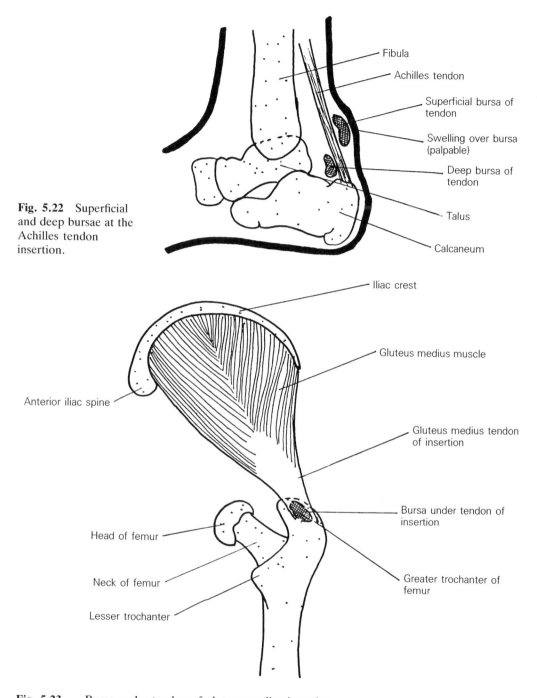

Fig. 5.22 Superficial and deep bursae at the Achilles tendon insertion.

Fibula

Achilles tendon

Superficial bursa of tendon

Swelling over bursa (palpable)

Deep bursa of tendon

Talus

Calcaneum

Iliac crest

Gluteus medius muscle

Anterior iliac spine

Gluteus medius tendon of insertion

Bursa under tendon of insertion

Head of femur

Neck of femur

Greater trochanter of femur

Lesser trochanter

Fig. 5.23   Bursa under tendon of gluteus medius insertion.

femoral pressure points but never for more than 15 minutes at a time (see Figs. 5.24 and 5.25). Such cases need hospitalisation as soon as possible. Mild cases of bleeding can be dealt with by pressure to the wound and elevation of the area.

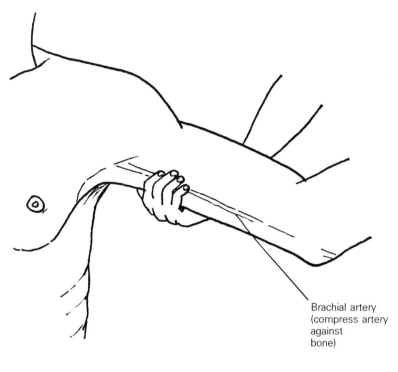

Fig. 5.24 Pressure point at brachial artery.

Brachial artery (compress artery against bone)

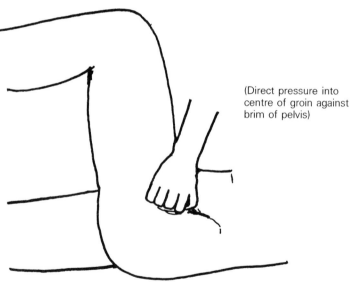

(Direct pressure into centre of groin against brim of pelvis)

Fig. 5.25 Pressure point at femoral artery.

5.17

Nerve injury

Nerve injuries may occur as a complication of fracture and/or dislocation − conditions requiring expert attention. Local bruising of a superficial nerve is not rare; the cause is usually a blow or a fall. Common sites are the ulnar nerve at the elbow (see Fig. 5.26) and the lateral popliteal nerve (see Fig. 5.27) as it passes around

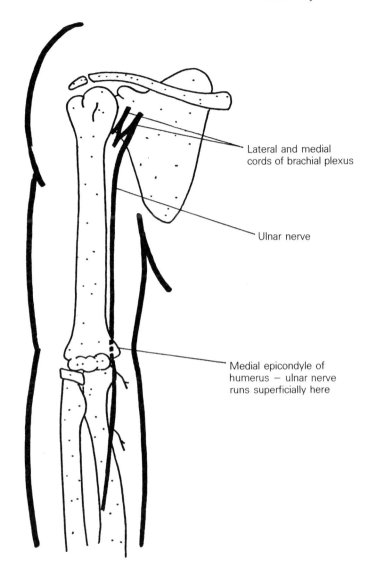

Lateral and medial
cords of brachial plexus

Ulnar nerve

Medial epicondyle of
humerus – ulnar nerve
runs superficially here

Fig. 5.26 Ulna
nerve. Common site
of injury at the elbow.

the head of the fibula on the outer part of the knee. Examination
may reveal local tenderness and possibly thickening of the sheath
of the ulnar nerve. The symptoms are usually felt at the lower end
of the nerve, for example ulnar nerve bruising will produce pins
and needles or possible paraesthesia in the fourth and fifth digits.
Recovery is usually complete but may take several weeks. Persistent symptoms will require the attention of a specialist. Nerves
may also be injured by stretching, for example when the neck is
forced into a position of extreme movement possibly in some
contact sport. Symptoms will be felt in any or even all parts of the
body; they usually subside with rest but may need expert treatment
and are beyond the scope of osteopathic treatment. Long-term

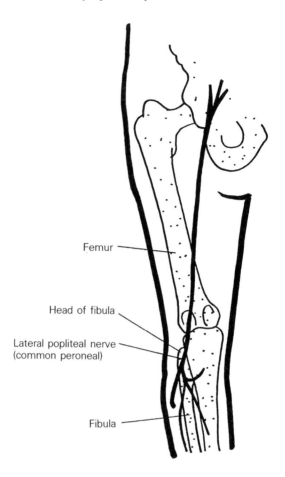

Femur

Head of fibula

Lateral popliteal nerve
(common peroneal)

Fibula

Fig. 5.27 Lateral
popliteal nerve.
Common injury at
lateral aspect of knee.

pressure from whatever source will produce nerve root type symptoms. The course of treatment to be followed will depend on a full examination and accurate diagnosis of the cause of the trouble − well within the scope of an osteopath.

Nerve damage to the brain in sport is often seen, i.e. *concussion*. The patient may not be unconscious but he may have difficulty concentrating or answering questions. The cause is a blow to the head with resultant bruising of the brain and should always be referred for expert treatment. Many cases of head and neck pain are seen in practice following concussion and will respond to osteopathic treatment. A full examination including the central nervous system is followed by correction of mechanical disorders.

There is one other condition seen quite commonly in athletes which results from nerve pressure and that is the development of a *neuroma*. The common site is between the first and second metatarsal heads just before the nerve divides to supply the adjacent sides of the great and second toes. The patient will complain of pain and possibly pins and needles on the adjacent surfaces of the first and second toes and there is unlikely to be a history of injury from any direct cause. The symptoms will have come on insidiously. Examination often reveals a palpable enlargement in the inter-osseous space. The symptoms can be exaggerated by compressing the metatarsal heads together and then shearing one on the other. Some cases can be relieved by a pad of chiropody felt placed under the neuroma, but many have to be excised.

Chapter 6   The Shoulder Girdle

It should be established straight away that any discussion of this anatomical region must encompass the shoulder girdle as a whole (see Fig. 6.1). It's remarkable range of mobility together with it's great strength can only be achieved by overall arthrological integrity, co-ordination of muscular action with capsuloligamentous support. A fault in any one of these mechanisms can result in dysfunction, pain, loss of mobility, weakness or mechanical derangement, or a combination of these. However, each of the joints concerned has to be considered individually to appreciate the overall girdle mechanics and therefore the possibilities for the various derangements.

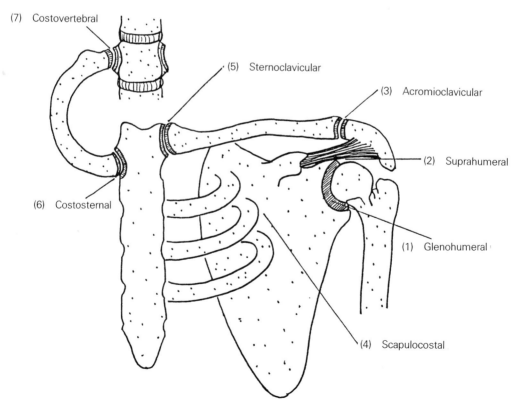

Fig. 6.1   Joints forming the shoulder girdle complex.

6.1

The glenohumeral joint

This is the articulation between the head of the humerus and the glenoid cavity of the scapula. The joint surfaces are incongruous; there is only a small area of opposition of the joint surfaces at any given point in the movement of the joint as the head of the humerus is much larger then the glenoid cavity, which is only marginally increased by the fibrous lip, 'the glenoid lip'. The joint is therefore dependent on muscular action for both primary movement and stability.

The capsule is attached around the glenoid cavity beyond the lip, and above to the root of the coracoid process so the long head of the biceps brachii muscle is surrounded in a capsular sheath of synovial membrane as it lies within the joint. The capsule is attached to the anatomical neck of the humerus except on the medial side where it passes downward for about 1 cm onto the shaft of the bone. The capsule is remarkably lax; when the arm hangs down, the superior part of the capsule is taut while the inferior part is loose and folded forming the axillar recess or axillary fold. When the arm is fully abducted the capsule is taut inferiorly and loose and folded superiorly. This laxity allows the gliding movement of the joint to take place. The synovial membrane of the capsule lines the capsule and is reflected onto the tendon of the long head of biceps within the joint.

The capsule is strengthened above by the coracohumeral ligament which arises from the tip of the coracoid process and blends into the capsule as far as the tubercles of the humerus. Anteriorly there are three weak glenohumeral ligaments which are horizontal folds of the capsule itself (see Fig. 6.2). Between the superior and middle glenohumeral ligaments is a weak spot, the 'foramen of Weitbrecht' which may be covered by a thin layer of capsule or may be a perforation connecting with the suprascapular fossa and through which anterior dislocation occurs. This communication is between the capsule and the bursa which lies between it and the tendon of the subscapularis muscle.

Other bursae are placed:

(1) between the infraspinatus tendon and the capsule which may communicate with the joint;
(2) between the deltoid and the capsule − the subacromial or subdeltoid bursa which does not communicate with the joint but lies under the acromion and the coracoacromial ligament;
(3) lying on the upper surface of the acromion;
(4) between the long head of the triceps and teres major;
(5) on either side of the tendon of latissimus dorsi (behind and in front of the tendon).

The capsule is strengthened by various muscles. Above by supraspinatus, below by the long head of triceps, in front by the

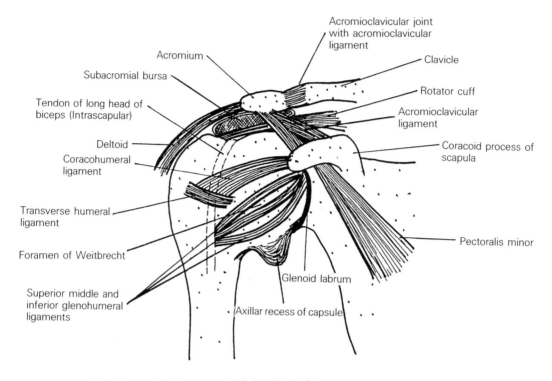

Fig. 6.2   Anterior aspect of shoulder joint.

tendon of subscapularis and behind by the tendons of infraspinatus and teres minor. With the exception of the long head of triceps, all these tendons blend with the capsule to some extent thus increasing their support. In addition, the long head of biceps reinforces the capsule anteriorly. Lying within the bicipital groove where it is held by the transverse humeral ligament, which is continuous above with the capsule of the joint, the tendon allows the humerus to slide along it as the dependent arm is moved away from the side of the body. Above, the joint is reinforced by the bony acromion process and the lateral end of the clavicle together with the ligaments of the acromioclavicular joint (see Fig. 6.3). This arrangement is so strong that dislocation can only occur anteriorly or posteriorly with some downward component.

6.2

The suprahumeral space

This is the area between the humeral head below, and the acromion process and the acromioclavicular joint above. It's position between two bony areas renders it vulnerable to direct trauma, for example pressure from above, especially if repeated. The space contains the subacromial bursa which reduces the effects of pressure. Under the bursa lies the tendon of supraspinatus which forms part of the

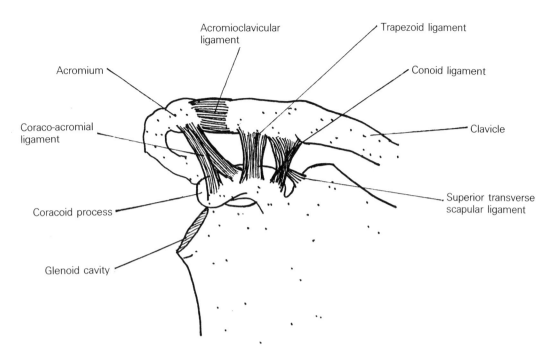

Acromioclavicular ligament

Trapezoid ligament

Acromium

Conoid ligament

Coraco-acromial ligament

Clavicle

Coracoid process

Superior transverse scapular ligament

Glenoid cavity

Fig. 6.3   Acromioclavicular joint, aspect from inside and below.

conjoint tendon of the rotator cuff muscles, namely supraspinatus, infraspinatus, teres minor and subscapularis. The conjoint tendon has a long insertion in the form of an arch into the humeral tubercles and the muscles serve to support the dependent arm.

This space is not a joint, strictly speaking, but movement must occur, for as the arm is abducted, the humeral head must not compress the structures within the space. The movement of the humeral head depends on fine muscular coordination.

6.3   **The acromioclavicular joint**

This is a plane articulation between the lateral end of the clavicle and the acromion process of the scapula. The capsule is weak, but is reinforced by strong ligaments superiorly and inferiorly, (the superior and inferior acromioclavicular ligaments). A cartilagenous disc is present until the fourth decade of life, after which it degenerates and the joint becomes more vulnerable to injury. The stability of the joint is largely maintained by the coracoclavicular ligament which ensures a constant relationship between the clavicle and scapula during all movements. The coracoclavicular ligament is divisible into two distinct parts. The trapezoid ligament arises from the upper medial margin of the coracoid process and extends to the trapezoid line of the clavicle. The conoid ligament arises from the base of the coracoid process and fans out to become attached to the conoid tubercle. Instability of the acromioclavicular joint can only occur if the coracoclavicular and superior acromioclavicular ligaments are severed or severely stretched.

6.4   **The sternoclavicular joint**

This is the saddle joint between the medial end of the clavicle and the superolateral portion of the manubrium sterni and the first costal cartilage. There is a meniscus within the joint which divides the joint cavity into two. The capsule is slack and thick and is attached to the periphery of the articular surfaces. It is reinforced by the anterior and posterior sternoclavicular ligaments. In addition, the interclavicular ligament passes from the upper part of the sternal end of one clavicle to the other. The costoclavicular ligament is short, flat and strong; it is attached below to the upper surface of the cartilage of the first rib and above to the under surface of the medial end of the clavicle. This ligament acts as a fulcrum for the sternoclavicular joint in all movements of the shoulder girdle (see Fig. 15.4).

6.5   **The scapulothoracic joint**

'The scapula floats in a sea of muscle on the posterior thoracic wall.' There are no formal articular surfaces but muscular action retains the anterior scapular surface in relation to the thoracic wall. (Occasionally there is a pseudoarthrosis between the scapula and the middle ribs but this is of no consequence.) Rotation of the scapula around the thoracic wall is essential to arm movement; for example, the medial scapular margin is raised as the arm is elevated.

6.6   **The costosternal, costotransverse and costovertebral joints**

These articulations are the mechanism whereby force from the appendicular skeleton (shoulder girdle) is transmitted to the axial skeleton (dorsal spine). These joints are therefore of great import-ance whenever there is some pathophysiological dysfunction of the mechanics of the shoulder girdle. The *costosternal joint* may be irritated or mechanically disturbed by the sternoclavicular joint above, via the first costal cartilage. The *costovertebral* and *costo-transverse joints* can be disturbed either primarily, or secondarily from shoulder girdle dysfunction or from mechanical problems of the cervical and/or thoracic spine. In the latter case, there can be an adverse effect on the shoulder girdle, especially on the keystone mechanism of the sternoclavicular joint. Thoracic outlet mechanics heavily influence shoulder girdle mechanics. Pain in the latter may originate in the former and vice versa. (For the anatomical review of the costovertebral and costotransverse joints, see section 15.7.)

The costosternal joints, excepting that of the first rib, are synovial joints, but this is only the articulations between the sternum and the true ribs. Each joint has a capsule which surrounds the articular surfaces; it is thin and is reinforced anteriorly and posteriorly by the costosternal ligaments which are attached to the relevant surface of each cartilage and to the adjacent part of the sternum. The movement which occurs at these joints is of a gliding type and of small range. The range of movement reduces as the costal cartilages become ossified in middle life when strains of these joints become more common and can have an adverse effect on the shoulder girdle mechanics.

6.7

Scapulohumeral rhythm

Full elevation of the arm, overhead, is achieved by a complex and synchronous coordination of all the joints of the shoulder girdle. Pure abduction at the glenohumeral joint is only possible to 90°, at which point the greater tuberosity of the humerus *opposes* the inferior aspect of the acromion and the coracoacromial ligament. To prevent this opposition, the rotator cuff muscles (see Fig. 6.4), via their conjoint tendon, contract to externally rotate and depress the humeral head, thereby allowing 120° of active abduction to

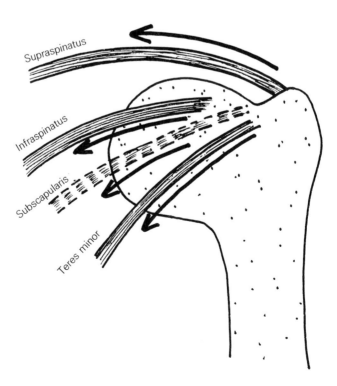

Fig. 6.4 Rotator cuff, direction of pull.

occur. The normal limb is capable of 180° abduction; the additional 60° is provided by scapular rotation around the thoracic cage, the raising of the inferior angle of the scapula and movement of the clavicle (discussed later in this section). Rotation of the scapula occurs at the scapulothoracic joint. The two prime movers are trapezius – the upper, middle and lower fibres – and the serratus anterior muscle. (Trapezius is described in section 14.2 and serratus anterior in section 15.1.) In active movements the middle fibres of trapezius act to fix an axis of rotation of the scapula at the acromioclavicular joint. Relative to this axis, the upper and lower fibres of trapezius together with serratus anterior, act as scapular rotators thus elevating the glenoid cavity upwards. This mechanism also serves to keep the scapula closely applied to the thoracic wall, until in full elevation the glenoid cavity lies directly underneath the humeral head.

In actuality, these actions of glenohumeral movement and scapular rotation occur simultaneously in the ratio of 2:1 to give a full range of 180° abduction of the limb.

The deltoid muscle acts directly on the glenohumeral joint, as an abductor. One other factor governing the efficiency of the action of the deltoid muscle is the arrangement of the coracoclavicular ligament which prevents rotation at the acromioclavicular joint. During active abduction this ensures that the deltoid muscle retains optimum length and therefore strength as it's acromial origin and humeral insertion remain at the same distance apart.

The last but by no means least, contribution to shoulder girdle movement is the action of the clavicle. This bone is an uneven S-shape between the medial two-thirds and the lateral one-third. It has a conjoint facet medially with the first rib at it's articulation with the manubrium sterni, forming the sternoclavicular joint, while laterally it articulates with the acromion process of the spine of the scapula – forming the acromioclavicular joint. The clavicle itself has several important ligamentous and muscular attachments which serve to stabilise the bone. In active elevation of the arm, scapular rotation occurs with complementary clavicular movement at the sternoclavicular joint (see Fig. 6.5). The first 30° occurs by elevation of the lateral end of the clavicle. The remaining 30° results from an axial rotation of the S-shaped crank of the bone along it's axis. During this movement, the joint is stabilised by the strong costoclavicular ligament which also provides a fulcrum for the clavicular excursion and for the shoulder girdle movements.

In conclusion, the integrity of all the mechanisms and their synchronous action are fundamental to efficient shoulder girdle mechanics. Failure of the mechanism may be due to direct tissue insult, injury, a subconscious protection of the hurt, or post-operative. Rotator cuff injury and/or dysfunction can be a tendinitis, a partial or total tear, and is dealt with separately. (Diagnostic

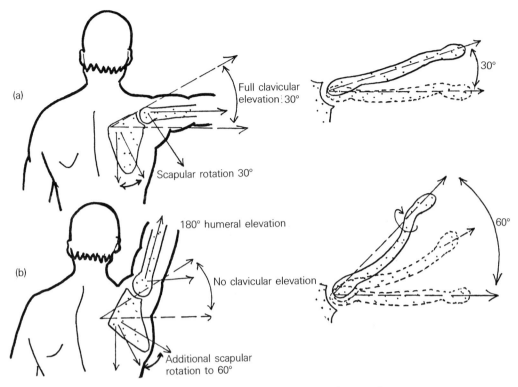

(a)

Full clavicular
elevation: 30°

30°

Scapular rotation 30°

180° humeral elevation

(b)

No clavicular elevation

60°

Additional scapular
rotation to 60°

Fig. 6.5   Scapular rotation as a result of clavicular rotation.

insight is gained by careful observation of loss of normal scapulo-humeral rhythm.)

Scapular control and rotation is also an integral part of scapulo-humeral rhythm. In addition to the principal muscles already mentioned, namely trapezius and serratus anterior, the rhomboids, levator scapulae and latissimus dorsi may be responsible for some scapula control and can help regain scapula and clavicular rotation.

A much ignored role in shoulder girdle movement is played by the clavicle. It is vulnerable to trauma which can affect the mechanics of the sternoclavicular joint, which in turn can compromise the mechanics of the whole shoulder girdle. The characteristic syndrome of a depressed or impacted medial end of the clavicle can result from injury to the bone and have far-reaching effects on the shoulder girdle integrity and is often overlooked, remaining undiagnosed and therefore untreated. This is dealt with later.

Muscles acting on the glenohumeral joint

The four muscles which comprise the rotator cuff are, the supraspinatus, infraspinatus, teres minor and subscapularis (see Figs. 6.6 and 6.7). These act together with deltoid to depress the humeral head during abduction of the arm.

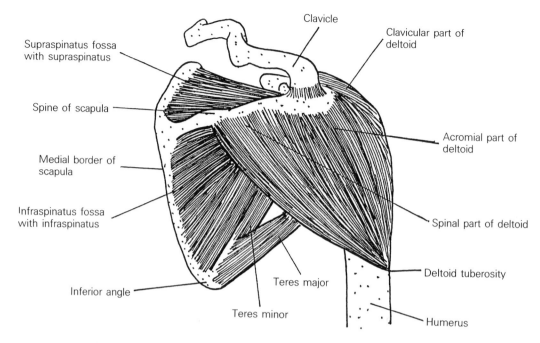

Supraspinatus fossa
with supraspinatus

Spine of scapula

Medial border of
scapula

Infraspinatus fossa
with infraspinatus

Inferior angle

Clavicle

Clavicular part of
deltoid

Acromial part of
deltoid

Spinal part of deltoid

Deltoid tuberosity

Teres major

Teres minor

Humerus

Fig. 6.6   Dorsal muscles of the shoulder, posterior aspect.

The *supraspinatus* arises from the supraspinous fossa (above the spine of the scapula) on the posterior surface. It passes deep to the coracoacromial ligament and has a tendinous attachment to the greater tuberosity of the humerus. The nerve supply consists of the suprascapular nerve, C4, C5 and C6.

The *infraspinatus* arises from the infraspinous fossa (below the spine of the scapula) on the posterior surface. It follows the direction of the supraspinatus to become attached to the greater tuberosity just below the supraspinatus muscle. Nerve supply is as for supraspinatus; i.e. suprascapular nerve, C4, C5 and C6.

The *teres minor* arises from the middle one-third of the lateral border of the scapula and passes upward and laterally to become inserted just below infraspinatus on the greater tuberosity of the humerus. Nerve supply is as for supraspinatus and infraspinatus, i.e. the suprascapular nerve, C4, C5 and C6 but via the axillary nerve.

These three muscles form the conjoined tendon prior to insertion.

The *subscapularis* arises from the whole of the anterior surface of the scapula and passes laterally to become attached to the lesser tuberosity of the humerus by means of a tendon (see Fig. 6.7). There is a bursa between the tendon and the neck of the scapula which is connected with the synovial cavity of the shoulder joint. The nerve supply consists of the upper and lower subscapular nerves, C5 and C6.

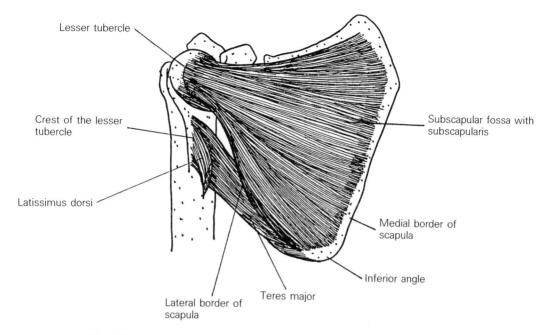

Lesser tubercle

Crest of the lesser tubercle

Latissimus dorsi

Subscapular fossa with subscapularis

Medial border of scapula

Inferior angle

Lateral border of scapula

Teres major

Fig. 6.7 Dorsal muscles of the shoulder, anterior aspect.

Between the subscapularis and the supraspinatus muscles there is a space through which the tendon of biceps (with it's sheath) passes. This is strengthened by the coracohumeral ligament but there is a weak spot between the tendon and the ligament which is frequently the site of a tear, longitudinally, of the rotator cuff. It is the region of arterial anastomosis between the osseous and muscular arteries, so relative ischaemia is possible there. Degenerative changes in the cuff are found at this site. Only in the recumbent position is there ample blood supply to the conjoint tendon which may be why symptoms of a cuff tear tend to be aggravated at night.

The *deltoid* muscle arises from three places and is divisible into three distinct parts. The clavicular fibres arise from the lateral one-third of the clavicle; the acromial fibres from the lateral margin and upper surface of the acromion, while the spinal fibres arise from the lower border of the spine of the scapula. They all converge to become inserted into the deltoid tuberosity on the lateral side of the shaft of the humerus. The nerve supply consists of the axillary nerve, C5 and C6. The anterior fibres can flex and internally rotate the arm; the middle fibres abduct the arm; the posterior fibres can extend and externally rotate the arm. When the muscle acts as a unit it abducts the arm but tends to lift the humeral head against the coracoacromial ligament. That is when the cuff muscles act to lower the humeral head to enable abduction above 90° to occur.

Muscles acting on the scapula

The prime movers of the scapula are trapezius and serratus anterior (see Figs. 14.14, 15.9 and 15.10). *Trapezius* arises from the ligamentum nuchae and the cervical spinous processes. These are the upper fibres which are inserted into the upper margin of the medial two-thirds of the spine of the scapula. They pull the scapula upward and internally rotate it about the acromioclavicular joint.

The middle fibres arise from the spinous processes of C7 to T3 and from the supraspinous ligaments and are inserted into the acromial tip of the clavicle, the acromial process and the superior lip of the spine of the scapula. These fibres act to 'fix' the scapula during abduction of the arm. They are relaxed during flexion of the arm.

The lower fibres arise from the spinous processes of T2 to T12 inclusive and from the supraspinous ligaments and pass upwards to become inserted into the spinal trigone and adjacent part of the spine of the scapula. They pull the medial border of the scapula medially and downwards. The combined action of the upper and lower fibres rotates the scapula around the acromioclavicular joint so that the medial border of the bone is lowered while the glenoid is raised. The nerve supply consists of the spinal accessory nerve, 11th cranial nerve (see also section 14.2).

The *serratus anterior* arises by fleshy slips from the outer surface of the upper nine ribs. It passes around the chest wall and is inserted into the costal surface of the medial border of the scapula and into the angle of the scapula. The muscle lies within the 'scapulocostal joint'. It pulls the scapula forward. Acting with the trapezius it rotates the scapula about the acromioclavicular joint thus raising the glenoid fossa. The nerve supply consists of the long thoracic nerve, C5, C6 and C7 (see also section 15.1).

Deep to the trapezius muscle lie the *levator scapula, rhomboid major* and *rhomboid minor* muscles which also attach the scapula to the spine but are not involved in scapulohumeral rhythm. They help to stabilise the scapula and are dealt with in section 14.2 (levator scapula) and section 15.1 (rhomboids).

Downward movement of the glenoid fossa is assisted by the action of *latissimus dorsi* and *pectoralis major* (see section 15.1). Latissimus dorsi depresses the arm downwards and internally rotates it. Pectoralis major pulls the arm downward from full elevation and internally rotates it.

Teres major arises from the dorsal surface of the inferior angle of the scapula. It's fibres pass upward and laterally to become inserted by means of a tendon into the medial lip of the bicipital groove of the humerus. The nerve supply consists of the lower scapular nerve, C5 and C6. It acts to rotate the humerus medially and draw it backwards. It helps to stabilise the humerus but is not involved in scapulohumeral rhythm.

Latissimus dorsi acts to pull the elevated arm downwards and medially rotates the adducted limb, but is not involved in scapulo-humeral rhythm. See section 15.1.

On the anterior surface, *pectoralis minor* assists in stabilising the scapula but it too is not involved in the scapulohumeral rhythm. (See section 15.1).

Muscles acting on the clavicle

The scapula and clavicle are elevated by the action of *trapezius*, principally, but the sternomastoid muscle also acts on the clavicle, although it's principal action is to rotate the head. Nevertheless it is a stabiliser of the clavicle. (See section 14.2).

The *subclavius* muscle arises from the junction of the first rib and it's costal cartilage by means of a thick tendon and is inserted by fleshy fibres into a groove on the under surface of the middle one-third of the clavicle. This is an important muscle as it braces the clavicle against the articular disc of the sternoclavicular joint during movements of the shoulder girdle. The nerve supply consists of C5 and C6 (see Fig. 6.8; also see section 15.1).

Muscles of the upper arm

The *biceps brachii* lies in the front of the arm (see Figs. 6.8 and 7.3). The long head arises from the supraglenoid tubercle, is enclosed in a sheath of the synovial membrane of the shoulder joint and arches over the head of the humerus. It emerges through an opening in the capsule and descends in the bicipital groove of the humerus where it is retained by the transverse humeral ligament (see section 6.1).

The short head arises from the coracoid process together with the origin of the coracobrachialis muscle. The two muscle bellies do not fully unite until the muscle is within about 7.5 cms of its insertion into the tuberosity of the radius. The nerve supply consists of the musculocutaneous nerve, C5 and C6. The biceps is principally a supinator of the forearm and flexor of the elbow. However, the long head helps to depress the humeral head during deltoid contraction.

The *coracobrachialis* muscle arises from the coracoid process in common with the short head of biceps. It is inserted into the middle part of the medial border of the shaft of the humerus between the origins of triceps and brachialis. The nerve supply is made up of the musculocutaneous nerve, C7. This muscle acts with the anterior fibres of deltoid to prevent lateral shift of the humeral head during abduction of the arm.

The *triceps* is situated on the posterior aspect of the arm (see

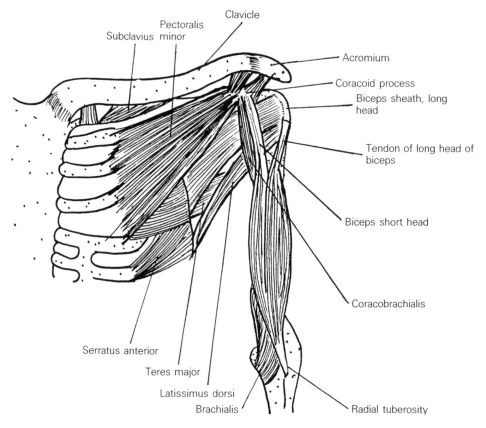

Fig. 6.8   Deep muscles of the upper arm, anterior aspect.

Fig. 7.4). The long head arises from the infraglenoid tubercle. The lateral head arises from the posterior surface of the shaft of the humerus and the medial head from the shaft of the humerus below the spiral groove. It is inserted into the olecranon, posteriorly. The muscle acts principally as an extensor of the elbow. The long head supports the inferior part of the capsule of the shoulder joint (glenohumeral joint) and assists in drawing the humeral head backwards when the arm is extended. The nerve supply consists of the radial nerve, C6, C7 and C8.

Anterior thoracic muscles

Pectoralis major − see section 15.1 − is divisible into two parts. The clavicular fibres flex the arm, acting with the anterior fibres of deltoid and with coracobrachialis. The sternocostal fibres act with latissimus dorsi and teres major to depress the arm. When the raised arms are fixed, for example by gripping an overhead object, the muscle helps to draw the trunk upward and forwards, for example during climbing or in certain gymnastics.

Pectoralis minor lies deep to pectoralis major – see section 15.1. It acts with serratus anterior to rotate the scapula forwards around the chest wall. Acting in conjunction with the rhomboids and levator scapulae it rotates the scapula to depress the point of the shoulder.

6.8

Muscle injuries

Muscle injury around the shoulder joint is not particularly common despite the fact that there is a great deal of muscular tissue present. The reason is that tendon injuries far outweigh muscular ones. *Wasting* can be seen and may affect the serratus anterior, deltoid or pectoral muscles.

Wasting of *serratus anterior* will lead to the classic 'winged' scapula. The winging is clearly seen if the athlete is asked to lean forward and push against a wall with straight arms. Active elevation of the arm is limited to 45° as the scapulohumeral rhythm is disturbed, but passive elevation is found to be full and pain-free. The condition may be secondary to a cervical disc injury at the level of C5, C6 and/or C7 or the long thoracic nerve may have been damaged peripherally, for example by a severe blow on the scapula. Usually the condition comes on for no apparent reason; there may be an ache in the shoulder girdle region which is not increased by movement. Recovery takes several months but can be assisted by giving the necessary exercises and osteopathic treatment as and where relevant. This will include the neck, thorax and shoulder girdle areas.

Wasting of the *deltoid* may be secondary to compression of the axillary nerve especially in a dislocation of the glenohumeral joint. Full elevation may be possible for the athlete provided he has strength in the supraspinatus muscle. If the arm is in the position of 90° abduction, extension will be impossible. Recovery takes several months, during which time the athlete should be encouraged to elevate his arm by using his supraspinatus. Osteopathic treatment will be needed to the neck, thorax and shoulder girdle to minimise mechanical faults resulting from the original injury.

If there is weakness of the biceps, supraspinatus and infraspinatus muscles as well as deltoid, and no history of dislocation, the C5 nerve root is implicated.

Wasting of the *pectoral* muscles may be secondary to rib injury or to interference of the nerve supply, C6, C7, C8 and T1. It can be more readily seen if the athlete is asked to raise both arms to the horizontal, in front, and then push his hands together when the weak side will be evident. Treatment consists of exercises and osteopathic treatment to the neck, thorax and shoulder girdle areas.

Injury to muscle fibres may result from some *direct force* or blow. In this case there will be a helpful history and bruising may be evident. Active and resisted movements will be painful, and passive stretching of the damaged fibres may also elicit pain. Treatment consists of soft tissue treatment as possible, ice packs, arnica to reduce bruising, and gentle osteopathic and active mobilisation. Recovery is usually within a few days, depending on the extent of the injury. Return to full athletic activity should not be before full recovery has taken place, or there is a high risk of further injury.

Intrinsic strains of muscles in this region are not commonly seen. They can, however occur anywhere, but are most frequently seen in the *deltoid, pectorals, subclavius, trapezius, rhomboids* and in *latissimus dorsi.* In each case there will be a history of some unusual or overstressful activity and localised pain on active and resisted movement. Passive stretch may be painful. These conditions respond well to deep soft tissue treatment and a rubifacient such as Tiger balm is helpful. Complete recovery must take place before full activity is resumed. Osteopathic treatment to all the anatomically related areas must be given as muscle injuries can occur if the mechanics of the relevant joints are impaired, thus placing additional stress on the muscle concerned, during contraction.

6.9   **Tendon injuries**

Tendinitis is seen commonly in older athletes, affecting the conjoint tendon of the rotator cuff. The area is ischaemic during normal daily activities − see page 85 − which may well predispose to degenerative changes in the tendon. Heavy use of the muscles will also predispose to these changes as will an increased thoracic kyphosis, whereby the scapula position is altered relative to the position of the humerus. Inefficiency of the rotator cuff mechanism to unlock the joint in elevation movements results in repetitive insults to the cuff tendon. These insults occur in the subacromial space where the tendon is pressurised by the acromion in cases of osteoarthritic change in the acromioclavicular joint, or clavicular rotation with facet locking. The athlete will complain of pain, usually described as an ache, radiating from the deltoid muscle towards it's insertion. It is a constant nagging ache, exacerbated by lying on the injured side. X-ray appearances are normal.

Complete tears of the conjoint tendon do occur, which will result in loss of active elevation beyond 90°, but are often difficult to differentiate from tendinitis.

Degenerative changes are commonly seen in the tendon in middle life, especially where there has been excessive use of the muscles concerned, for example in racquet sports, weight lifting or in heavy manual workers. These changes can impair the rotator cuff mechanism, rendering it inefficient in unlocking the joint during elevation of the arm. Rotator cuff tears can occur as a result of a fall or blow, or can develop as a chronic result of repeated insult to the cuff tendon. A tear can occur at any point along the tendon but they are most often seen under the acromion. Damage to the tendon can be on the deep or superficial surface. Long-term cases may show calcification of the tendon which will be visible on X-ray.

A painful arc of movement (see Fig. 6.9) is present when there is *impingement* of a structure within the subacromial space, either because the structure is inflamed (i.e. oversized due to swelling) or the space is reduced due to some bony fault, for example elevation of the humeral head which can result from insufficiency of the rotator cuff muscles to depress it. The structures which can be impinged are the conjoint tendon and the subacromial bursa but it is likely that the bursa becomes irritated when the tendon is damaged. A *bursitis* here without the tendon being involved could result from a direct blow but the two conditions are more likely to occur together. The causes of a painful arc are: osteoarthritic changes in the acromioclavicular joint, when the arc will be painful towards the full range of elevation; inflammation of the conjoint tendon when the painful arc will be at the start of abduction (usually), and anterior carriage of the whole of the shoulder girdle, when the painful arc can be at any point in the range of abduction.

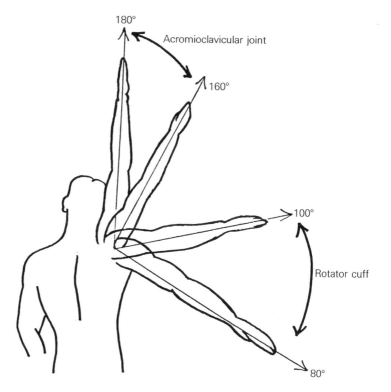

Fig. 6.9 The painful arc of movement.

Hypertonicity of the rotator cuff muscles results from damage to the conjoint tendon, this being of a protective nature. Paradoxically the protective contraction makes the tendon more vulnerable in an attempt to restrict movement, not less so.

The exact clinical picture is difficult to assess as it is so variable. *Reverse scapulohumeral rhythm* is common in subacromial pathologies which can cause variations in the painful arcs which are seen in clinical practice. So each case has to be carefully observed and individually assessed according to the exact dysfunction found. Whatever the cause of a painful arc, relief can only be gained if the irritation is removed. Abnormalities in the scapulohumeral rhythm can be improved by osteopathic treatment. Rest will reduce the inflammation of the impinged structure, but a complete tear of the conjoint tendon will require surgical treatment. Following this, osteopathic treatment to the neck, thorax and the shoulder girdle will be beneficial together with any corrective exercises. The athlete must not return to full activity until healing is complete.

Should a tendinitis affect the infraspinatus muscle, there will be the painful arc of movement, and pain will be felt on resisted external rotation as well.

If the tendon of subscapularis is affected there will be a painful arc of movement and pain on resisted internal rotation as well. Tendinitis of the biceps tendon usually affects the tendon where it is palpable. There will be pain on resisted supination of the forearm and on resisted flexion of the elbow. The condition responds well to soft tissue treatment and to ultrasound, with ice packs application.

6.10

Musculotendinous junction injuries

Injury to the rotator cuff muscles at the site of the musculotendinous junction is seldom seen, the tendons themselves being the common site of injury.

The musculotendinous junction of *pectoralis major* is sometimes damaged especially in any sporting activity which involves pushing forward. The athlete will complain of pain at the site of the injury which is painful and swollen on palpation. Resisted adduction with medial rotation of the arm will cause pain. Deep soft tissue treatment to the injured fibres resolves the condition and ice packs help to reduce the inflammation.

The musculotendinous junction of the *biceps* muscle is sometimes injured especially if the sport has overstressed elbow flexion. Supination can be excessive in tennis players who place a great deal of top spin on the backhand and by so doing can injure this musculotendinous junction. The damaged area is palpable and can be felt to be swollen, and resisted supination of the forearm is painful as is elbow flexion. Deep soft tissue treatment, ice packs and ultrasound are the treatments of choice. Osteopathic examination and treatment of the shoulder girdle, thorax and elbow may be necessary to completely resolve the condition. Possibly a change of style of the backhand stroke may be advisable.

6.11

Bone injury

The clavicle and scapula are relatively superficial, so they are both vulnerable to direct injury, especially in contact sports or as a result of a fall. Bruising would then occur; the bone would be painful and a tender swollen area would be palpable. Any anti-inflammatory treatment such as ice packs will reduce the swelling and pain recovery is swift. If the humerus is injured directly, the surrounding muscles will also be injured.

It is possible for the supraclavicular nerve and vessels to be damaged, but this is not common. Similarly, the suprascapular nerve may be damaged by direct injury, but it is well protected as it runs through the suprascapular notch, by the suprascapular ligament. However, it is possible for damage to the nerve to interfere with the function of the supraspinatus and infraspinatus muscles.

Fracture of the *clavicle* is caused by a fall onto the outstretched hand or onto the point of the shoulder and usually happens in the middle one-third of the bone due to it's shape. The athlete will complain of pain, locally, which is worse on active arm movements. The deformity is obvious as the lateral portion of the bone is drawn downwards by the weight of the arm while the medial portion is held up by the sternomastoid muscle. The athlete will hold his arm across his chest and support it with the other hand. Malunion is common, leaving the bone shortened, which in turn affects the angle of the arm and commonly interferes with the scapulohumeral rhythm. To minimise this, the shoulder should be held in a figure of eight support, thus stretching the clavicle while healing takes place, for about three weeks. During this time active movements of the shoulder must be carried out to prevent residual stiffness. This injury is common in cyclists, jockeys and those who partake of contact sports.

Fracture of the *scapula* occurs with falls onto it or possibly in contact sports. The coracoid process may be fractured by falling onto the shoulder. All shoulder movements will cause pain, but despite the pain can be carried out actively. Treatment is to wear a sling for comfort and support. These fractures show on X-ray. Osteopathic follow up treatment, after bony union, is designed to eliminate any residual problems in the surrounding tissues.

The common sites of fracture of the *humerus* are the shaft, where the fracture may be transverse or spiral, and less commonly the neck or even the greater tuberosity. Fracture of the shaft, if transverse or oblique, results from a fall usually onto the elbow with the arm abducted. A spiral fracture usually results from a fall onto the outstretched hand when the humerus is subjected to a twisting stress. These fractures are treated with a wrist sling. It is possible for the shaft to fracture if it is struck violently, for example a fall off a horse striking the arm on a solid object. There will be pain, swelling, tenderness and loss of normal movement and a history of injury. Osteopathic treatment is necessary to the shoulder girdle, neck and thorax following union, as there will probably be residual problems resulting from the original injury and from the imposed rest of the arm during the healing phase.

6.12 Epiphysitis

This occurs at the proximal humeral epiphysis in adolescents who overstress the area, particularly with repeated throwing, hence the fact that the condition is known as 'little league shoulder', from it's association with baseball. It can also occur in any other throwing sport and in tennis players who overstress the epiphysis during adolescence. The athlete will complain of acute pain in the shoulder if he attempts to throw a ball (or anything else). This is followed by an ache in the surrounding area. The condition resolves with rest but no throwing must be permitted until the condition has completely resolved, which may take several months. Osteopathic treatment is indicated to all the surrounding tissues, as described above, following fractures.

6.13 Joint and ligament injury

The three articulations of the shoulder girdle, the glenohumeral joint, the acromioclavicular joint and the sternoclavicular joint are all relatively unstable as they allow a very wide range of movement in the girdle as a whole. The supporting ligaments, therefore, are relatively lax and so can become stretched easily. If the supporting ligaments are sufficiently stretched, *dislocation* of the joint can occur. Dislocation can be with or without fracture. Dislocation occurs when sufficient force is applied to overwhelm the muscular and capsuloligamentous apparatus.

The *glenohumeral joint* is protected above the bony arch of the acromion, acromioclavicular joint and the clavicle, so dislocation does not occur upward, but takes the least line of resistance. Anterior dislocation accounts for 90% of cases and posterior for only 10%. The anterior part of the capsule is protected only by the glenoid labrum and the three capsular thickenings, the superior, middle and inferior glenohumeral ligaments, between which are two unprotected foraminae, of which the upper is the weaker. It is here through the foramen of Weitbrecht that dislocation occurs most frequently. The humeral head then comes to rest in a position below the coracoid process. Very occasionally the humeral head may position below the clavicle or the glenoid, or posteriorly under the scapular spine.

Dislocation is invariably caused by a fall with the arm raised and outstretched; it is possible from a fall onto the point of the shoulder, or if the arm is pulled outward and backwards by another player. The athlete will give a history of injury. He will complain of a substantial amount of pain. There will be gross deformity of the shoulder profile with loss of the normal fullness. There will be loss of mobility and the arm may be held away from the trunk. X-rays will show an anterior dislocation but a posterior dislocation will only show clearly on an axillary view. Techniques of reduction are beyond the scope of this book and the injury should be dealt with in a hospital.

Statistically a primary dislocation in the second or third decade is more likely to become recurrent later on.

Post-traumatic healing is poor, especially of the capsule. A common sequel of dislocation is the so-called 'Broca defect' – a notch on the posterolateral aspect of the humeral head near the margin of the articular surface. This is caused by the forced impaction of the humeral head on the glenoid rim during dislocation. It can be seen on X-ray and is important because if the Broca defect and the glenoid rim are opposed, a self-dislocating leverage is exerted on the humeral head, levering it out of position again, thus leading to an increased possibility of recurrent dislocation. Special X-rays are needed to determine the presence of the defect which will guide the surgeon; he may just repair the capsule or he may shorten the subscapularis tendon to prevent the dislocating action of the notch.

Some dislocations occur without gross trauma and are classified as 'habitual dislocations'. They are most often seen in young females and the surgical results are not as good in these cases. The traumatic dislocation repairs well following surgery and after rehabilitation the athlete can usually return to contact sports following a suitable interval of time. Once the athlete is deemed fit, it is common to find a protective picture similar to the 'impacted clavicle' (see later in this section) with unresolved muscle spasm. Osteopathic treatment aimed at restoring the scapulohumeral rhythm is then needed for full efficiency of the shoulder.

Residual pain following reduction of a dislocation is rare, but if present, suggests a cuff tear or possibly an avulsion of the greater tuberosity. The latter will show on X-ray.

Dislocation of the *acromioclavicular joint* follows damage to the acromioclavicular ligament and the coracoclavicular ligaments. The cause is usually a fall onto the outstretched arm, elbow, or point of the shoulder so that the joint is forced inward and upward. The dislocation may be total or partial depending on the degree of ligamentous damage and may occur with or without fracture. The history will be helpful. Obvious deformity is seen and all shoulder movements are painful. X-rays confirm the diagnosis. Reduction can sometimes be achieved by manipulating the displaced portion of the clavicle and retaining it with a pressure pad and bandage around the elbow joint which is flexed to a right angle. The results, however, are not good, but the residual deformity does not impair shoulder movement much. Only gross residual instability warrants surgery. Osteopathic treatment is aimed at restoring the scapulo-humeral rhythm.

Less frequently the *sternoclavicular joint* dislocates as a result of some violent force on the point of the shoulder. Should the medial end of the clavicle displace posteriorly, it can pressurise the trachea and great vessels of the neck. Usually the medial end of the clavicle displaces anteriorly and is obvious as a deformity. The joint is the fulcrum for the elevation of the shoulder, and if it is unstable, the scapulohumeral rhythm will be disturbed. The athlete complains of pain which may be in the region of the shoulder rather than the sternoclavicular joint but the injured joint will be painful on pressure. The history of injury will be helpful. Most cases are treated by rest only, but posterior displacements of the clavicle require expert attention. Osteopathic rehabilitation and treatment is aimed yet again at restoring the scapulohumeral rhythm.

The medial end of the clavicle may become impacted or depressed. This is caused by a minor fall or by repeated minor traumata to the clavicular joints, such as occurs in many sports, for example throwing. The clavicle gives the impression of being driven down-wards and medially into the sternum, producing a subluxation of the sternoclavicular joint. The proximity of the medial end of the clavicle to the first costal articulation means that not only is there a loss of joint space at the sternoclavicular joint, but the position also intrudes upon the facet of the first rib. This reduces the normal mobility of the sternoclavicular joint and the excursion of the first rib. A common maintaining factor is spasm of the subclavius muscle. This, together with the presence of a rudimentary meniscus within the joint gives rise to the possibility of a facet lock occurring. In addition, at rest the clavicle sits anatomically axially rotated if the medial end is depressed; under normal circumstances this only occurs with scapular movement and has the effect of raising the lateral end of the clavicle due to the crank-like shape of the bone. The result of this is a 'stepping' at the acromioclavicular joint (see Fig. 6.10) and a fullness at the sternoclavicular joint. This mechanical disturbance gives rise to a disturbance of the normal scapulohumeral rhythm; it may be a primary lesion or secondary to pain and dysfunction elsewhere in the shoulder girdle.

The athlete will present complaining of a possible variety of symptoms. Examination will reveal asymmetry of the sternal ends

'Stepping'

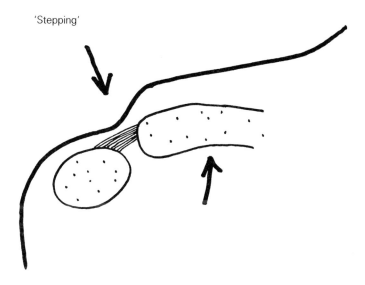

Fig. 6.10 'Stepping' at acromioclavicular joint.

of the two clavicles, observed when the athlete is standing, sitting and lying supine. There will be a fuller feel to the medial end of the clavicle. The subclavius muscle will be tender and hypertonic. There will be tenderness over the co-facets of the clavicle and the first rib. There will be tenderness over the coracoclavicular ligaments often accompanied by hypertonia of pectoralis minor. There will be relative elevation of the lateral end of the clavicle. There may be pain and tenderness at the acromioclavicular joint; this is often the presenting symptom. There will be a compromise of the costoverterbral articulations, especially the first and second ribs via the scalenes and the C7 to T2 vertebral joints. There will be unilateral spasm of the sternocleidomastoid muscle. The shoulder girdle will be carried relatively anterior on the affected side with internal humeral rotation and therefore possible hypertonia of the latissimus dorsi muscle.

Treatment of this condition is aimed at restoration of normal structural integrity. All muscle spasm and hypertonia has to be relieved and the acromioclavicular, sternoclavicular and glenohumeral joints normalised. Treatment to the spinal areas may be necessary from the neck (sternocleidomastoid) to as far as the pelvis (latissimus dorsi). Only when all the extraneous stresses are removed can the coordinated muscle action in the region be adequate, and pain-free function of the shoulder girdle take place.

The sports which may cause this syndrome to occur are those which may lead to a fall onto the shoulder or outstretched arm, for example the martial arts, equestrian events and body contact sports. In addition, the shoulder may be jarred in sports which require a harness such as parachuting, hang-gliding or where a seat belt is worn. Postsurgically the athlete may carry the arm in the 'wounded limb' posture which can result in this condition, as can immobilisation of the arm in a sling or collar and cuff.

The *glenoid labrum* is often damaged in anterior dislocation of the shoulder, but can occur without instability of the glenohumeral joint in activities such as throwing, boxing and in racket sports. The athlete will complain of a deep pain especially when the arm is elevated and a sensation of instability or locking on certain movements. There is seldom a history of injury. Examination reveals normal or near normal active, passive and resisted movements. The joint is sensitive to palpation and a click may be felt on passive movement. Firm diagnosis can only be made on arthroscopic examination, so expert referral is required. Rehabilitation will include exercises and osteopathic treatment to all the surrounding tissues.

6.14

Mobility injury

Stiffness of the shoulder may be muscular and result from some unusual activity. The athlete will give a history of some unusual activity, possibly of a lifting or throwing type; the stiffness occurs on the day following such activity. Examination reveals hypertonia of the surrounding muscles which causes pain if contracted. Passive movement of the joint is usually only marginally impaired. Resisted movements will cause pain.

This type of injury responds well to rest from excessive use but the joint should be put through it's full range of movement repeatedly to avoid a 'frozen shoulder' developing. Use of a rubifacient such as Tiger balm helps to improve the muscular condition.

The so-called 'frozen shoulder' is all too commonly seen in practice. The condition causes pain which is exacerbated by attempted use of the joint in the early stages, but later there is no pain if the joint is not moved (usually). All active and passive movements are limited and painful and there is frequently muscular guarding. In the late stages there may be muscular wasting due to disuse. The pathological changes within the joint are adhesion formation within the capsule. This may be secondary to contracture of the biceps or conjoint tendons, adherence of the folds of the capsule in the anterior part of the joint, irritation of the subdeltoid bursa causing adhesions to form, or more likely in athletes the condition may result from some abuse to the musculature of the shoulder girdle.

The condition is considered to be self-limiting with spontaneous recovery eventually, but this is by no means certain and there may well be residual problems of efficiency and mobility which could impede athletic activity. The clavicular joints are often involved and not functioning correctly, while the scapulohumeral rhythm is impaired. The condition is often made worse by the athlete's reluctance to use the joint, thus encouraging stiffness.

The condition is most frequently seen in middle life, probably because there is an ischaemic factor. It may come on following an injury as striking the joint or pulling it, but the cause is often obscure.

The diagnosis is obvious as all movements are limited and painful. Treatment in the early inflammatory stage is to reduce the inflammation and ice packs applied six times a day are needed. If the condition is treated this way early enough, full mobility may well be regained in about two weeks. If however adhesions have already formed, then treatment will be needed to stretch these in order to regain full mobility of the joint. The surrounding joints will also need treating, as well as the whole of the spine and ribs, because of the anatomical relationships. This can be a distressing condition but the athlete must be encouraged to use the arm as much as possible, without strain, within the discomfort range. He should not cause himself pain as this may increase the inflammation.

Recovery depends on the degree of capsulitis present but can take several months. Manipulation under anaesthetic is sometimes necessary in severe cases. Following this, osteopathic treatment is needed to all the surrounding areas to ensure correct function of the whole shoulder girdle before full sporting activity can be resumed.

Recurrent dislocation is dealt with under section 6.13.

Instability of the shoulder joint is sometimes seen but no dislocation has actually occurred. There is *hypermobility* of the humeral head within the glenoid cavity during use of the joint. The athlete will complain of pain possibly during or after sport and the condition is seen most frequently where throwing is involved, or an implement such as a racquet or stick is used. Repeated use of the arm above the head as in volley ball may also precipitate the condition. The athlete may feel that the joint feels unstable if he raises the arm above his head.

Examination reveals a positive 'apprehension test'. If the capsule is stretched anteriorly, the athlete will resist movement beyond a certain point, if his arm is abducted and externally rotated while he is supine. A similar reaction is obtained if the arm is abducted and internally rotated when the capsule is stretched posteriorly.

Mild cases can be improved by strengthening exercises to the shoulder girdle musculature, but severe cases may require surgically stabilising as the possibility of dislocation is a risk.

The scapulohumeral rhythm should be normalised by osteopathic treatment as any defect in this could be a causative factor. Should there be any interference of the nerve supply to the supporting muscles, this could also be a contributory factor, so osteopathic attention must also be paid to the relevant spinal regions.

6.15   **Bursitis**

Although there are several bursae around the shoulder, only the subdeltoid bursa tends to become inflamed. Bursitis elsewhere is extremely rare although the supra-acromial bursa is occasionally damaged by some direct injury.

Subacromial bursitis is seldom a primary condition. It is usually secondary to a conjoint tendon problem, or to some dysfunction of the clavicular joints. In each case the subacromial space is reduced, so irritation of the bursa becomes possible. Inflammation of the conjoint tendon may be followed by calcification which not only increases the girth of the tendon but also causes direct irritation of the bursa.

The athlete will complain of pain especially on use of the shoulder joint and there may be a residual ache following use. Examination will reveal pain on abduction and there will be a painful arc of movement as the bursa becomes pressurised against the acromion process.

Treatment will depend on the primary cause of the problem. It may be necessary to attend to the faulty clavicular mechanics or to the conjoint tendon problem. In the acute phase it is unlikely that much improvement will be achieved by ice packs as the cooling effect will probably not reach down to the bursa. An injection into the bursa may prove effective as an anti-inflammatory. Rest from all irritating activity is essential but movement of the shoulder through it's pain-free range is essential, as a capsular problem might develop. Osteopathic treatment is needed to restore normal scapulohumeral rhythm.

6.16   **Referred pain**

When consideration is made of any shoulder complaint, initial differential diagnosis of all possible causes must be made. Pathologies of a number of structures can give rise to pain in the region of the shoulder.

Neurogenic pain from some brachial plexus problem is probably the most common cause; this can originate from the anterior cervical roots at the uncovertebral joints, the apophyseal joints, a cervical disc or the thoracic outlet in relation to the scalenes or the first rib.

Visceral pain may be referred to the shoulder from the gall bladder, bronchus, apex of a lung or possibly from cardiogenic origin. In these cases no abnormality will be found in the shoulder on examination and the athlete should be referred for further investigation if the pain persists.

Chapter 7   The Elbow

7.1

Joints of the elbow

The elbow is a compound joint, consisting of three joints all within the same capsule (see Fig. 7.1). There is an articulation between the lower end of the humerus and the ulna – the humero-ulnar joint, one between the lower end of the humerus and the radius – the humeroradial joint and one between the radius and the ulna – the superior radio-ulnar joint. In addition, there is a continuous fibrous joint between the whole of the shaft of the radius and the ulna which prevents parallel displacement of these bones and transmits pressure stresses from one bone to the other. This 'interosseous membrane' is so strong that the bones tend to fracture before it's fibres are torn, during overstrain of the forearm (see Fig. 7.2).

The *humero-ulnar joint* is a hinge joint; the movements which occur are flexion and extension. Flexion is brought about by contraction of brachialis, brachioradialis and biceps brachii muscles (see Fig. 7.3).

Brachialis arises from the anterior aspect of the lower half of the humerus and is inserted into the ulnar tuberosity. The nerve supply consists of the musculocutaneous nerve, C5 and C6. *Brachioradialis* arises from the lateral supracondylar ridge of the humerus and is inserted into the styloid process of the radius. The nerve supply consists of the radial nerve, C5 and C6. The *biceps* muscle acts on the shoulder joint as well as the elbow and arises from the supraglenoid tubercle and from the coracoid process and is inserted into the tuberosity of the radius. The nerve supply consists of the musculocutaneous nerve, C5 and C6 (see section 6.7).

Flexors of the elbow

Brachialis, brachioradialis and biceps brachii are the flexors of the elbow. Some minor assistance is given by flexor muscles of the wrist which arise above the elbow joint.

Flexion is normally limited by the apposition of soft parts and tension in the triceps muscle. (See also Fig. 6.8.) Extension is brought about by contraction of the triceps brachii muscle. It arises from the infraglenoid tubercle of the scapula, the radial groove of the humerus and from an area lateral to the groove from the dorsal surface of the humerus. It is inserted by means of a strong tendon into the olecranon process of the ulna (see Fig. 7.4). The nerve

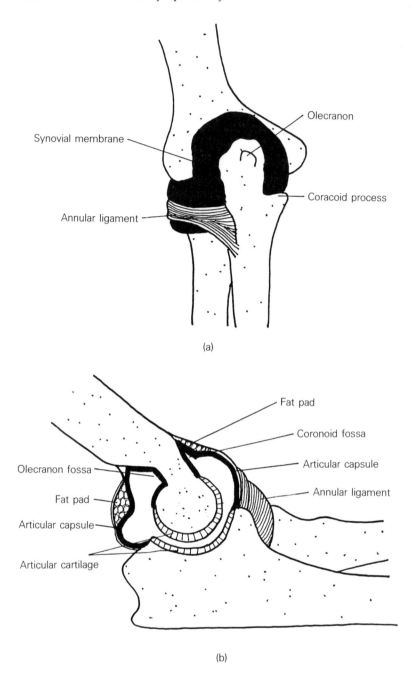

Fig. 7.1 Sagittal section of the left elbow joint. (a) Posterior aspect; (b) medial aspect.

supply consists of the radial nerve C6, C7 and C8. (There is a small and comparatively insignificant muscle which acts with triceps – anconeous m. but it's main function seems to be to tense the capsule of the elbow joint.)

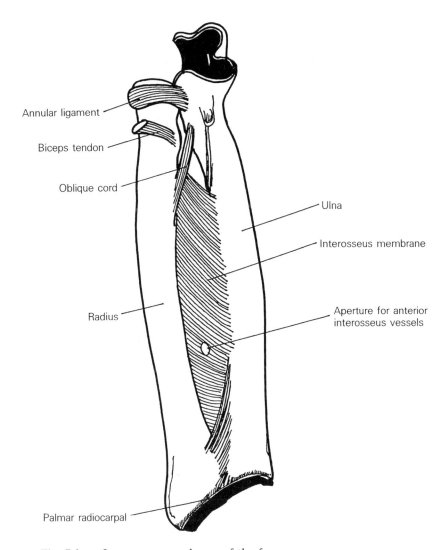

Annular ligament

Biceps tendon

Oblique cord

Radius

Palmar radiocarpal

Ulna

Interosseus membrane

Aperture for anterior
interosseus vessels

Fig. 7.2   Interosseus membrane of the forearm.

Extensors of the elbow

Triceps brachii is the extensor of the elbow. Extension is limited
by the opposition of bony parts (the olecranon process on the
olecranon fossa), tension in the anterior part of the capsule and
anterior ligament and by tension in the flexor muscles. If extension
is forced beyond a certain stage the capsule will be torn and the
joint dislocated or the olecranon will fracture and the capsule tear.

The total range of flexion is approximately 140°. The total range
of extension is approximately 160°.

The *humeroradial joint* is formed between the capitulum on the
lateral aspect of the humerus and the concave fovea on the superior

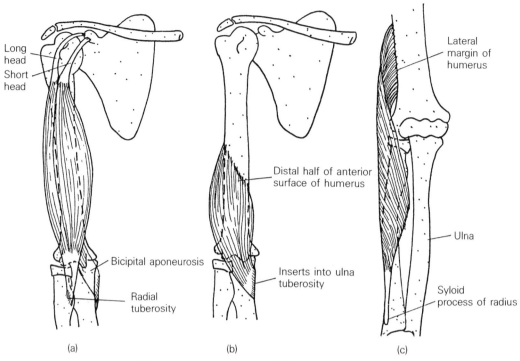

Fig. 7.3   (a) Biceps brachii muscle; (b) brachialis muscle; (c) brachioradialis muscle.

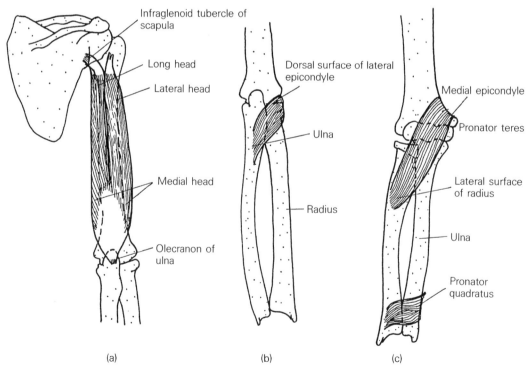

Fig. 7.4   Posterior aspect of (a) triceps brachii muscle and (b) anconeus muscle; (c) anterior aspect of pronator teres muscle and pronator quadratus muscle.

surface of the head of the radius. It is a ball-and-socket joint where the radial head rotates on the capitulum. The *superior radio-ulnar joint* is a pivot joint which allows the radial head to rotate around the ulna. The movements which occur at these two joints are pronation and supination (see Fig. 7.5).

Pronation is the movement which rotates the forearm so that the palm of the hand is facing backwards (patient upright). The radius rotates around the ulna (the bones cross over each other). It is brought about by contraction of the following muscles − pronator teres, flexor carpi radialis, extensor carpi radialis longus (with forearm flexed), pronator quadratus, brachialis and palmaris longus − in order of efficiency.

Pronator teres arises from the medial epicondyle of the humerus and from the intermuscular septum and from the coronoid process of the ulna, and is inserted by means of a flat tendon into the middle of the lateral surface of the shaft of the radius. The nerve supply consists of the median nerve C6 and C7.

Flexor carpi radialis arises from the common flexor tendon on the medial epicondyle of the humerus and is inserted into the palmar surface of the base of the second metacarpal (and sometimes into the third metacarpal) (see Fig. 7.6). The nerve supply consists of the median nerve, C6, C7 and C8. This muscle also flexes the wrist.

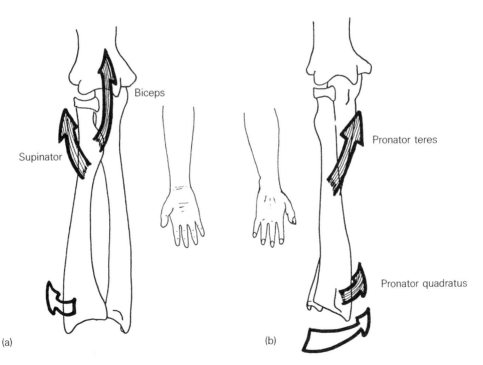

(a)

Biceps

Supinator

(b)

Pronator teres

Pronator quadratus

Fig. 7.5   (a) Supination; (b) pronation.

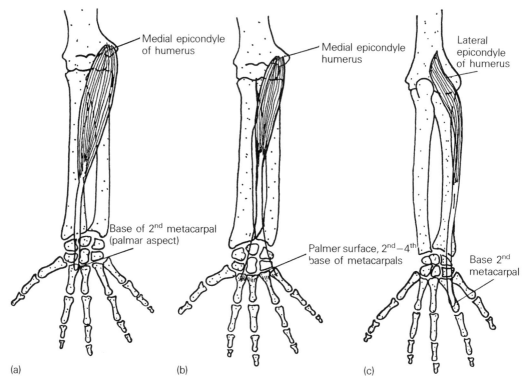

Medial epicondyle
of humerus

Medial epicondyle
humerus

Lateral
epicondyle
of humerus

Base of 2nd metacarpal
(palmar aspect)

Palmer surface, 2nd–4th
base of metacarpals

Base 2nd
metacarpal

(a)   (b)   (c)

Fig. 7.6   (a) Flexor carpi radialis; (b) palmaris longus; (c) extensor carpi radialis longus.

Extensor carpi radialis longus arises from the lower one-third of the lateral supracondylar ridge of the humerus and is inserted by means of a tendon into the dorsal surface of the base of the second metacarpal (see Fig. 7.6). The nerve supply consists of the posterior interosseous nerve C6 and C7. The tendon passes under the extensor retinaculum at the wrist immediately behind the styloid process of the radius.

Pronator quadratus arises from the oblique ridge on the lower part of the anterior surface of the shaft of the ulna and the medial part of the lower one-quarter of that bone and is inserted into the lower one-quarter of the anterior border and shaft of the radius. The nerve supply consists of the anterior interosseous branch of the median nerve, C6 and C7.

Brachialis, see flexors of the elbow.

Palmaris longus arises on the medial side of the flexor carpi radialis from the common flexor tendon and passes in front of the flexor retinaculum at the wrist to be inserted mainly into this structure (see Fig. 7.6). It is not always present. The nerve supply consists of the median nerve, C8.

Pronation is limited by the crossing of the radius over the ulna.

The total range of pronation is 90° and any forced movement beyond that will cause damage to the radio-ulnar joint of a ligamentous type, but is unlikely, as the shoulder joint will internally rotate.

Supination is the opposite of pronation when the radius and ulna lie parallel and the palm of the hand faces forward. It is brought about by contraction of biceps brachii, supinator, abductor pollicis longus and brachioradialis muscles − in order of efficiency.

Biceps brachii, see flexors of the elbow. It's action is stronger when the elbow is flexed.

Supinator arises from the epicondyle of the humerus, the supinator crest of the ulna and from the collateral and annular radial ligaments (see Fig. 7.7). It is inserted into the radius between the radial tuberosity and the attachment of pronator teres. It encircles the radius and supinates the forearm in all positions of flexion and extension of the elbow. The nerve supply consists of the radial nerve C5 and C6.

Abductor pollicis longus arises from the dorsal surface of the ulna distal to the supinator crest and from the dorsal surface of radius and the interosseous membrane between and is inserted into the base of the first metacarpal (see Fig. 7.7). As it's name implies,

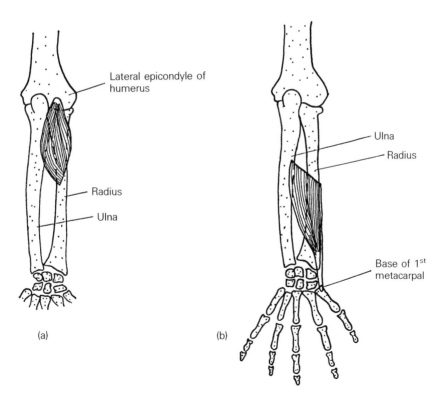

Fig. 7.7   (a) Supinator; (b) abductor pollicus longus.

it also abducts the thumb and assists in wrist flexion. The nerve supply consists of the radial nerve C5 and C6.

Brachioradialis muscle, see flexors of the elbow.

Supination is limited by tension on the annular ligament when the radius and ulna lie parallel and by tension in the pronator muscles. The normal range is 90° and any forced supination beyond this will cause the inferior radio-ulnar ligament to become stretched and this may eventually lengthen and weaken − see section 8.1.

Ligaments of the elbow

The ligaments of the elbow reinforce the capsule. The lateral ligament is attached above to the lateral epicondyle of the humerus and below to the annular ligament (see Fig. 7.8).

The *posterior ligament* is attached to the humerus immediately behind the trochlea and below to the upper lateral part of the olecranon, to the ulna behind the radial notch and to the annular ligament. The medial or ulnar collateral ligament is a thick triangular band which runs from the medial epicondyle of the humerus (see Fig. 7.9). The anterior fibres are attached to the coronoid process and the posterior fibres to the olecranon. The ulnar nerve runs immediately posterior to the latter fibrous bundle.

The *annular ligament* is attached to the ulna and encircles the head of the radius and is very strong.

When the elbow is in the supinated position, and extended,

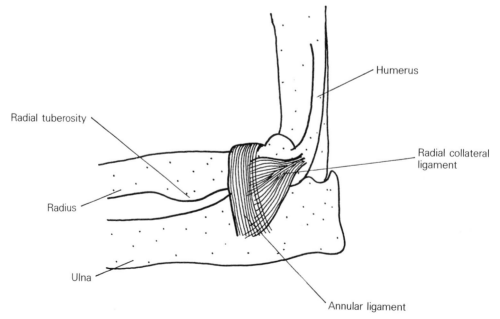

Fig. 7.8   Radial collateral and annular ligaments of the left elbow, lateral aspect.

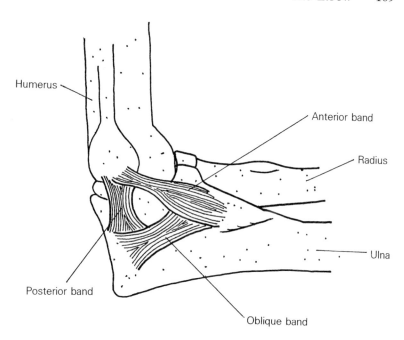

Humerus

Anterior band

Radius

Ulna

Oblique band

Posterior band

Fig. 7.9 Medial ligament (ulna collateral ligament) of the left elbow, medial aspect.

there is an obtuse angle between the upper arm and the forearm. This can vary and is more marked in women; it is known as the 'carrying angle'.

7.2

Skin injuries around the elbow

Abrasions are common in this region usually following a fall. *Bruising* may also be present and the history will reveal the cause. Below the skin and over the olecranon there lies a bursa which may become inflamed following a blow on that area. It can become very large and alarm the patient but will usually resolve and only occasionally requires aspiration. All pressure must be kept from it and ice packs applied. Abrasions are cleaned and dressed and will usually heal swiftly. The only complication to be aware of is a possible injury to the ulnar nerve as it passes around the medial epicondyle where it lies in a groove in the bone. If this nerve is damaged there may be loss or impaired sensation in the skin of the fourth and fifth fingers. There may be inability to adduct the thumb and flex the ring and little fingers and inability to spread out the fingers owing to damage to the nerve supply to the dorsal interossei.

7.3

Muscle injuries around the elbow, including tendons, musculotendinous injuries

The *biceps* muscle is commonly injured (see Fig. 7.10), most frequently proximally — see Chapter 6. However it is impossible to

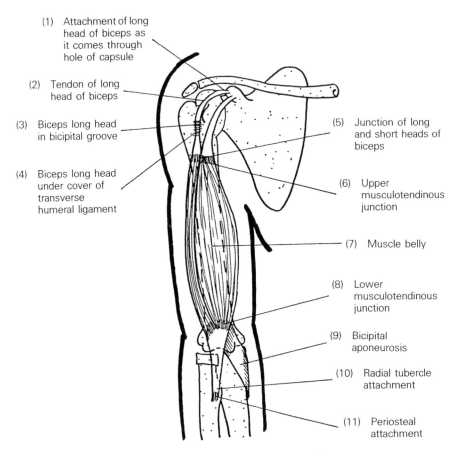

(1) Attachment of long head of biceps as it comes through hole of capsule

(2) Tendon of long head of biceps

(3) Biceps long head in bicipital groove

(4) Biceps long head under cover of transverse humeral ligament

(5) Junction of long and short heads of biceps

(6) Upper musculotendinous junction

(7) Muscle belly

(8) Lower musculotendinous junction

(9) Bicipital aponeurosis

(10) Radial tubercle attachment

(11) Periosteal attachment

Fig. 7.10   Common sites of injuries to biceps brachii.

give a definite line of demarcation between the shoulder and elbow. This muscle may be injured at the long head, within the belly, at the lower musculotendinous junction or at the point of insertion into the radial head. The patient will complain of pain which is exacerbated by certain movements especially flexion of the elbow and supination in some degree of flexion – for example in sports where a bat or racket is used. The elbow joint is found to be normal in passive movements (there may be some discomfort on full passive extension). Resisted flexion is painful. Resisted supination is also painful, but resisted flexion with the forearm fully pronated is not painful. If the lesion is within the belly of the muscle, this will be the site of pain on the above tests. An area of local tenderness, usually in the deep fibres will be found and must be palpated for by pinching the belly of the muscle between finger and thumb. Palpation from the anterior aspect of the muscle is not usually helpful.

Deep soft tissue treatment to the injured area and correction of any mechanical faults within the elbow and shoulder joints is essential as the problem may well be secondary to such a fault. As the muscle is innervated from the C5 and C6 levels, this area must also be checked for any possible mechanical involvement. The patient may assist treatment by applying some rubifacient to the area to improve the blood supply and the muscle should not be excessively used during the healing period.

Injury to the musculotendinous junction is dealt with later. Should the lesion be at the insertion the symptoms will present there and resisted movements will give rise to pain at that level. Careful palpation will reveal the local lesion and pain will also be felt on full passive extension of the elbow joint. The patient may well say that the pain came on after some excessive lifting possibly in the gym, and such activity should be restricted until the pain has stopped. Treatment is deep friction to the area but it is painful and may take several weeks. All other possible contributory factors as for a belly tear must be dealt with if found.

Weakness of the *biceps* may be secondary to some lower motor neuron disorder or possibly a cervical spine problem which has affected the nerve supply to the muscle. In this case there will also be weakness of the extensors of the wrist and/or abductors of the arm. Many biceps problems occur as a result of faulty mechanics at the shoulder joint especially where the humeral head is held anteriorly, for example following an old fracture of the clavicle where the bone has become shorter than it was before. Such an anterior rotation of the shoulder will result in shortening of the biceps, thus leaving it vulnerable to any sport which requires stretch on the muscle.

The *brachialis* muscle flexes the elbow joint in all positions of pronation and supination. Resisted flexion in full pronation will be painful if there is a lesion of this muscle. The injured area may be difficult to find if it lies under the biceps tendon. As this muscle is subject to myositis ossificans it is wise to routinely X-ray before carrying out soft tissue treatment. The injured fibres will respond to this form of therapy in the absence of myositis ossificans. Again as a safeguard to both the osteopath and the patient it is not wise to treat this muscle actively unless there is full extension of the elbow joint. Rest may well be the treatment of choice and all flexion of the elbow should be avoided until the condition has resolved. Myositis ossificans is almost invariably a complication of fracture and will be dealt with later – see section 7.

Injury to the *triceps* muscle is uncommon but if it occurs the lesion is usually at the musculotendinous junction – see later. Weakness of the triceps muscle may occur following pressure on the radial nerve, for example from a crutch, or from interference of the seventh cervical root when neck movements will be limited.

Injury to the *supinator* muscle is rare except following direct injury to the forearm. Active and resisted supination will be painful (the latter in full extension of the elbow to rule out a lesion of the biceps). The local lesion is usually palpable between the two bones of the forearm (in supination). Friction to the area is beneficial and the mechanics of the elbow and inferior radio-ulnar joints must be checked. There is often some degree of hypersupination and chronic stretch of the inferior radio-ulnar ligament.

The *pronator* muscles are seldom injured and resisted pronation is found to be most commonly painful when a 'Golfer's elbow' is found. If there is a lesion in the pronator muscles it is palpable and will respond well to deep soft tissue treatment and rest during the recovery period.

Tennis elbow is very common in sportspersons. It results from any repetitive movement which involves gripping a small handle, for example a badminton racket. (It is most often caused by the use of a screwdriver, hammer or even paintbrush.) The injury is to the extensor muscles of the wrist and/or hand, but the pain is felt at the origin of these muscles, i.e. at the elbow. The patient will complain of pain often sudden in origin and felt at the lateral aspect of the elbow. There is localised tenderness. The exact site may be at the common extensor tendon, in the musculotendinous junction or within the muscle belly (see Fig. 7.11). Pain is felt on gripping and exaggerated by resisted extension of the wrist. There is seldom any loss of mobility at the elbow (unless active movement is limited by pain). The exact location of the injury can be found by careful palpation. The common age of the patient is between 40 and 60 years of age but I have seen the problem in a patient as young as 20. In tennis players it seems probable that the injury is caused by excessive top spin on the backhand, whereby there is forced and repetitive hypersupination. This results in the inferior radio-ulnar ligament becoming chronically stretched and there will be excessive passive movement between the lower ends of the radius and ulna. This must always be checked in all cases of tennis elbow, because the problem will recur if this excessive movement is not stopped.

It is for this reason that the Medisplint is effective as it supports the inferior radio-ulnar joint as well as giving local support to the common extensor origin. A support to the elbow alone in such cases is relatively ineffective. Treatment to the local lesion by means of deep soft tissue treatment and to the belly of the affected muscle, and correction of any mechanical problem at the elbow and possibly the wrist, will give relief. The wearing of a Medisplint is beneficial and will reduce the chance of recurrence. The mechanical fault most commonly seen is a posterior fixation of the radial head and this must be corrected. Play should only be resumed when resisted extension of the wrist is no longer painful when wearing a Medisplint. It is also essential that the tennis racket is checked by an expert to be sure that the handle is not undersized

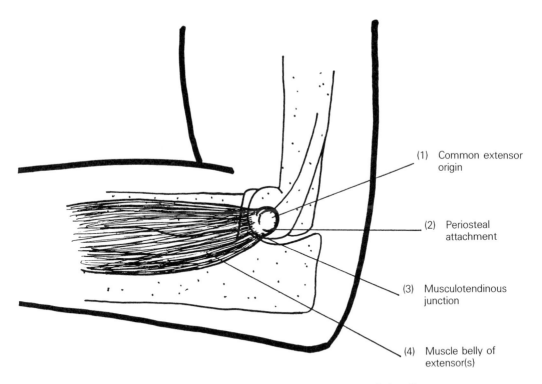

(1) Common extensor origin

(2) Periosteal attachment

(3) Musculotendinous junction

(4) Muscle belly of extensor(s)

Fig. 7.11   Common sites of pain at the lateral aspect of the elbow.

and that the tension of the strings is neither too great nor too slack.

Golfer's elbow is a strain of the common flexor origin at the elbow and is less common than tennis elbow (see Fig. 7.12), and is less disabling. The patient will complain of pain at the medial aspect of the elbow usually insidious in origin. He is often a golfer. Examination reveals a full painless range of movement at the elbow but pain is elicited on resisted flexion of the wrist. The lesion is palpable and tender and responds well to localised soft tissue treatment. There may well be some limitation of passive lateral shift in the elbow which must be corrected to minimise the chance of recurrence. The patient's golf clubs should be checked by an expert for the correct size of handle, and play should not be resumed until resisted flexion of the wrist is no longer painful, possibly when wearing a support around the upper part of the forearm.

Repeated trauma to either the common extensor or flexor origins may lead to the development of an ossified body at the site of injury. This will act as an irritant to the tendon. If present it may or may not be palpable and if suspected from the history, X-rays will reveal its presence. Surgical removal is then necessary.

In cases of tennis or golfers elbow, the mechanical integrity of

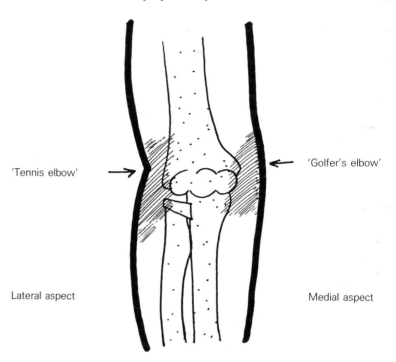

'Tennis elbow' →

← 'Golfer's elbow'

Lateral aspect

Medial aspect

Fig. 7.12 Tennis elbow and golfer's elbow, anterior aspect.

the lower cervical and upper dorsal spine must be checked as there may well be a contributory factor in this area.

The common sites for a *musculotendinous lesion* are the biceps, triceps, common flexor and common extensor origins. Pain will be elicited at these sites on the relevant resisted movements but it is necessary to determine if the lesion is muscular or musculotendinous in order to give an accurate prognosis. Any lesion at a musculotendinous junction will take longer to resolve, as the blood supply to the area is less plentiful than to the muscular part of the muscle. Similarly the recuperative period is longer if the lesion is at the tenoperiosteal junction and in such cases an injection can accelerate healing but must always be given by an expert who is capable of palpating the exact site and injecting there. Otherwise excessive scar tissue may result with possible restriction of movement later.

7.4

Bone injuries

Fractures around the elbow joint are comparatively common, usually as a result of a fall onto the hand or onto the elbow itself. All fractures cause pain, swelling, tenderness, bruising, abnormal movement and possibly some visible deformity. There is a history of a fall or severe blow.

The lower end of the humerus may fracture either from a fall onto the hand or from a direct blow. It may be a straight or spiral fracture, in the latter case the bone may be visibly shortened. A fall onto the elbow in an adult drives the olecranon upwards and the condyles split apart. In a child, a fall onto the hand with the elbow flexed causes a supracondylar fracture with posterior displacement while there is anterior displacement if the elbow is straight. The lateral condyle may fragment in a child. In an adult the capitulum and trochlea may be broken off and displaced proximally. In adolescents the medial epiphysis may detach with or without dislocation. The head of the radius may fracture in either children or adults; in children the fracture is invariably transverse while in adults it is often vertical and frequently missed. The olecranon may fracture into several fragments following a fall onto it or from a direct blow, or it may fracture transversely, usually from a fall onto the hand. The radius and ulna may both fracture together, usually from a fall onto the hand or only one of them may fracture, but this is less common. Any severe fall should alert the osteopath to the possibility of fracture and the necessary X-rays should always be taken, if only as a precaution. All fractures require expert treatment and should be referred. Complications of elbow fracture are involvement of the radial and ulnar nerves and possibly of the radial artery all of which lie in close proximity to the joint.

Myositis ossificans is a complication of fracture of the elbow where there is deposition of bony tissue within the muscle. It is found to occur in the brachialis muscle. The exact cause is unknown but it may well be due to trauma to the muscle at the time of fracture. Some authorities, however, maintain that the condition comes about when the original fracture is not rested sufficiently in flexion. Whatever the cause there is little doubt that the condition may be worsened by active manipulation of the brachialis muscle and any osteopathic treatment to this muscle should only be carried out once it is established that no bony deposition is present. Once the condition has passed the active stage, there will be limitation of flexion, extension and rotation and the condition will not respond to osteopathic treatment. X-rays will reveal the condition.

7.5 Epiphysitis

This is not a common problem at the elbow but I have seen it in adolescents where the elbow has been subjected to overuse, for example in young gymnasts and in cases where there has been too much stress on the joint by virtue of excessive gripping as in hockey or tennis players. The condition responds to rest.

7.6 Joint and ligament injuries

Synovitis is a generalised inflammation of the whole joint usually following prolonged stress but it occurs in some athletes for no apparent reason. The patient complains of pain which is worse when he tries to use the joint. The onset is usually insidious and for no apparent reason. Examination reveals some swelling and warmth and there is limitation of all movements, active and passive at the extremes. X-rays appear normal. The condition is treated by rest, cold packs and movement within the painless range only. Once the acute phase has passed, the joint is put through its full range and any mechanical fault rectified by osteopathic means. The condition is seldom recurrent but it may be a complication of some other condition such as gout or rheumatoid arthritis and these conditions should be looked for by blood analysis if recurrence occurs.

Dislocation of the elbow joint occurs with fracture. Dislocation of the head of the radius can occur as a result of a severe pronation strain without fracture of the ulna when the radial head will displace backwards. It can be corrected by strong supination but will require immobilisation while the ligaments heal. Dislocation of the radial head can be congenital and is then usually bilateral when an X-ray reveals that the head is dome-shaped; thus an X-ray will differentiate a congenital dislocation from an acquired dislocation. Following stabilisation, the elbow joint must be mechanically sound from a functional point of view before normal activity is resumed and osteopathic treatment is aimed to restore normal mechanics.

A *loose body* may occur within the joint usually following trauma. This will result in possible locking in certain movements and will show on an X-ray if it is radio opaque. Removal is required. A loose body may also result from degenerative change within the joint and is suspected if there is degeneration with locking.

Degeneration is not common in the elbow joint as it is not a weight bearing joint, but it can occur following old injury. A generalised (active) arthritic condition may be due to either rheumatoid arthritis or gout.

Damage to a ligament may occur if the joint is stressed beyond its normal range of movement. The patient will complain of pain especially at the extreme of movement which puts that ligament on *stretch*. There will be a history of overstretch possibly from a fall. Passive stretch of the ligament will cause pain. The commonest ligament to become stretched is the medial ligament following an abduction strain of the joint, for example in judo. Pain is elicited on passive abduction and there may well be an increased carrying angle. This is a difficult condition to treat. Any further abduction strain must be avoided and exercises to strengthen the muscles which arise from the common flexor origin will help. The joint must be checked for any mechanical fault and the appropriate treatment given. The annular ligament is subject to overstretch and the radial head may become locked posteriorly. This can be corrected and normal movement of the head is restored. Loss of a full range of lateral shift within the elbow joint is often seen in elbow conditions and will lead to additional stress on various ligaments. Correction of this fault is essential if normal function of the joint is to be achieved.

7.7

Mobility injury

The elbow is subject to *stiffness* often following trauma such as an old fracture but it is not particularly limiting in function and most athletes can accommodate for any minor inconvenience caused. However, the possibility of an active condition must always be considered such as tuberculosis, rheumatoid arthritis or gout.

There is one other mobility injury which is peculiar to the elbow joint. In children the radial head may be marginally displaced downwards or upwards, a 'pulled radius' or the reverse, a 'pushed radius'. The child will complain of some degree of pain in use of the joint and there may be some limitation of both active and passive pronation and supination. Palpation will reveal that the radial head is somewhat tender and there is an increased space between the radial head and the capitulum of the humerus in a pulled radius whereas the space is palpably reduced in a pushed radius. Both conditions respond well to corrective articulation which should be carried out carefully and gently until normal mechanics are restored. A pulled radius is said to be caused by a pull on the forearm such as a parent pulling the child along. A pushed radius is most commonly found following a fall onto the hand and should only be considered once the possibility of fracture has been eliminated by X-ray.

Chapter 8   The Wrist and the Hand

8.1

The inferior radio-ulnar joint

This articulation occurs between the head of the ulna and the ulnar notch of the lower end of the radius. It is a pivot joint, enclosed in a capsular ligament which is lined with a synovial membrane, and the capsule is slightly thickened in front and behind. Movement takes place in pronation and supination of the forearm. In pronation the radius crosses the ulna obliquely, taking the hand with it while in supination the movement is reversed. The main pronator is the *pronator teres* muscle, and the supinator assisted by biceps (when the elbow is flexed) contracts to supinate the joint (see Chapter 7).

8.2

The wrist, hand and thumb

This area involves 27 bones and over 20 joints which are moved by 33 muscles, so detailed anatomy is not possible here. The wrist joint is the articulation between the distal end of the radius − the head of the radius − and the articular disc, attached to the ulna, and the proximal row of carpal bones, together with the midcarpal joint which is the articulations between the proximal and distal rows of carpal bones (see Fig. 8.1).

The capsule of the *radiocarpal* joint is distinct from the capsules of the midcarpal joints and is reinforced anteriorly, posteriorly medially and laterally. The capsule, lined by synovial membrane of the midcarpal joint is distinct from that of the other carpal joints. The distal row of carpal bones also articulate together but any movement of the wrist will involve movement of each and every tiny joint in the area. The whole construction of the wrist forms an arch which is concave anteriorly, and the posterior ligaments are stronger on the dorsal surface than the palmar ones on the front. The movements which occur at the wrist are flexion, extension, abduction and adduction while all four enable circumduction, in combination.

The *carpometacarpal* joint of the thumb is a saddle-shaped joint formed between the trapezium and the base of the first metacarpal, and has a wide range of movement. The capsule is thick but loose and the lining synovial membrane is distinct from that of the other carpometacarpal joints. The capsule is reinforced by anterior and posterior ligaments. The movements which occur at this joint are flexion, extension, abduction and adduction. Opposition is the

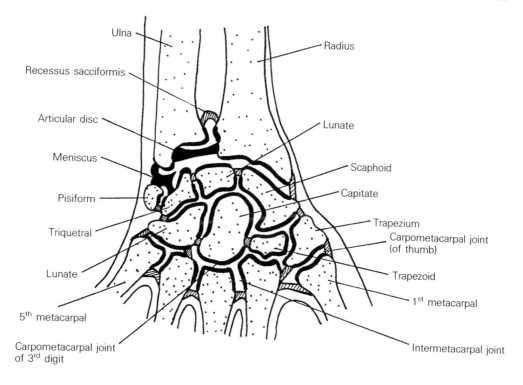

Ulna

Recessus sacciformis

Articular disc

Meniscus

Pisiform

Triquetral

Lunate

5th metacarpal

Carpometacarpal joint
of 3rd digit

Radius

Lunate

Scaphoid

Capitate

Trapezium

Carpometacarpal joint
(of thumb)

Trapezoid

1st metacarpal

Intermetacarpal joint

Fig. 8.1 Distal radius and ulna, the wrist joints.

movement whereby the tip of the thumb approximates the tip of one of the fingers and is a combination of flexion and medial rotation. Circumduction is extension, abduction, flexion and adduction consecutively in that order.

The joints of the second, third, fourth and fifth metacarpal bones with the carpus are plane joints and have a common capsule. The lining synovial membrane is continuous with that of the intercarpal joints. Movement only occurs at these joints when other more flexible joints nearby are moving. This is known as accessory movement.

The second, third, fourth and fifth also articulate with their neighbouring metacarpal, the synovial membrane being continuous with that of the carpometacarpal articulations. Here too, movement is accessory.

The *metacarpophalangeal* joints are condyloid; each has its own separate capsule lined by synovial membrane. Each capsule is strengthened on the palmar, lateral, and medial surfaces and in addition there is a deep transverse ligament of the palm which connects the adjacent metacarpophalangeal joints, second to fifth inclusive. The movements which occur at these joints are flexion, extension, abduction and adduction.

The *interphalangeal* joints are of the hinge type. Each has a capsule and synovial membrane and reinforcing ligaments on the palmar aspect and on both sides of the joint. The movements which occur are flexion and extension with some small degree of accessory rotation.

Flexion of the wrist occurs on contraction of the following muscles, flexor carpi radialis, flexor carpi ulnaris and palmaris longus with some assistance from flexor pollicis longus and the abductor pollicis longus.

Flexor carpi radialis originates from the common flexor origin on the medial epicondyle of the humerus and from the intermuscular septum. Halfway down the forearm it becomes a long tendon which passes through a canal in the lateral part of the flexor retinaculum and occupies a groove on the trapezium which is lined there by a synovial sheath. The tendon inserts into the palmar surface of the second metacarpal giving a slip to the third metacarpal. The nerve supply consists of the median nerve, C6 and C7.

Flexor carpi ulnaris (see Fig. 8.2) arises by two heads which are connected by a tendinous arch. The larger head arises from the medial margin of the olecranon and the upper two-thirds of the posterior border of the ulna by an aponeurosis common to it and the extensor carpi ulnaris. The smaller head arises from the common flexor tendon on the medial epicondyle of the humerus. A long tendon forms halfway down the muscle and is inserted into the pisiform bone. The nerve supply consists of the ulnar nerve, C8 and T1.

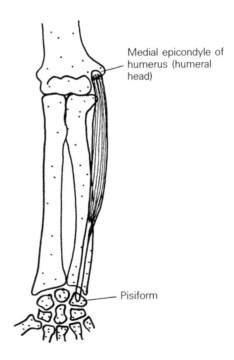

Medial epicondyle of humerus (humeral head)

Pisiform

Fig. 8.2 Flexor carpi ulnaris.

Palmaris longus has already been described under the flexors of the elbow (see section 7.1).

Extension of the wrist occurs when the following muscles contract, extensor carpi radialis longus, extensor carpi radialis brevis, extensor carpi ulnaris with some assistance from extensor digitorum, extensor digiti minimi, extensor indicis and extensor pollicis longus.

Extensor carpi radialis longus arises mainly from the lower one-third of the lateral supracondylar ridge of the humerus with a few fibres from the common extensor origin. A flat tendon forms one-third of the way down the forearm, runs along the lateral border of the radius, under the extensor retinaculum where it lies in a groove on the back of the radius immediately behind the styloid process. It is inserted into the radial side of the dorsal aspect of the second metacarpal. The nerve supply consists of the radial nerve, C6 and C7.

The *extensor carpi radialis brevis* (see Fig. 8.3) is shorter than the previous muscle; it arises mainly from the common extensor tendon and from the lateral ligament of the elbow joint. A flat tendon forms about halfway down the forearm which runs parallel to the extensor carpi radialis longus, and medial to it, to be

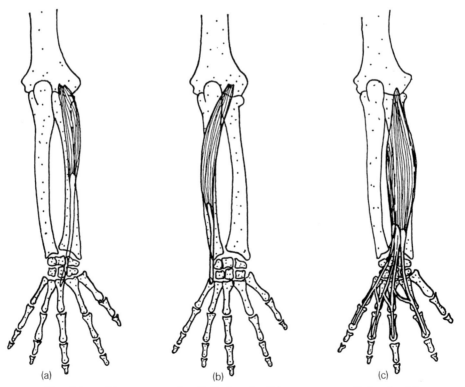

(a)   (b)   (c)

Fig. 8.3   Extensor carpi radialis brevis; (b) extensor carpi ulnaris; (c) extensor digitorum.

inserted into the base of the third metacarpal giving a small slip to the second. As the two extensor muscles pass under the extensor retinaculum they share a common sheath. The nerve supply consists of the posterior interosseous nerve, C6 and C7.

The *extensor carpi ulnaris* (see Fig. 8.3) arises from the common extensor tendon and from an aponeurosis common to it and the flexor carpi ulnaris. Its tendon runs in a groove between the head and the styloid process of the ulna, and passing through a separate compartment of the extensor retinaculum is inserted into the tubercle on the ulnar side of the base of the fifth metacarpal bone. The nerve supply consists of the posterior interosseous nerve, C7 and C8.

Adduction of the wrist comes about as a result of the combined contraction of flexor carpi ulnaris and extensor carpi ulnaris – i.e. both working together.

Abduction occurs when flexor carpi radialis acts with the extensors carpi radialis longus and brevis with some assistance from abductor pollicis longus and extensor pollicis brevis.

Movements of the wrist are limited by the tension which builds up in the ligaments which are being stretched and by increased tension in the opposing muscles.

The *flexor retinaculum* is a strong fibrous band which lies on the anterior surface of the wrist. It is attached to the pisiform bone and the hook of the hamate, medially, and to the scaphoid and the trapezium, laterally. It forms a tunnel on the front of the wrist by virtue of the curve (concave anteriorly) of the bone structure of the wrist. Under the flexor retinaculum pass several flexor tendons (all except the flexor carpi ulnaris) within a tendon sheath, and the median nerve (see Fig. 8.4).

The *extensor retinaculum* is a strong fibrous band which extends across the back of the wrist. It is attached on the lateral side to the anterior border of the radius and to the ridges on the posterior surface of that bone, and medially it is attached to the styloid process of the ulna, the triquetral and the pisiform bones. Under this retinaculum there are six tunnels for the passage of the extensor tendons; each passage has a synovial sheath (see Fig. 8.4).

In the palm of the hand is another specialised fascial sheet, namely the *palmar aponeurosis* (see Fig. 8.5). It is continuous with the flexor retinaculum and the central part is very tough forming a protection to the probable pressures to the palm of the hand. The central portion is bound to the skin by dense fibro-areolar tissue but the medial and lateral portions are far less dense.

The movements which take place at the first carpometacarpal joint (the base of the thumb) are flexion, extension, abduction, adduction and opposition. Circumduction is a combination of these. Flexion is brought about by contraction of flexor pollicis brevis, flexor pollicis longus and opponens pollicis.

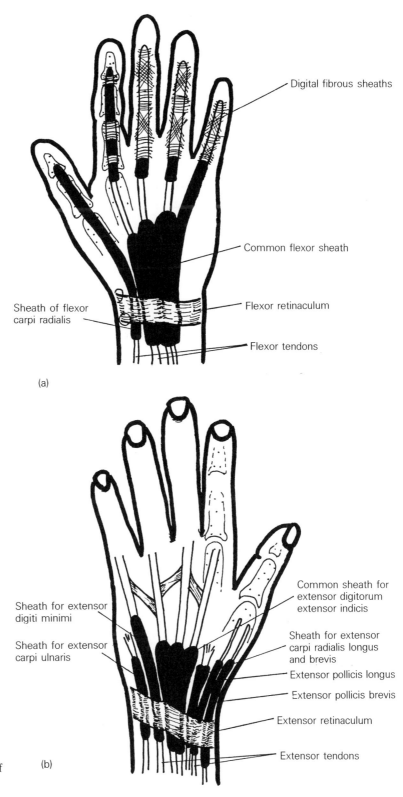

Fig. 8.4 (a) Flexor retinaculum and tendon sheaths; (b) extensor retinaculum and tendon sheaths, of the left hand.

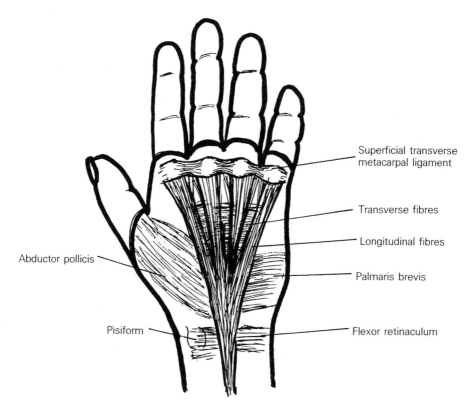

Superficial transverse
metacarpal ligament

Transverse fibres

Longitudinal fibres

Abductor pollicis

Palmaris brevis

Pisiform

Flexor retinaculum

Fig. 8.5   Palmar aponeurosis.

Flexor pollicis brevis arises from the flexor retinaculum and from the crest of the trapezium and passes along the radial side of the flexor pollicis longus to be inserted into the base of the proximal phalanx of the thumb. The nerve supply consists of the median nerve, C8 and T1.

Opponens pollicis arises from the flexor retinaculum and from the crest of the trapezium and is inserted into the whole length of the lateral border and the lateral half of the palmar surface of the first metacarpal. The nerve supply consists of the median nerve, C8 and T1.

Flexor pollicis longus arises mainly from the anterior surface of the shaft of the radius and from the common flexor tendon. A flattened tendon passes behind the flexor retinaculum and is inserted into the palmar surface of the distal phalanx of the thumb. The nerve supply consists of the median nerve, C8 and T1. Figure 8.6 illustrates the above flexor muscles.

Extension occurs when extensor pollicis longus and extensor pollicis brevis and abductor pollicis longus contract. Extensor pollicis longus arises from the lateral part of the middle one-third of the shaft of the ulna. It forms a tendon which passes through its own

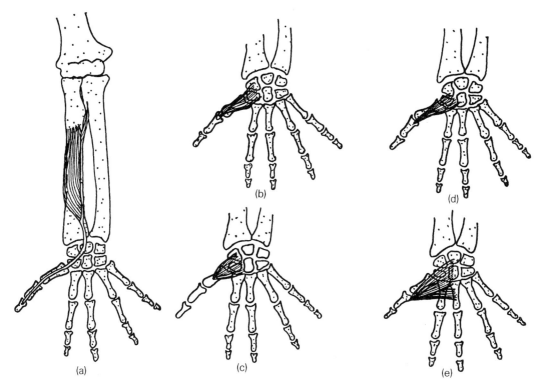

Fig. 8.6   (a) Flexor pollicis longus; (b) abductor pollicis brevis; (c) opponens pollicis; (d) flexor pollicis brevis; (e) adductor pollicis.

compartment of the extensor retinaculum where it lies in a narrow groove on the back of the lower end of the radius. It then crosses the two extensor carpi radialis muscles and forms the medial side of the so-called anatomical snuff box at the base of the thumb. The tendon is finally inserted into the posterior surface of the distal phalanx of the thumb. The nerve supply consists of the posterior interosseous nerve, C7 and C8.

Extensor pollicis brevis arises from the lower one-third of the shaft of the radius on its posterior surface. It's tendon passes through a groove on the lateral side of the lower end of the radius and is inserted into the dorsal surface of the base of the proximal phalanx of the thumb. The nerve supply consists of the posterior interosseous nerve, C7 and C8. Figure 8.7 illustrates the above extensor muscles.

Abductor pollicis longus arises just above extensor pollicis brevis on the radius and it's tendon passes with that of extensor pollicis brevis to be inserted into the base of the first metacarpal bone on it's radial side. The nerve supply consists of the posterior interosseous nerve, C7 and C8.

Abduction is brought about by contraction of abductor pollicis

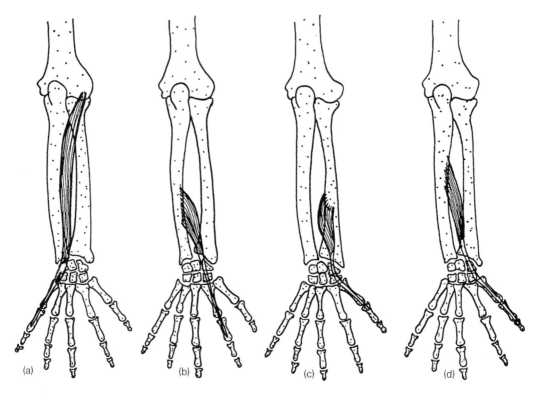

Fig. 8.7   (a) Extensor digiti minimi; (b) extensor indicus; (c) extensor pollicis brevis; (d) extensor pollicis longus.

brevis and abductor pollicis longus. Abductor pollicis brevis forms the radial part of the thenar eminence. It originates mainly from the flexor retinaculum and is inserted by a thin flat tendon into the base of the proximal phalanx of the thumb. The nerve supply consists of the median nerve, C8 and T1. Abductor pollicis longus has already been described as an extensor of the thumb.

Adduction occurs when the adductor pollicis muscle contracts. This muscle arises by two heads. The oblique head arises from the capitate and trapezoid bones and from the bases of the second and third metacarpal bones. The transverse head arises from the distal two-thirds of the palmar surface of the third metacarpal bone. The two heads converge into a tendon which is inserted into the ulnar side of the base of the proximal phalanx of the thumb. The nerve supply consists of the ulnar nerve, C8 and T1.

Opposition is brought about by the contraction of opponens pollicis and flexor pollicis brevis both of which have been described as flexors of the thumb.

The movements of the thumb are limited either by the opposition of soft parts or by tension building up in the opposing muscles and supporting ligaments. The movements give a wide range to the joints and intricate movements become possible.

The joints of the fingers are basically capable only of flexion and extension. Two muscles are responsible for flexion. The *flexor digitorum sublimis* arises mainly from the common flexor tendon, but a few fibres arise from the upper part of the anterior border of the radius. Four tendons pass under the flexor retinaculum, each passing to a different finger finally to be inserted into the sides of the shaft of the middle phalanx. Before its insertion each tendon splits to allow the passage of the tendon of the flexor digitorum profundus. From this arrangement it is seen that this muscle flexes the finger at the middle joint and not at the proximal joint. The nerve supply consists of the median nerve, C7, C8 and T1.

Flexor digitorum profundus as its name implies is a deeper muscle in the forearm (see Fig. 8.8). It arises from the upper three-quarters of the shaft of the ulna from its medial and anterior borders. This muscle also ends in four tendons which run behind

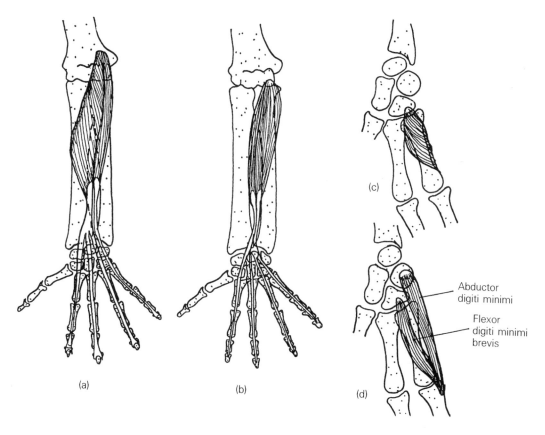

Fig. 8.8   (a) Flexor digitorum superficialis; (b) flexor digitorum profundus; (c) opponens digiti minimi; (d) abductor digiti minimi and flexor digiti minimi brevis.

the flexor retinaculum deep to the tendons of the flexor digitorum sublimis (see Fig. 8.9). At the level of the proximal phalanx, each tendon passes through the openings in the tendons of the flexor digitorum sublimis to become inserted into the distal phalanx of each finger on its palmar surface, at the base of the bone. From this arrangement it can be seen that this muscle flexes the finger at the distal joint but it comes into action after flexor digitorum sublimis has flexed the middle joints. The nerve supply consists of the median nerve laterally and the ulnar nerve medially, C8 and T1.

Extension of the finger joints is due to action of extensor digitorum muscle (see Fig. 8.7). Anatomists separate the main bulk of this muscle from extensor digiti minimi but both muscles have similar action. It arises from the common extensor tendon and becomes four tendons by two-thirds of the way down the forearm, which pass under the extensor retinaculum in a common sheath. The tendons are then inserted into the base of both the middle and distal phalanges on the dorsal surface. The nerve supply consists of the posterior interosseous nerve, C7 and C8.

In addition there are four small muscles of the palm on the medial side (see Fig. 8.8). *Palmaris brevis* arises from the flexor retinaculum and is inserted into the skin on the ulnar border of the hand. Contraction deepens the hollow of the palm and wrinkles the skin over the hypothenar eminence. The *abductor digiti minimi* arises from the pisiform bone and is inserted into the ulnar side of

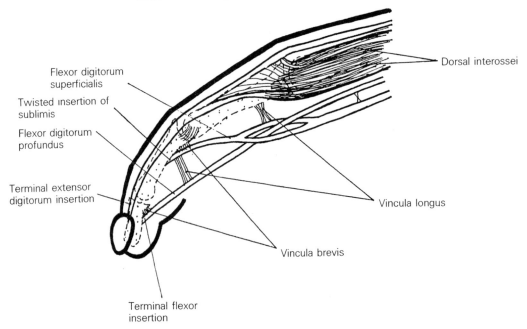

Fig. 8.9   Tendons of attachments of flexor digitorum superficialis and profundus muscles.

the base of the proximal phalanx of the little finger, and acts as an abductor of the little finger. *Flexor digiti minimi* arises from the hook of the hamate bone and is inserted into the base of the proximal phalanx of the little finger, so is able to flex the proximal phalanx of this digit. The *opponens digiti minimi* also arises from the hook of the hamate and is inserted into the whole length of the ulnar margin of the fifth metacarpal bone. Its action is to draw the little finger forwards and laterally, so deepening the palm of the hand. All these four small muscles are supplied by the ulnar nerve, C8 and T1.

The *interosseous* muscles of the hand occupy the spaces between the metacarpal bones (see Fig. 8.10). Those on the dorsal side of the hand arise from the adjacent sides of the metacarpal bones and are inserted into the bases of the proximal phalanges below. They abduct the fingers away from the axis of the hand, i.e. the middle finger. Those on the palmar side of the hand are smaller and adduct the fingers towards the axis of the hand. The nerve supply of all the interosseous muscles is the ulnar nerve, C8 and T1.

The *lumbrical* muscles act in conjunction with the interossei and are four small fleshy structures (see Fig. 8.10). They arise from the tendons of the flexor digitorum profundus and are inserted into the bases of the proximal phalanges and the dorsal expansion of the extensor digitorum muscle as it covers the dorsal surface of the finger. They flex the metacarpophalangeal joints. The two medial muscles are supplied by the ulnar nerve, C8 and T1 and the lateral two by the median nerve, C8 and T1.

8.3

Skin and muscle injuries of the hand and wrist

Skin injury to the hand is common and expert treatment should be obtained for any severe cut or abrasion, especially if damage to

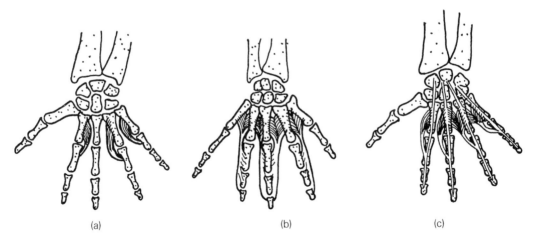

(a)   (b)   (c)

Fig. 8.10   (a) Palmar interossei; (b) dorsal interossei; (c) lumbrical muscles.

some underlying structure, for example the median nerve or an artery, is suspected. Callous formation is also frequently seen and can be a problem especially if the callous splits. Most minor skin injuries will heal well and swiftly with sterile dressing.

Sometimes a foreign body becomes embedded in the hand. If it can be removed easily and the lesion dressed, all well and good, but if there is any doubt, the case should be despatched to hospital.

Muscle injuries in the hand are comparatively rare. The commonest muscle to be injured is one or more of the *interossei*. The injury may be from some direct force, for example striking the hand on some object, or possibly the muscle injury is secondary to a fracture of a metacarpal bone. Occupationally the interossei can be damaged, for example from overvigorous fingering by a pianist or violinist. A simple strain will respond extremely well to deep soft tissue treatment. The patient will complain of pain in the relevant interdigital space which may have come on suddenly or slowly depending on the cause. The pain will be exaggerated by use of the hand especially where fine movements are involved. Clinical examination will reveal a tender area between the metacarpal(s) and there will be pain on resisted abduction with the fingers flexed if, as is more common, one of the dorsal interossei is injured. (Pain will be felt on adduction if one of the palmar interossei is injured.)

Occasionally one of the *thenar* muscles is injured, usually from an abduction strain of the thumb, for example by falling with the thumb in that position. The patient will complain of pain in that area and give a history of injury; the pain will be exacerbated by resisted abduction. Deep soft tissue treatment is very beneficial and the thumb must be checked for any mechanical fault. If rest is required, the thumb can be strapped in semi-abduction so that movement of the rest of the hand is not restricted. Pain in the thenar muscles is very common as a result of osteoarthritic changes in the thumb joint. Many people over 40 suffer from this.

Weakness of the *interosseous* muscles is often seen when there is a lesion of the first thoracic root. Weakness of the thenar muscles may be secondary to osteoarthritic changes in the thumb or to the presence of a cervical rib. This can be suspected if the contour of the lower cervical/horizontal fibres of trapezius is abnormal. The rib, if present can be palpated and confirmed on X-ray if bony. Palsy of the radial nerve, for example from pressing the inner arm over the back of a hard chair can give rise to weakness of extension of the wrist but there will also be weakness of the flexors of the elbow. See Fig. 4.3.

Weakness of the thenar muscles is also seen in about one-third of cases of carpal tunnel syndrome which will be dealt with in section 8.11.

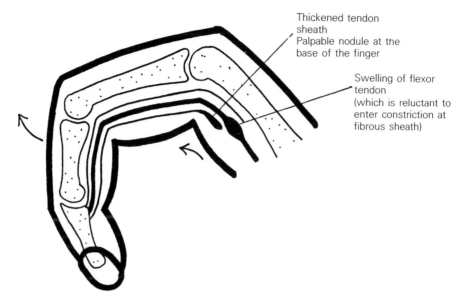

Thickened tendon
sheath
Palpable nodule at the
base of the finger

Swelling of flexor
tendon
(which is reluctant to
enter constriction at
fibrous sheath)

Fig. 8.11   Trigger finger.

8.3

Tendon injuries

Tendon injuries at the wrist are common simply because there are
so many tendons. Most of these tendons lie within a tendon sheath,
the exceptions being flexor carpi ulnaris and the two extensor carpi
radialis muscles. These three, therefore may be subject to a true
tendinitis; all the other muscles are likely to suffer from tenosynovitis.
Tenosynovitis is an inflammation of the synovial sheath surrounding a
tendon. The patient will complain of pain in the area of the
inflammatory condition which is made worse when he uses the
muscle affected. The history is often of overuse, and frequently the
athlete may have taken part in some unusual activity for him. The
condition is commonly seen in oarsmen especially after training in
rough water. Canoeists may suffer similarly. The common sites are
the extensor tendons and less so the flexors and the tendons of the
thumb. Clinical examination will reveal pain on one or more active
movements and pain on the opposite passive movement. There is a
local tender area around the affected tendon and fine crepitus may
be elicited there.

As this is essentially an overuse condition, logically rest is an
important part of treatment. Deep soft tissue treatment is often
helpful together with stretching of the relevant muscle fibres. The
surrounding joints must be checked for any abnormality of function.
Should the condition not respond to this conservative treatment,
an injection may resolve the trouble and only occasionally is surgery
required. Exercises are contraindicated as the condition is a result

of overuse. Some cases of tenosynovitis at the wrist are as a result of direct trauma, such as a blow in body contact sports.

A *trigger finger* is the result of a swelling on any of the flexor tendons (see Fig. 8.11). The usual site is just proximal to the metacarpophalangeal joint and is most often seen in the thumb, third or fourth finger. The patient will complain of a palpable swelling which is usually quite painless. If the swelling becomes large it catches within the tendon sheath when the finger is fully flexed. At that point the patient will be unable to actively extend the finger and will have to release it by using his other hand. At the point of release the patient will be aware of a sharp snap. This condition is most often seen in fencers. Surgery may be needed if the swelling becomes too obstructive.

A tendon may *rupture*. This is seen when the finger is extended and then subjected to a flexion force such as that from a cricket ball. This is known as a 'Mallet' finger. There are, therefore, two opposing forces within the finger and since the force of the ball is greater, the extensor tendon gives way. Frequently it detaches the small portion of bone into which it is inserted. The pain is due to the blow and there may be immediate swelling, and local tenderness on the base of the phalanx. Treatment should be as soon as possible. Clinical examination reveals that the distal joint can be fully flexed but only extended for half of its normal range although this is full passively. An X-ray will reveal bony detachment if there is any and the treatment is the same for either condition. The injured finger should be fixed in full flexion on the palm of the hand by strapping. In this way the distal part of the tendon is fully relaxed since the distal joint is held in extension while the tendon is held taut proximally as the proximal interphalangeal joint is flexed. This position is maintained for four weeks by which time union will have taken place. This injury is also seen in netball, football and volleyball where there is a probability that a ball may strike the end of a finger − the most likely one being the longest, i.e. the middle finger. (See Fig. 5.11).

A *ganglion* is a swelling in or around a tendon sheath. To an athlete it can cause a degree of disability out of all proportion to its size. It is invariably rounded and mobile within the sheath. Pressure on the ganglion will often disperse it or the patient may be encouraged to try the all-time remedy of dropping the family bible onto it! Acupuncture seems to be the treatment of choice if simple pressure does not disperse it. The common site is around the posterior aspect of the wrist especially on the radial side, but a ganglion can occur anywhere. Some therapists believe that a ganglion is more likely to develop following a sprain to the wrist.

8.5   **Musculotendinous injuries**

As there are few musculotendinous junctions around the wrist, these strains are not often seen. However, it is worth mentioning that abductor pollicis brevis and extensor pollicis brevis may be subject to such an injury in *abduction strains* of the thumb. There will be pain felt by the patient on active use i.e. abduction of the thumb, and passive adduction will also cause pain. An area of localised tenderness is palpable. Deep friction and avoiding abduction will help the injury to heal.

8.6   Bone injuries

The commonest fracture of the wrist is the *Colles' fracture*. It is caused by falling on the wrist while it is in extension. The radius fractures about an inch above the wrist and the styloid process of the ulna is often fractured too. This results in the so called 'dinner fork deformity'. There is a history of a fall and the patient is in great pain and unable to move the joint. The deformity is obvious. Treatment has to be from an expert. Following bony union there will be some mechanical problems within the wrist and possibly also the elbow and even the shoulder and neck depending on the force of the fall. All these areas must be treated osteopathically to ensure full efficient mobility. Any resultant weak muscles must be given the necessary rehabilitation exercises.

The same injury in a child may cause a fracture separation of the lower radial epiphysis. Both conditions are diagnosable on X-ray. The scaphoid bone may be fractured from a fall on the hand or in boxing. There is pain and swelling and some loss of movement but this fracture is commonly overlooked and X-rays may appear normal, so a diagnosis of a sprain may be given. Repeated X-rays, including oblique views are essential to form a correct diagnosis. Treatment is necessary by an expert. Following union, osteopathic treatment is required to normalise the mechanics. This is a serious fracture as in some cases there is bone necrosis when the dead fragment may have to be excised and this will weaken the wrist somewhat.

A *Bennett's fracture* occurs at the base of the thumb with or without dislocation. It is not rare in boxers. There is pain, localised swelling and tenderness and the fracture shows on X-ray. Again, expert treatment followed by osteopathic treatment after union has occurred should render full power and mobility.

Fracture of any metacarpal bone is usually the result of a punch and therefore may occur not only in boxing but in any body contact sport where the contestant becomes overenthusiastic! There will be the usual signs of fracture and treatment is as for other fractures of the area.

The proximal phalanx may fracture when some hard implement is being held and the hand is struck by a hard object, for example in hockey or cricket. Treatment is as for the fractures already described. The Mallet finger has already been described under tendon injury (see section 8.4).

Fracture of a terminal phalanx may occur in sports such as volleyball, handball or basketball where the finger is struck by the ball especially along its long axis.

Throwers wrist is a condition where an exostosis forms on the dorsal surface of the second and/or third metacarpals at the base. Repeated hyperextension of the wrist during activities such as putting the shot helps the athlete to accelerate its projection. The irritation of this repeated action causes an exostosis to form which may obstruct hyperextension of the wrist and may need to be removed surgically.

The only other common injury to bone among athletes is bruising which will be caused by a blow. This must never be assumed and a diagnosis of bruising can only be made once the presence of a fracture has been ruled out. Arnica is then the treatment of choice together with cold packs until the swelling subsides.

8.7   Epiphysitis

This is not common in the wrist and hand but it can occur in sports where weight is taken on the hand, for example in gymnastics. It will usually occur at the lower end of the radius and will recover with rest. It is possible for the epiphysis to become displaced − see Colles' fracture in section 8.6.

8.8   Joint and ligament injuries

Any of the ligaments of the wrist or hand may be traumatised if sufficiently stressed, for example by a fall or during body contact sports. In judo the injury can happen when the hold on an opponent's clothing is forcibly broken. Diagnosis can only be made once the presence of a fracture has been excluded. Such strains will normally resolve with a light strapping and rest but there may be residual faults in the mechanics of the area which will need treatment once the swelling has subsided.

Sprains of the finger joints are common usually in body contact sports where some force has been applied at an angle to the finger. Once a fracture has been found to be absent, the injured finger should be strapped to its neighbour and active movement encouraged. Once the acute phase has passed examination will reveal a loss of lateral shift in the joint which must be restored by osteopathic technique as soon as possible. The finger should return to normal in about twelve weeks.

Strain of the inferior radio-ulnar joint is not rare in racket sports and has been dealt with in section 7.3 under tennis elbow.

Dislocations are not rare in this area and are caused by a force which the joint cannot withstand, for example the thumb may be forced into abduction by a hard ball. This is a common site for dislocation and a fracture must be excluded by X-ray. The joint will be painful and swollen and possibly bruised. Movement will cause pain and will be limited in at least one direction. Passive movement will feel unstable and the joint will feel deformed. Traction will usually reduce the dislocation but it may be unstable due to ligamentous damage and may require expert treatment. If the joint feels stable after reduction it should be supported in a firm strapping for four weeks, after which active correction to any residual mechanical faults can be carried out.

Subluxation can occur especially at the scaphoid or lunate, usually caused by a fall. There will be localised tenderness and some swelling over the bone, which is persistent. X-rays reveal a gap between the scaphoid and the lunate and expert treatment is necessary.

The palmar fascia may be subject to progressive contracture, so called *Dupuytren's contracture*. It is considered to be caused by repeated minor trauma to the area and it is possible that it may develop in oarsmen. The fascia shortens usually starting at the base of the fourth finger. Initially the condition can be relieved by progressive stretching but in many cases the fingers cannot straighten and surgical intervention becomes necessary. If present it would handicap use of the hand in sport.

8.9   Facet locking

This is extremely common in the wrist and hand probably because the area has so many tiny joints and is subjected to so many minor stresses. Osteopathic examination of each and every small joint will reveal any abnormality, and correction of any fault will render the joints completely mobile again. The patient will complain of discomfort when using the facet locked joints especially for fine movements. Many of these conditions are associated with abnormal function of the elbow joints, thus affecting the muscular integrity of the wrist and hand. These joints and possibly the shoulder and associated spinal areas must be checked. Any correction must be carried out, as the wrist and hand are mechanically the distal extension of the upper limb.

8.10   Mobility injury

Stiffness of the wrist and hand is usually associated with degenerative change or rheumatoid arthritis. The former occurs in older athletes especially those who have traumatised the area by many years of use. Rheumatoid arthritis, on the other hand, tends to affect younger people, more commonly women. Although the flexibility can be increased by osteopathic treatment, the conditions should be recognised, if present. Stiffness may also result from injury such as fracture. These cases will benefit enormously from osteopathic treatment aimed to increase joint mobility.

Recurrent dislocation and subluxation does not seem to occur in the hand and wrist. Seldom is hypermobility found on examination, probably because the area is not normally weight bearing. Loose bodies are uncommon but will lead to locking if present. Occasionally a loose body is found outside the joint but it is seldom of consequence as it is unlikely to interfere with normal movement.

8.11

Vascular and neurological involvement

The radial or ulnar artery may be injured when a fracture occurs and will be dealt with by the specialist who attends the patient. Obstruction of the circulation to the hands occurs, especially in long distance cyclists. It can be due to holding the shoulders taut thus obstructing the subclavian vessels, in which case osteopathic treatment to the cervicodorsal area and the first and second ribs together with relaxation of the shoulder girdles when cycling should relieve the symptoms. Alternatively it may be due to excessive weight being placed on the hands on the handlebars which must be corrected as a postural fault.

Radial nerve palsy has already been mentioned – see section 8.2.

Compression of the median nerve in the carpal tunnel is most likely to occur in women between the age of 40 and 50. The symptoms are pain and paraesthesia in the distribution of the median nerve and the symptoms are worse at night. There is pressure on the nerve which is in a restricted space; any enlargement of any of the neighbouring tendons can give rise to the condition or there may be contraction of the fibres of the flexor retinaculum itself. The symptoms can be relieved by placing the wrist in a cock-up splint – this is virtually diagnostic as it differentiates the condition from a cervical disc lesion. Osteopathy has been known to give relief if it is aimed at stretching the fibres of the flexor retinaculum. Any tenosynovitis, if present, should also be treated. If however the symptoms persist, surgical release of the retinaculum may be necessary. The condition is thought to be caused by repeated pressure on the retinaculum in some cases, such as that from handlebars on a bicycle or motor cycle.

Symptoms of nerve root pressure may occur in the wrist or hand from a cervical spine condition. It is then likely that there will be some symptoms in the spine and the pain is unlikely to be isolated to the wrist or hand alone. The symptoms may well be reproduced by movement of the spine and there may be a history which implies spinal involvement.

Chapter 9   The Hip and the Thigh

9.1   **General**

The hip joint is the articulation between the head of the femur and
the cup shaped fossa — the acetabulum — in the pelvis (see Fig.
9.1). The femur is the longest and strongest bone in the body. The
hip joint is very strong and so loses some flexibility by comparison
with the shoulder. It is a ball-and-socket joint; the capsule is both
strong and dense and is attached to the margin of the acetabulum
and to the base of the neck of the femur. The depth of the
acetabulum is increased by the presence of a fibrocartilagenous
rim, the labrum. The joint is synovial. In front, the iliofemoral
ligament reinforces the capsule; it is attached to the inferior iliac
spine above and to the trochanteric line of the femur below. It is
often called the Y ligament. The pubofemoral ligament runs from
the superior ramus of the pubis and blends with the Y ligament
below. Behind the joint the ischiofemoral ligament runs from the

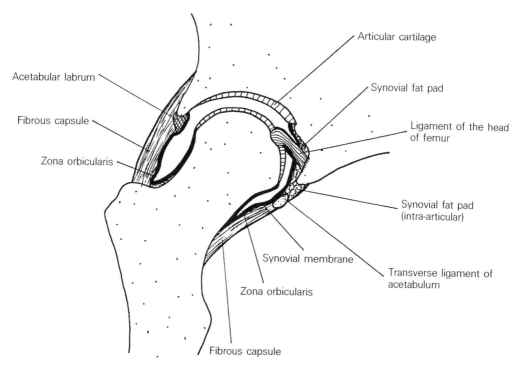

Fig. 9.1   Coronal section of the hip joint.

ischium below and behind the acetabulum and is attached to the base of the greater trochanter. The ligament of the head of the femur runs from the head of the femur to each side of the lower part of the acetabulum and varies greatly in strength from one person to another (see Fig. 9.2). The whole joint is surrounded by muscles.

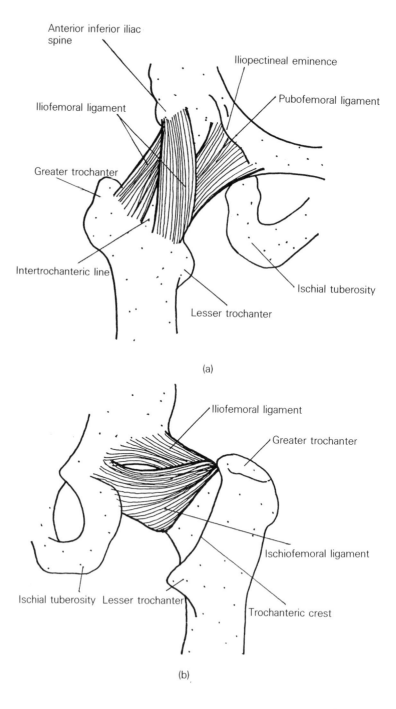

(a)

(b)

Fig. 9.2 Ligaments of the hip joint. (a) Anterior aspect; (b) posterior aspect.

The movements which occur are flexion, extension, abduction, adduction and medial and lateral rotation. Circumduction is a combination of these movements.

Flexion is brought about by psoas and iliacus assisted by pectineus, rectus femoris and sartorius muscles.

Extension is brought about by gluteus maximus assisted by the hamstrings.

Abduction depends on contraction of gluteus medius and gluteus minimus assisted by tensor fascia lata and sartorius.

Adduction is brought about by the three adductor muscles, longus, brevis and magnus, assisted by pectineus and gracilis.

Medial rotation is brought about by the action of tensor fascia lata, and the anterior fibres of gluteus medius and gluteus minimus. It is a weak movement.

Lateral rotation on the other hand is a powerful movement and is brought about by contraction of the obturators, the gemelli, quadratus femoris and piriformis.

The flexor muscles

Physiologically psoas and iliacus act together (see Fig. 9.3). *Psoas* arises from the anterior surface of each transverse process in the lumbar area and from the anterior surfaces of the bodies and intervening discs of T12 to L5 inclusive. *Iliacus* arises from the upper two-thirds of the iliac fossa, the iliac crest and from the upper surface of the lateral mass of the sacrum. Both muscles are inserted into the lesser trochanter of the femur, iliacus lying lateral to psoas. To maintain upright posture in the hip joints there has to be perfect balance between these two flexors (and rectus femoris) and the extensors of the hip. It is reasonable, therefore, to classify these muscles as principally postural muscles. The nerve supply to psoas is L2 and L3, and to iliacus is the femoral nerve L2 and L3. As the tendon of psoas crosses the pubic bone, a large bursa lies between it and the hip joint and occasionally communicates with the hip joint.

The *rectus femoris* arises from the anterior inferior iliac spine and from a groove above the acetabulum. It forms part of the quadriceps and is inserted into the patella; its action is chiefly as an extensor of the knee. The nerve supply consists of the femoral nerve L2, L3 and L4. See Figs. 9.4 and 9.5.

The *pectineus* arises from the pectineal line on the pubis and passes downwards, backwards and laterally to be inserted just below the lesser trochanter of the femur (see Fig. 9.6). The nerve supply consists of the femoral nerve, L2 and L3.

The *sartorius* is the longest muscle in the body (see Fig. 9.7). It arises from the anterior superior iliac spine and runs downwards and medially to be inserted into the upper part of the medial

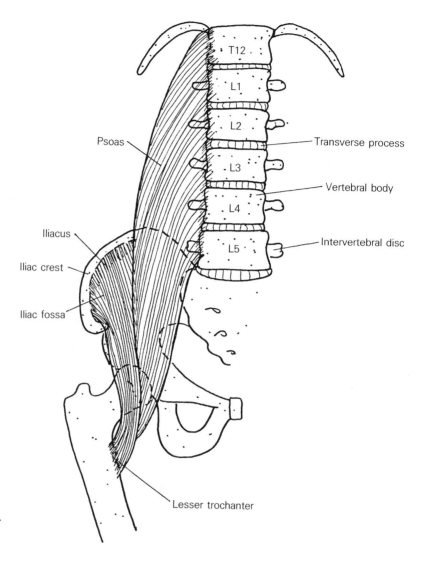

Fig. 9.3 Psoas major and iliacus muscles.

aspect of the shaft of the tibia in front of gracilis and semitendinosus. The muscle forms the roof of the subsartorial canal in the upper part of the thigh through which passes the femoral artery. The nerve supply consists of the femoral nerve, L2 and L3.

Flexion is limited by the apposition of soft parts and by tension in the gluteus maximus.

The extensor muscles

The movement is brought about by the action of gluteus maximus, assisted somewhat by the hamstrings (see Fig. 9.8). *Gluteus maximus* is a thick, fleshy muscle which forms the prominence of the buttock. It arises from the iliac crest, the posterior superior iliac spine and

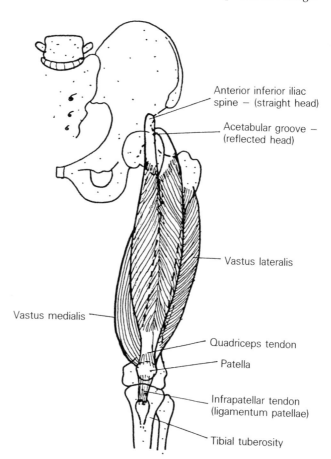

Anterior inferior iliac
spine — (straight head)

Acetabular groove —
(reflected head)

Vastus lateralis

Vastus medialis

Quadriceps tendon

Patella

Infrapatellar tendon
(ligamentum patellae)

Tibial tuberosity

Fig. 9.4 Quadriceps femoris. Rectus femoris, vastus medialis and vastus lateralis muscles.

from the posterior surface of the lower part of the sacrum and coccyx. The fibres run downwards and laterally and are inserted into the greater trochanter of the femur by means of a tendon. There is a bursa between the tendon and the bone. The nerve supply consists of the inferior gluteal nerve, L5, S1 and S2.

The *hamstrings* are principally flexors of the knee (see Fig. 9.9). However, there is a common tendon of origin of the long head of the *biceps femoris* and *semitendinosus* which arises from the ischial tuberosity. Together with the *semimembranosus* muscle these pass down the posterior aspect of the thigh to be inserted just below the knee joint. The nerve supply consists of the sciatic nerve L4, L5, S1, S2 and S3. Extension is limited by tension in the iliofemoral ligament.

Abduction

This movement is brought about by the action of gluteus medius and gluteus minimus, assisted somewhat by the action of tensor fascia lata and sartorius (see Fig. 9.8).

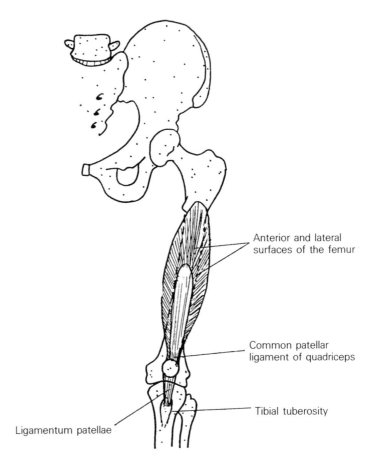

Anterior and lateral
surfaces of the femur

Common patellar
ligament of quadriceps

Tibial tuberosity

Ligamentum patellae

Fig. 9.5 Vastus
intermedius portion of
the quadriceps muscle.

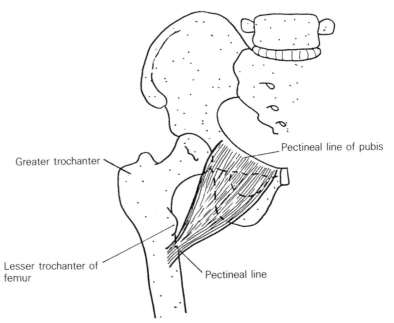

Pectineal line of pubis

Greater trochanter

Lesser trochanter of
femur

Pectineal line

Fig. 9.6 The
pectineus muscle.

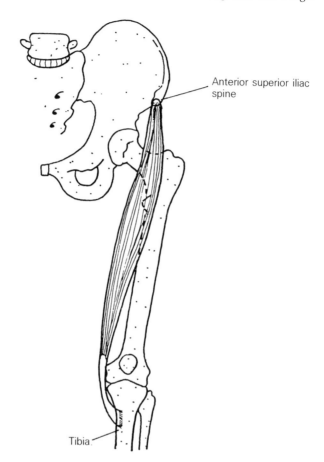

Anterior superior iliac
spine

Tibia

Fig. 9.7 The
sartorius muscle.

Gluteus medius arises from the iliac crest between the anterior
and posterior gluteal lines (see also Fig. 5.23). Its posterior one-
third is covered by the gluteus maximus. The fibres are inserted
into the greater trochanter by means of a tendon under which lies
a bursa. The nerve supply consists of the superior gluteal nerve,
L4, L5 and S1.

Gluteus minimus lies immediately under gluteus medius (see Fig.
9.8). It also arises from the iliac crest and is inserted into the
greater trochanter by means of a tendon under which lies a bursa.
The nerve supply consists of the superior gluteal nerve, L4, L5 and
S1. These two muscles act together but are anatomically separated
by fascia. They are very important in the maintenance of posture.

The tensor fascia lata arises from the anterior 5 cm of the iliac
crest and from the anterior superior iliac spine and is inserted into
the iliotibial tract (see Fig. 9.10). This structure passes down the
lateral aspect of the thigh to be inserted into the lateral condyle of
the tibia. It is a strong fascial sheath which supports the soft tissues
on the lateral aspect of the thigh and helps to give the contour to

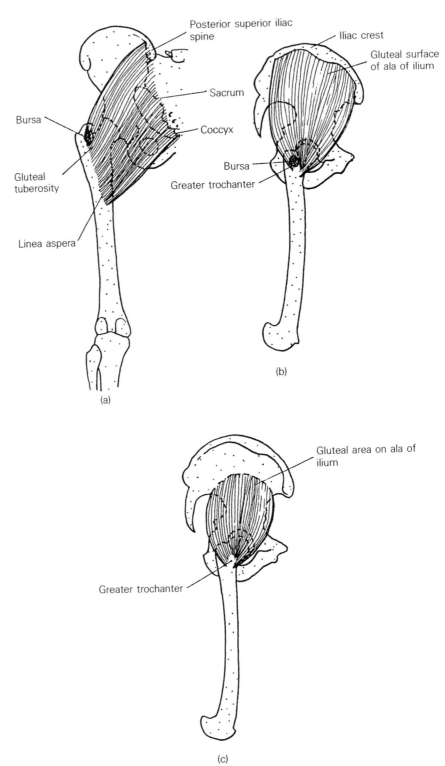

Fig. 9.8   (a) Gluteus maximus; (b) gluteus medius; (c) gluteus minimus.

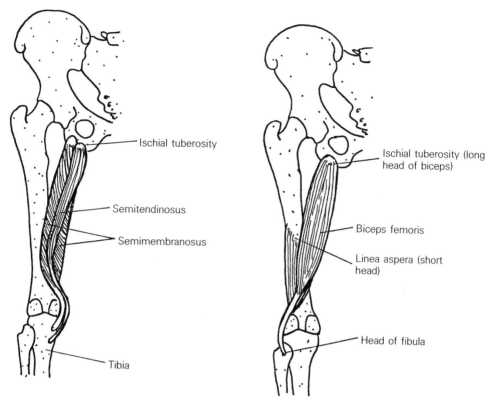

Ischial tuberosity

Semitendinosus

Semimembranosus

Tibia

Ischial tuberosity (long head of biceps)

Biceps femoris

Linea aspera (short head)

Head of fibula

Fig. 9.9   The hamstring muscles, semitendinosus, semimembranosus and biceps femoris.

this area. The nerve supply to the tensor fascia lata is the superior gluteal nerve, L4, L5 and S1.

Sartorius has already been described as a flexor of the hip.

Abduction is limited by tension in the adductor muscles and in the pubofemoral ligament.

Adduction

This movement is brought about by the action of adductor longus, adductor brevis and adductor magnus assisted by pectineus and gracilis (see Figs. 9.10 and 9.11). *Adductor longus* arises by a flat narrow tendon from the front of the pubis in the angle between the crest and the symphisis. It expands into a fleshy belly and passes downwards, backwards and laterally to be inserted into the middle one-third of the linea aspera of the femur between the vastus medialis and the other two adductors. Adductor longus is the most superficial of the three adductors. The nerve supply consists of the obturator nerve, L2 and L3.

Adductor brevis lies behind pectineus and adductor longus. It

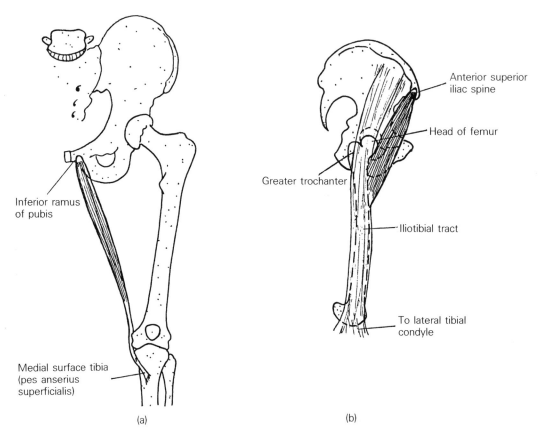

Inferior ramus
of pubis

Medial surface tibia
(pes anserius
superficialis)

(a)

Anterior superior
iliac spine

Head of femur

Greater trochanter

Iliotibial tract

To lateral tibial
condyle

(b)

Fig. 9.10   (a) Gracilis; (b) tensor fascia lata muscles.

arises by a tendon from the inferior ramus of the pubis between
the obturator internus and gracilis muscles. The fibres pass backwards, downwards and sideways and are inserted into the femur
along a line from the lesser trochanter to the linea aspera. The
nerve supply consists of the obturator nerve, L2, L3 and L4.

Adductor magnus is a large muscle. It arises from the inferior
ramus of the pubis and from the ramus and tuberosity of the
ischium. The fibres from the pubis are inserted into the medial
margin of the greater tuberosity of the ilium. Fibres from the
ramus of the ischium pass downwards and laterally and become
inserted into the linea aspera and the medial supracondylar line.
The fibres which arise from the ischial tuberosity pass almost
vertically and are inserted into the adductor tubercle, by means of
a tendon. This tubercle lies on the medial condyle of the femur.
This part of the muscle acts as a hamstring. The nerve supply for
the 'hamstring' portion is supplied by the sciatic nerve, L4 and L5,

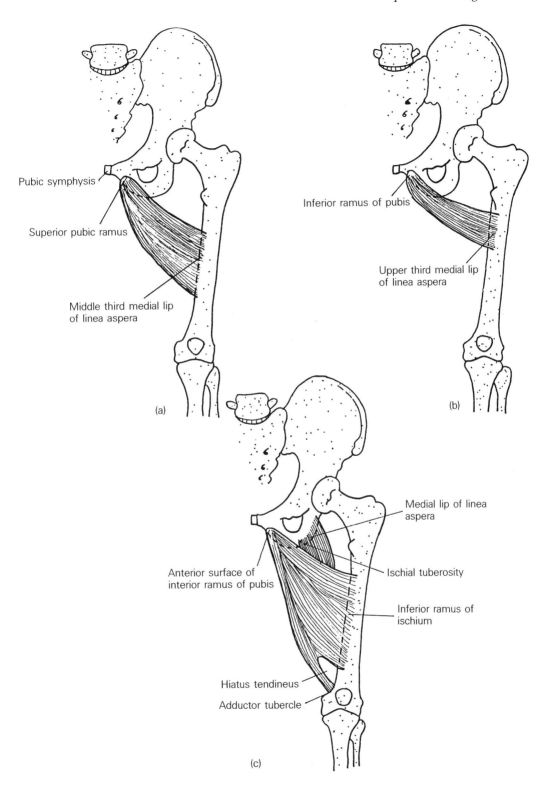

Pubic symphysis

Superior pubic ramus

Middle third medial lip
of linea aspera

(a)

Inferior ramus of pubis

Upper third medial lip
of linea aspera

(b)

Medial lip of linea
aspera

Ischial tuberosity

Inferior ramus of
ischium

Anterior surface of
interior ramus of pubis

Hiatus tendineus

Adductor tubercle

(c)

Fig. 9.11   The adductor muscles. (a) Longus; (b) brevis; (c) magnus.

but the 'true adductor' part of the muscle is supplied by the obturator nerve, L3 and L4.

Pectineus has already been described under flexors of the hip.

Gracilis is a thin ribbon-like muscle. It arises from the whole length of the inferior ramus of the pubis and the adjacent part of the ramus of the ischium. The fibres run vertically downwards and end in a rounded tendon which curves round the medial condyle of the tibia and becomes inserted into the upper part of the medial aspect of the shaft of the tibia immediately behind sartorius. It has a bursa between its tendon and the medial ligament of the knee. Its nerve supply is the obturator nerve, L2, L3 and L4.

Adduction is limited by contact with the opposite limb. However, if the hip is flexed, it is limited by tension in the abductors and in the ligament of the head of the femur.

Medial rotation

This movement is a weak movement. It takes place by the action of tensor fascia lata, and the anterior fibres of gluteus minimus and gluteus medius. It is limited by tension in the lateral rotator muscles.

Lateral rotation

This by contrast is a very powerful movement. It is brought about by the action of obturator internus, obturator externus, the gemelli, quadratus femoris and the piriformis muscles (see Fig. 9.12).

Obturator internus arises from the pelvic side of the obturator foramen. The fibres converge towards the lesser sciatic foramen and make a right-angled bend over the grooved surface of the ischium between the spine and tuberosity. The tendon then passes through the lesser sciatic notch, across the hip joint (where it receives the fibres of the gemelli) and is inserted into the medial surface of the greater trochanter. A bursa is present between the tendon and the hip joint. Its nerve supply is L5, S1 and S2.

The *gemelli* are accessories of obturator internus. The superior one arises from the ischial spine and the inferior gemellus from the ischial tuberosity. The fibres blend with the tendon of the obturator internus at the level of the hip joint.

Obturator externus arises from the outer surface of the obturator foramen. The fibres converge and pass backwards, upwards and laterally and end in a tendon which passes across the back of the neck of the femur to be inserted into the trochanteric fossa of the greater trochanter. Its nerve supply is the obturator nerve, L3 and L4.

Quadratus femoris lies under adductor magnus. It arises from

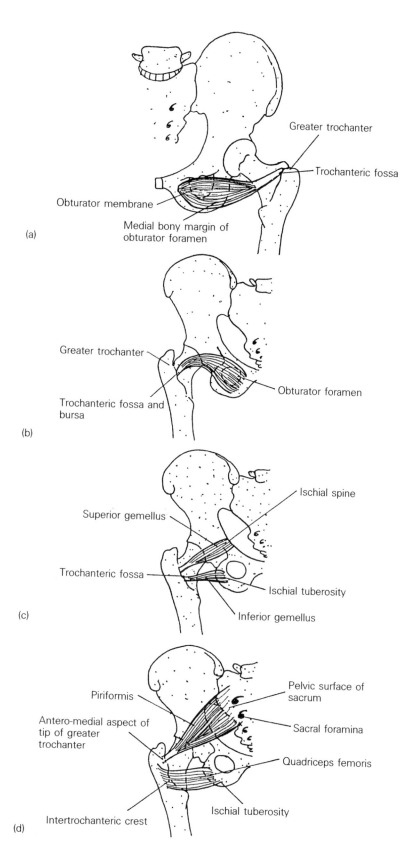

Fig. 9.12 (a) Obturator externus, anterior aspect; (b) obturator internus, posterior aspect; (c) the superior and inferior gemellus, posterior aspect; (d) piriformis and quadratus femoris, posterior aspect.

the ischial tuberosity and the fibres pass laterally to be inserted into a tubercle on the upper part of the trochanteric crest of the femur. A bursa is often present between the tendon of this muscle and the lesser trochanter. Its nerve supply is L4, L5 and S1.

The *piriformis* muscle arises within the pelvis from the anterior surface of the sacrum and from the upper part of the sacrotuberous ligament. The muscle fibres pass through the greater sciatic foramen and run parallel to the obturator internus in the buttock. It is inserted by a tendon into the greater trochanter, behind and above the obturator internus. In the interval between piriformis and the superior gemellus lie several important structures, namely blood vessels and the sciatic nerve, which may pass through the muscle itself in about 10% of people. Its nerve supply consists of S1 and S2.

Lateral rotation is limited by tension in the medial rotators and in the iliofemoral ligament of the hip joint.

9.2   **Muscle injuries**

Muscular injury in this area is very common indeed. Many such injuries are caused by direct (extrinsic) trauma when there will be a history of a blow or fall but many come on for no apparent reason other than stress during sport. The best way to describe muscle injuries in this area is to go through the muscles in the order in which they have been described.

Strain of the *iliopsoas* is not common but may occur in some body contact sports or where violent kicking is involved. The patient will give a history of pain which has become steadily worse and is aggravated by running or kicking actions. The pain may be felt above the hip joint and will be described as 'a deep pain'. It is difficult to palpate the fleshy part of this muscle but the diagnosis may be suspected if there is pain on resisted flexion of the hip when the hip is flexed to the right angle. This is to exclude the action of rectus femoris. The condition is usually associated with some mechanical problem within the lumbar spine (note the origin of psoas) which will require treatment. Gentle stretching of the muscle fibres is beneficial and rest from all activities which involve hip flexion until recovery has taken place. The commonest site of injury is in fact at the musculotendinous junction − see section 9.3.

Pectineus is often strained in extreme flexion with adduction of the hip joint such as performed by dancers. There will be localised tenderness and treatment consisting of deep soft tissue is beneficial. The part should be rested until pain subsides. Sartorius is seldom injured but is often found to be painful on palpation where there is an anterior rotation of the innominate − a classical strain of the sacro-iliac joint. There is also sensitivity at the insertion of this muscle.

The *gracilis* muscle may be painful and sensitive to palpate. Palpation is easy as the muscle is superficial in the thigh. Flexion of the hip with medial rotation is the usual cause of injury, such as an awkward kick at the ball in football. Horse-riding can also injure the muscle. The athlete will be aware of when and probably how he injured the muscle; resisted flexion with medial rotation of the hip joint will cause pain. If the lower fibres are damaged, the possibility of a bursitis between the tendon of insertion of the muscle and the medial ligament of the knee joint must be remembered and treated if present.

Most flexion strains of this area will involve the lumbar spine rather than the hip joint and possibly the sacro-iliac joints, as hip flexion is limited by tension building up within the very strong gluteus maximus before the flexors are traumatised. However, the possibility of a hernia causing pain in the front of the hip must always be considered.

The upper part of the *quadriceps* can be damaged in which case resisted flexion of the hip will cause pain. In this case, pain will be more marked when resisted extension of the knee is tested with the patient prone, to keep the hip extended. Deep soft tissue treatment to the affected area will help resolve the injury but if the surrounding mechanics are impaired there is an increased likelihood of recurrence. In the case of a quadriceps injury the hip, knee, pelvis and lumbar spine must be checked and any necessary corrections made.

Injury to the *gluteal* muscles is common either from overuse or from direct force. The area will be painful, even possibly on walking. If gluteus maximus is injured, the pain will be exaggerated by resisted extension of the hip or if the other muscles are affected resisted abduction will increase pain. Deep soft tissue treatment and the application of ice packs is the treatment of choice and the condition usually resolves quickly. Again the mechanics of the hip, pelvis and spine must be checked.

Adductor strains are extremely common. They frequently come about as a result of direct trauma, for example a kick, but can also be caused by excessive use, for example in horse riding, the so-called 'rider's strain'. There will be an area of pain and localised tenderness and possible bruising. Active adduction will cause pain as will passive abduction and resisted adduction. The injury responds well to local soft tissue treatment. The risk of recurrence must be lessened by making sure that all the surrounding joints are working correctly.

Piriformis is often seen in a state of hypertonia which seems to be a complication of a pelvic and/or lumbar spine disorder. Because of its anatomical relationship to the sciatic nerve there may be symptoms of sciatic irritation. Pain will be felt in the area of the muscle which is deep but easily palpable and there will be increased pain on resisted lateral rotation of the hip. The muscle responds well to deep inhibitory type soft tissue treatment and it is essential to make sure that the sacrum and pelvic areas are functioning properly; any necessary correction must be performed.

If one *obturator* muscle is hypertonic, the other one is usually in the same condition. They seem to act as 'muscle guards' in conditions of the hip joint and are seldom if ever injured except possibly as a result of pelvic injury.

The *iliotibial* band may be subjected to a muscle pull at the level of tensor fascia lata. This is most commonly seen in fencers and is a difficult condition to treat. If the injury is at the muscular level, it will respond to soft tissue treatment. However, this structure is more often damaged within its fibrous component and soft tissue treatment seems relatively ineffective. Ultrasound may well be the treatment of choice or acupuncture.

Muscle injuries in the thigh are very often seen in the *hamstrings*; these will be dealt with under the knee joint (see section 10.4).

<table>
<tr><td>9.3</td><td>

Tendon injuries

</td></tr>
</table>

These are also quite common around the hip joint and tend to be seen more often in older athletes. Because of the enormous forces applied avulsion from the bony attachment is not rare.

The common tendons to be injured are the piriformis, the rectus femoris and the adductors.

The patient will complain of pain on use of the muscle and there will be a palpable area of tenderness over the tendon. Resisted movements which stress the muscle will increase the pain. Ultrasound to the affected fibres is helpful and stretching of the muscular component gradually. Many tendon injuries respond best to local infiltration and the muscle should be rested until resisted movement no longer produces pain.

It is not uncommon for a tendon to become *avulsed* from its attachment in this area of the body. The common sites for this to happen are the *adductor* tendons of origin from the pubis in particular, and the *hamstrings* from the ischial tuberosity. Surgical treatment may be necessary. Alternatively there may be a degree of ossification around the bony attachment which can cause problems. On occasions, the symptoms seem to be due to inflammation at that site but some do not respond to anti-inflammatory treatment and require specialist attention. The hamstrings are commonly affected in hurdlers and the adductors in footballers and fast bowlers who need to make stretching movements and tighten the adductors as they do so. This appears to be due to repeated minor traumata. In some cases the symptoms can be relieved by stretching the muscular fibres and lessening the pull on the tendon attachment. It is always worth trying before resorting to surgery, and sometimes stretching the muscle under anaesthetic resolves the problem.

9.4   **Musculo-tendinous injuries**

These are not common around the hip area but the one which is so often overlooked is damage to the musculotendinous junction of psoas. The patient will complain of pain in the groin which is worse on running; it may have been present for a long time, probably varying in intensity. Resisted flexion with the hip at a right angle will exacerbate the symptoms. An area of localised tenderness is palpable just below the inguinal ligament and just medial to the inner border of sartorius. The condition responds well to deep soft tissue treatment to the injured fibres.

9.5   **Bone injuries**

The bone structure of this area is particularly strong so is not subject to a great deal of injury; however a direct force of sufficient intensity will cause bony damage. The bone may be bruised or may fracture. The common site for a fracture of the femur is at the neck of the bone which may occur following a fall. The patient will be in severe pain and unable to bear weight and there will probably be obvious deformity of the leg. This is a stretcher case.

Stress fractures are not particularly rare in this area. The neck of the femur may be subject to a stress fracture in cases of overuse and especially in young people. It has been said that a stress fracture is 'produced by too much activity too soon or too much activity all at once'. They occur, therefore in 'weekend athletes' who have been particularly energetic without preparing properly. The patient may well be able to weight bear but it may cause discomfort. All movements of the hip joint are likely to be normal (although mildly uncomfortable). There may be some muscular guarding especially in the obturator muscles. Any jarring of the hip is painful as is any activity such as running. An X-ray is diagnostic and the condition requires specialist treatment.

A stress fracture of the pubic ramus may also occur especially in sports such as football. There will be a dull ache in the area of the fracture which will be worse if the patient attempts to run. The area may be somewhat swollen and tender. If suspected, an X-ray is essential to differentiate the condition from a tendon injury or avulsion in the same area. Usually no specialist treatment is necessary but the athlete must rest to allow healing to take place. Resisted movements may also exacerbate the pain if the stress fracture is at the point of attachment of a muscle.

Perthe's disease occurs in the hip joint of children usually aged between 4 and 8, but is sometimes seen in children up to the age of 13. The child will complain of a slight ache or there may be no discomfort at all but he will walk with a slight limp which the parent will have noticed rather than the child. On examination all movements may be full and pain-free but there is an apparent slight shortening of the leg on standing examination. X-rays will reveal a flattening of the head of the femur; this is a necrotic condition and the degree of deformity varies greatly. Some cases seem to lay down new growth efficiently and there is not always permanent damage to the femoral head.

Paget's disease may give rise to pain around the hip joint, especially in the femur. The patient complains of an ache rather than pain and the bone appears bent on inspection. It is also likely to feel thicker than normal and the skin over the thigh will be abnormally warm. This condition is rare under the age of 50, but it could present as an athletic injury, for example in a keen middle-aged golfer.

9.6   Epiphysitis

The upper femoral epiphysis may become displaced in adolescents. There is either a history of one major injury, usually a fall, or there is a history of several repeated 'sprains' usually caused by minor exertion only. Some authorities think that there is an inherent weakness in the area for this to occur. The patient complains of pain which may be in the groin, thigh or knee and a limp is evident. Movement may be normal or only slightly reduced − medial rotation and abduction being those most affected. X-rays will show the defect and specialist treatment is necessary. Avulsion may occur in adolescents along the epiphyseal line, for example the iliac crest. All nagging pain in adolescents should be thoroughly investigated and never dismissed.

It is also essential to remember that pain is often referred to the knee, from the hip and vice versa, especially in young persons.

9.7   Ligament and joint injury

The ligaments around the hip joint are seldom injured as they are very strong. A muscular injury is more likely to occur. The ligament of the head of the femur is known to detach but the trauma to cause it has to be great, for example an accident while motor racing. There is pain which is worse on use of the hip and may refer to the groin, front of thigh or even the knee. After any serious injury extensive X-rays are taken and this condition should not therefore be missed.

Dislocation of the hip is usually congenital and therefore not a condition likely to be found in athletes. However, traumatic dislocation of the hip is possible if the foot is fixed and traction applied to the leg, for example a fall from a horse with the foot fixed in the stirrup. The history would alert the practitioner as would the obvious extreme pain and deformity. Specialist treatment is necessary but after the joint has stabilised there is likely to be mechanical problems within the affected leg, the pelvis and the lumbar spine if not in other parts of the body as well. These will all respond favourably to osteopathic treatment.

A *loose body* can occur in the hip joint. The patient will complain of sudden severe pain while walking or running which may be in the front of the thigh and run down as far as the knee. At this point, the hip tends to let the patient down. The episode may be repeated with the next step or not for several weeks. As the loose body is unlikely to be of bone, it will probably not show on X-ray and the condition is difficult to diagnose with certainty. Osteopathic treatment is unlikely to help as it cannot remove the loose body.

A generalised *synovitis* can affect the hip joint and is usually a result of overuse. The patient will complain of an ache rather than pain, which is worse when he uses the joint. To jump would definitely be painful. All active and passive movements are marginally limited but resisted movements are normal. X-rays are also normal. The condition usually resolves in a few days with rest but the possibility of some underlying disease must be considered if the symptoms persist.

Degenerative changes are common in the hip joint especially in athletes over 50 years of age. Repeated trauma to one hip may precipitate the condition, for example a batsman at cricket who has pounded his front leg many thousands of times over the years. Old injury of a more violent type, for example a fracture, will also tend to lead to osteoarthritic change prematurely. The patient will complain of mild pain around the hip in the early stages but is more likely to have noticed that he has difficulty cutting his toe nails. He will develop a characteristic limp. In the early stages, osteopathic treatment to improve the range of movement and relax any hypertonic muscles is very helpful. Exercises to maintain the fuller range of movement are essential and should be done daily without fail. I have seen some of these hips remain static over a period of years this way. Advanced cases are better referred for an orthopaedic opinion with a view to possible joint replacement as are those with a great deal of pain. Stiffness may also be a sign of other pathological conditions such as early osteomyelitis of the femur which is not as rare as one might think.

9.8   **Bursitis**

This condition is particularly persistent. The likely sites are under the tendon of insertion of gluteus maximus, under the tendon of iliopsoas in the groin and under the tendon of insertion of piriformis or of obturator internus into the greater trochanter. The patient will complain of pain which is quite localised to the site of the bursal swelling and is exacerbated by use of the relevant muscle. The origin of the hamstrings from the ischial tuberosity is another possible site for this condition. The bursa is usually palpable but may be difficult to find unless the palpation is deep to the overlying structures. Symptoms tend to persist and treatment is usually to infiltrate the bursa. This often seems to be a magic cure for the patient!

9.9   **Referred pain**

The hip joint receives innervation from the third lumbar level as does the knee joint. Hence pain originating in one of these joints can refer to the other. Pain from the hip can also refer from the groin down the front of the leg almost to the ankle as this is the dermatome supplied by L3. There is a small area of the buttock supplied by L3, namely the upper inner quadrant so pain can refer there too.

Pain can be referred to the hip from the knee, or from the level of L3 where a possible lesion may be present. This lumbar level must be checked out in all cases of hip pain.

9.10   **Neurological involvement**

The sciatic nerve is closely related to the hip joint, particularly to the piriformis muscle in the buttock. Hypertonia of this muscle can give rise to irritation of the sciatic nerve and pain may be referred to any point of distribution of that nerve. The patient will complain of pain in the posterior aspect of the lower extremity which he feels originates in the buttock. When questioned he affirms that he has no low back pain (but that does not necessarily mean that there is no associated problem in the lumbar area). Resisted lateral rotation of the hip may well increase the pain and pressure over piriformis, in the middle, will usually produce symptoms in the leg. This condition responds well to relaxatory soft tissue treatment and the symptoms usually subside gradually as the muscle condition improves. Some persistent conditions of piriformis are associated with disturbances within the sacral and pelvic joints which need to be checked out.

Chapter 10   The Knee Joint

10.1   **Knee joint**

The knee joint is the articulation between the lower end of the femur and the upper end of the tibia (see Fig. 10.1). The patello-femoral joint complicates the anatomy of the area and will be considered separately. The *knee joint* is a hinge joint partly sub-divided by two semilunar fibrocartilages placed between the femur and the tibia — the meniscii or 'cartilages'. These are attached to the tibia. The articular surfaces of the knee are not congruent and are more adapted to one another by the meniscii whose function is emphasised by the fact that they regenerate following surgical excision.

If the knee joint is subjected to excessive stress following removal of a meniscus the articular cartilage will suffer permanent damage, yet the joint can be used actively without any sign of instability during the regenerative phase.

It is interesting that in lower mammals the knee joint is separated into two distinct joints each with it's own synovial membrane, and only in higher mammals is it one continuous joint.

The *capsule* is complicated, being partly deficient and partly replaced by strong expansions of surrounding muscles. Posteriorly the fibres run vertically from the femoral condyles above and the intercondylar notch to the tibial condyles below and blend above with the heads of the gastrocnemius muscle, and are strengthened by the posterior oblique ligament. Medially the capsule blends with the medial ligament. Laterally the fibres are attached to the femur above the origin of the popliteus muscle and pass downward to the lateral condyle of the tibia covering that muscle. The lateral ligament is separated from the capsule by a small pad of fat. Anteriorly the capsule is attached to the tibial condyles below while above it blends with the expansions of the vastus medialis and vastus lateralis muscles which are attached to the margins of the patella and the patellar ligament. They extend backwards on each side as far as the collateral ligament and are attached to the condyles of the tibia, forming the medial and lateral patellar reti-naculum. Above the patella, the capsule communicates with the suprapatellar bursa. Laterally the capsule is strengthened by the iliotibial tract and medially by the sartorius and semimembranosus muscles. See Fig. 10.2.

The *synovial membrane* of the knee is the most extensive in the

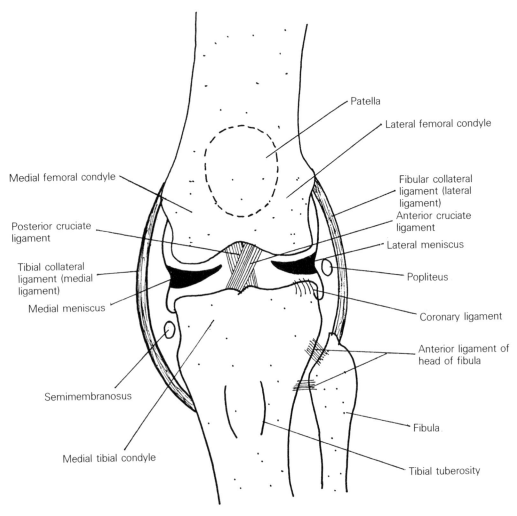

Fig. 10.1   Coronal section of the knee joint.

body (see Fig. 10.3). Above and in front, it communicates with the suprapatellar bursa. Below and in front, it is separated from the patella by a pad of fat — the infrapatellar pad, on either side of which the synovial membrane projects into the knee joint as a fringe-like fold named the alar fold, the two converging to form the infrapatellar fold which passes to the intercondylar notch. Posteriorly there is a fold of synovial membrane between the lateral semilunar cartilage and the tendon of the popliteus muscle while on either side it lines the capsule of the joint. It also covers the anterior and posterior cruciate ligaments in front and on either side but is reflected from the sides of the posterior cruciate ligament posteriorly onto the adjacent parts of the capsule. There is also a bursal recess between the cruciate ligaments from the lateral side of the knee. These complicated reflections of the synovial membrane

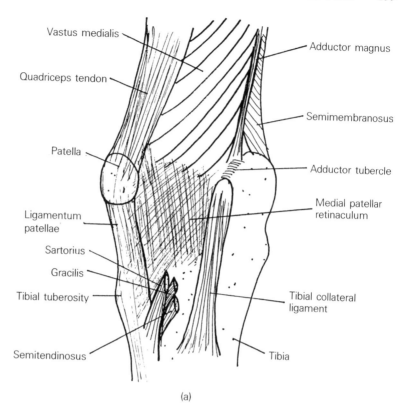

Vastus medialis

Adductor magnus

Quadriceps tendon

Semimembranosus

Patella

Adductor tubercle

Medial patellar
retinaculum

Ligamentum
patellae

Sartorius

Gracilis

Tibial tuberosity

Tibial collateral
ligament

Semitendinosus

Tibia

(a)

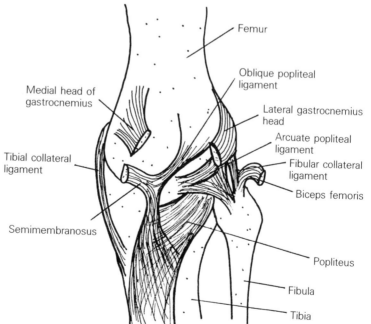

Femur

Oblique popliteal
ligament

Medial head of
gastrocnemius

Lateral gastrocnemius
head

Arcuate popliteal
ligament

Tibial collateral
ligament

Fibular collateral
ligament

Biceps femoris

Semimembranosus

Popliteus

Fibula

Tibia

Fig. 10.2
Reinforcements of the
capsule of the right
knee joint. (a)
Anterior aspect; (b)
posterior aspect.

(b)

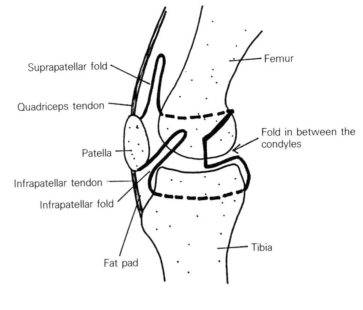

Section through
condyles

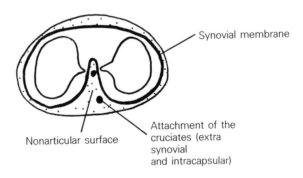

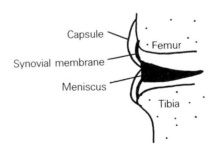

Fig. 10.3 Folds of
the synovial
membrane.

increase the surface area considerably and become involved in synovial irritations of the joint when the swelling can therefore be extensive and widespread.

The *oblique posterior ligament* is attached above to the lateral condyle of the femur. It consists of a strong bundle of fibre derived from the tendon of the semimembranosus muscle and is sometimes known as the ligament of Winslow. The arcuate ligament also attaches to the lateral femoral condyle and passes downwards to blend with the capsule, straddling the popliteus tendon.

The *medial ligament* is attached above to the medial epicondyle of the femur immediately below the adductor tubercle and passes to the medial surface of the shaft of the tibia. It is crossed by the tendons of sartorius, gracilis and semitendinosus where a bursa intervenes. The ligament is attached to the edge of the medial meniscus.

The *lateral ligament* is a strong rounded cord which is attached to the lateral epicondyle of the femur above and to the head of the fibula below. It is not attached to the capsule of the joint nor to the lateral meniscus. It is largely covered by the tendon of insertion of the biceps femoris muscle deep to which a bursa may be present. See also Fig. 10.1.

The *cruciate ligaments* are very strong. The anterior cruciate is attached to the medial part of the interior portion of the inter-condylar area of the tibia and passes upward, backwards and laterally crossing the posterior cruciate ligament, to become attached to the posterior part of the medial surface of the lateral condyle of the femur. The posterior cruciate ligament is stronger than the anterior. It arises from the posterior part of the intercondylar area of the tibia and the lateral meniscus and passes upwards, forwards and medially to attach to the medial condyle of the femur. The coronary ligaments are portions of the capsule of the knee joint which attach the meniscii to the anterior part of the tibial condyles (see Fig. 10.4).

The *meniscii* consist of dense collagenous tissue containing neither blood vessels nor nerves and are flatter towards the centre than around the periphery (see Fig. 10.4). Each covers approximately two-thirds of the corresponding articular surface of the tibia. They serve to deepen the articular surface of the tibia to conform more nearly with the femoral condyles. The medial meniscus is nearly semicircular in shape and it is important to remember that it is attached to the medial ligament of the knee joint thus reducing it's mobility and increasing the chance of injury. Damage to the medial meniscus is twenty times more common than to the lateral. The lateral meniscus is almost circular and is not attached to the capsule nor to the lateral ligament of the knee joint.

There is a large number of *bursae* around the knee joint some of which communicate with the joint itself (see Fig. 10.5).

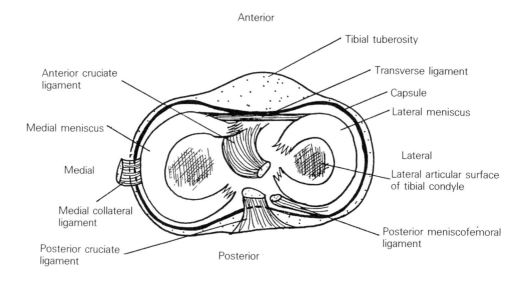

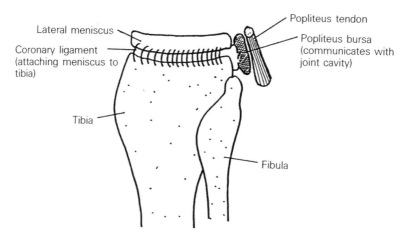

Fig. 10.4   Meniscii, coronary ligaments and popliteus bursa. (a) Superior aspect of right tibia; (b) lateral aspect.

Anteriorly there are four bursae: the *prepatellar* bursa lies between the lower part of the patella and the skin, the deep *infrapatellar* bursa between the upper part of the tibia and the ligamentum patellae (this sometimes communicates with the joint), the *superficial infrapatellar* bursa between the lower part of the tibial tubercle and the skin, and the *suprapatellar* bursa between the femur and the deep surface of the quadriceps muscle. This is a very large bursa and always communicates with the knee joint.

Laterally there are four bursae: one lies between the lateral head of the gastrocnemius muscle and the capsule of the joint (with which it may communicate), one between the tendon of

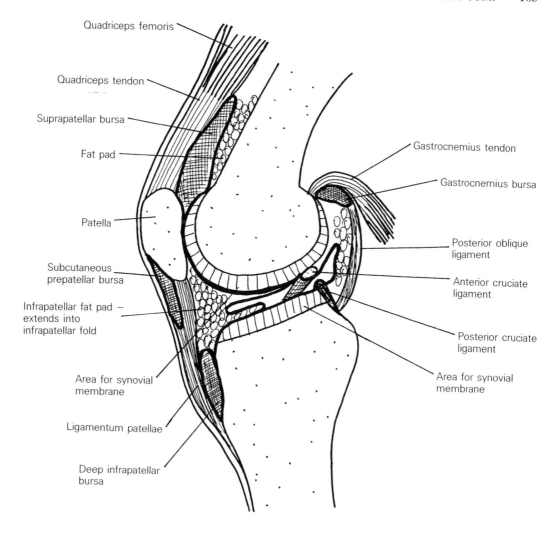

Quadriceps femoris

Quadriceps tendon

Suprapatellar bursa

Fat pad

Patella

Subcutaneous prepatellar bursa

Infrapatellar fat pad — extends into infrapatellar fold

Area for synovial membrane

Ligamentum patellae

Deep infrapatellar bursa

Gastrocnemius tendon

Gastrocnemius bursa

Posterior oblique ligament

Anterior cruciate ligament

Posterior cruciate ligament

Area for synovial membrane

Fig. 10.5   Bursae at the knee joint, sagittal section.

biceps femoris and the lateral ligament, one between the tendon of popliteus and the lateral ligament, and another between the tendon of popliteus and the lateral condyle of the femur.

Medially there are five bursae: one lies between the medial head of gastrocnemius and the capsule (and frequently communicates with the joint), one lies between the tendons of sartorius, gracilis and semitendinosis and the medial ligament (sometimes known as the tibial intertendinous bursa), one lies between the medial ligament and the tendon of semimembranosus, one between the tendon of semimembranosus and the medial condyle of the tibia, and one between the tendons of the semimembranosus and semitendinosus muscles (which may communicate with the joint).

The frequency of occurrence of bursae around the knee joint and their vulnerability to direct injury leads to bursitis being a commonly seen condition and it is necessary to diagnose which bursa is affected if it is to be treated satisfactorily. The exact location and the ability to palpate accurately are essential to the osteopath.

The active movements of the knee are flexion, extension, and medial and lateral rotation both of which can only occur when the knee is flexed. This is because both collateral ligaments are taut in the position of extension; during extension the femoral condyles glide backwards on the meniscii and tibia and the axis of movement shifts forward. Conversely during flexion the posterior part of the tibial articular surfaces approximate the posterior parts of the femoral condyles and the collateral ligaments are relaxed in full flexion. That is why injury to the knee is commoner in flexion than extension. See Fig. 10.6 for common sites of tenderness at the knee.

Flexion and extension occur around a moving axis which moves forward during extension. There is 5° of lateral rotation at the extreme of extension so the movements of flexion and extension are not 'pure' as in the elbow joint.

Flexion is brought about by contraction of the hamstring muscles, namely biceps femoris, semitendinosus and semimembranosus, with assistance from popliteus and gastrocnemius.

Extension occurs when the quadriceps muscle contracts.

Medial rotation is brought about by contraction of popliteus, semimembranosus and semitendinosus with some assistance from sartorius and gracilis.

Lateral rotation is brought about by the action of biceps femoris. *Biceps femoris* arises by two heads. The long head has it's origin from the ischial tuberosity in common with the semitendinosus. The short head arises from the linea aspera of the femur, from the middle third of the lateral lip. The two heads unite to form a large fleshy muscle which is inserted by means of a tendon into the head of the fibula (see Fig. 9.9). Between the tendon of insertion and the lateral ligament of the knee joint is a bursa (sometimes known as the inferior subtendoneal bursa). The long head of the biceps also acts on the hip joint – as an extensor. The action of the muscle produces lateral rotation as well as flexion. The nerve supply for the long head consists of the tibial nerve, L5, S1 and S2 and for the short head the common peroneal nerve, S1 and S2.

Semitendinosus arises by a common head (with biceps, see above) from the ischial tuberosity and forms a tendon just below the middle of the thigh which lies on the surface of semimembranosus. The tendon curves round the medial condyle of the tibia, passes across the medial ligament of the knee joint (from which it is separated by a bursa with sartorius and gracilis) and is inserted

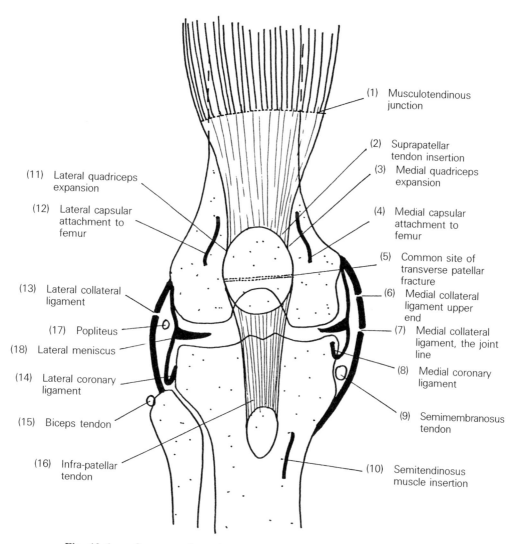

(1) Musculotendinous junction

(2) Suprapatellar tendon insertion

(3) Medial quadriceps expansion

(4) Medial capsular attachment to femur

(5) Common site of transverse patellar fracture

(6) Medial collateral ligament upper end

(7) Medial collateral ligament, the joint line

(8) Medial coronary ligament

(9) Semimembranosus tendon

(10) Semitendinosus muscle insertion

(11) Lateral quadriceps expansion

(12) Lateral capsular attachment to femur

(13) Lateral collateral ligament

(17) Popliteus

(18) Lateral meniscus

(14) Lateral coronary ligament

(15) Biceps tendon

(16) Infra-patellar tendon

Fig. 10.6   Common sites of tenderness at the knee.

into the upper part of the medial surface of the shaft of the tibia behind sartorius and below gracilis. The nerve supply consists of the tibial nerve, L5, S1, S2.

The *semimembranosus* also arises from the ischial tuberosity above and lateral to the origin of biceps and semitendinosus. It is closely related to the semitendinosus muscle with which it is some-times fused. Inferiorly the tendon of insertion divides into three parts; the first runs anteriorly to be inserted into the medial tibial condyle; the second is inserted into the fascia of the popliteus muscle while the third part continues into the posterior wall of the capsule of the knee joint as the oblique popliteal ligament. Before the tendon divides, there is a bursa between it and the tendon of the medial head of gastrocnemius. The nerve supply consists of the tibial nerve, L5, S1 and S2. Semimembranosus and semitendinosus produce medial rotation at the knee joint with flexion (unlike biceps which produces lateral rotation).

The *popliteus* muscle forms the floor of the lower part of the popliteal fossa. It arises by a strong tendon which is intracapsular, from the lateral condyle of the femur and is inserted into the medial two-thirds of the triangular area above the soleal line on the posterior part of the shaft of the tibia. It is thought that this muscle acts as a flexor of the knee as flexion starts from full extension – i.e. before the hamstrings act. Its nerve supply consists of the medial popliteal nerve, L4, L5 and S1.

The *gastrocnemius* muscle forms the bulk of the calf. It arises by two tendons, one from each condyle of the femur. Approximately halfway down the calf the muscle blends with the soleus and the two form the tendo calcaneus which is inserted into the middle of the posterior surface of the calcaneum. There is a bursa beneath the medial head of origin and a fibrocartilagenous sesamoid beneath the lateral head of origin. Together with soleus this muscle is the principal plantarflexor of the foot and provides the propelling force in walking, running and jumping. The gastrocnemius also flexes the knee joint. It's nerve supply consists of the medial popliteal nerve, S1 and S2.

The *plantaris* muscle is an accessory to the gastrocnemius and is not always present. It arises from the lateral supracondylar line and from the oblique posterior ligament of the knee joint. It blends with gastrocnemius and soleus to be inserted into the posterior part of the calcaneum. Its nerve supply is as for gastrocnemius.

Extension of the knee depends on contraction of the quadriceps muscle which consists of four distinct portions, namely rectus femoris, vastus lateralis, vastus medialis and vastus intermedius.

Rectus femoris arises from the anterior inferior iliac spine and from the upper margin of the acetabulum (see Figs. 9.5 and 9.6). It occupies the middle of the front of the thigh and runs vertically downwards to be inserted into the base of the patella. It also acts on the hip.

Vastus lateralis arises from the lateral surface of the greater trochanter, the intertrochanteric line, the gluteal tuberosity and from the lateral lip of the linea aspera. It is the largest part of the quadriceps and is inserted into the lateral part of the patella. Its nerve supply consists of the femoral nerve, L2, L3 and L4.

Vastus medialis arises almost entirely from the medial lip of the linea aspera and is inserted into the medial border of the patella and the quadriceps femoris tendon while it sends an expansion to reinforce the capsule of the knee joint. Its nerve supply consists of the femoral nerve, L2, L3 and L4.

Vastus intermedius arises from the front and lateral surfaces of the upper two-thirds of the shaft of the femur and is inserted into the lateral border of the patella (see Fig. 9.6). Its nerve supply consists of the femoral nerve L2, L3 and L4.

The four muscles join to form a common tendon of insertion which inserts into the patella. Distal to the patella the tendon continues as the patellar ligament which is inserted into the tibial tuberosity. Some of the superficial fibres run across the patella while the deep fibres are inserted into it's upper and lateral margins. Some of the fibres of rectus femoris and vastus medialis form the medial patellar retinaculum while those of vastus lateralis together with some from rectus femoris, form the lateral patellar retinaculum. The retinacula pass distally around the patella to the tibial condyles.

Medial rotation is brought about by semitendinosus and semi-membranosus − see flexor muscles.

Lateral rotation is brought about by biceps femoris − see flexor muscles above.

In addition there are three accessory movements which can be assessed passively in the knee joint. A wide range of rotation can be obtained when the knee is flexed to 90° and in this position there is a shift obtainable of the tibia on the femur forward and backward called the A−P shift. In extension the tibia can be shifted medially and laterally on the femur, this is called the lateral shift. In addition, the femur and tibia can be separated slightly by traction in either flexion or extension but this movement is easier to assess in extension.

Flexion is limited by the opposition of soft parts. The range of movement is 140° actively and 160° passively when full flexion is achieved as the heel touches the buttock. In active flexion the collateral ligaments are relaxed.

Extension is full at 180°, i.e. the leg is straight. There is normally a further 5−10° of extension possible passively. Extension is limited by tension in the collateral ligaments.

Medial rotation occurs up to 30° (only with the knee flexed to 90°). During this movement the cruciate ligaments become twisted around each other thus limiting the movement.

Lateral movement has a range of up to 45°. During this movement the cruciate ligaments become unwound and the movement of extension is limited by tension in the medial collateral ligament. Because of the oblique position of the two cruciate ligaments, in every position of the knee joint, one or other is always fully or partially tensed thus maintaining great stability of the joint, i.e. the cruciates maintain stability when the collaterals relax.

10.2   **The patellofemoral joint**

This joint is the articulation between the posterior surface of the patella and the medial and lateral condyles of the femur. The patella can be considered a sesamoid bone within the tendon of the quadriceps muscle, modified to form a joint with the femur. The articular surface of the patella is only imperfectly congruent with the corresponding parts of the femur. In flexion and extension the patella moves in a saggital plane. When the quadriceps contract i.e. in extension, the patella is pulled up by the muscular contraction. As the condyles of the femur move posteriorly in relation to the condyles of the tibia and as the patella is bound by ligaments to the tibia, so the patellar movement must follow the relative movement of the tibia. In rotation the same relative movement occurs, in this case in a frontal plane. Thus during medial rotation the patella is dragged laterally and medially during lateral rotation. The joint is a synovial joint totally separate from the knee joint. The patella also serves as a protective guard to the anterior surface of the knee joint which would be extremely vulnerable to direct injury were the patella not present.

No movement takes place except in conjunction with the knee joint.

10.3   The superior tibiofibular joint

This articulation is a plane joint between the lateral condyle of the tibia and the head of the fibula. The articular surfaces are flat and the joint is of the synovial type. The capsule is attached to the articular surfaces on the margins. It is strengthened by an anterior ligament in front and a posterior ligament behind which is covered by the tendon of the popliteus muscle. Passive movement occurs as the fibular head glides backward and forward on the tibial condyle. The joint is important to osteopaths when considering the mechanics of biceps femoris which is inserted into the fibular head and acts as a flexor and lateral rotator of the knee joint.

10.4   Muscle injuries around the knee

The *quadriceps* muscle is often injured either by a direct or an indirect (intrinsic) force. If the injury was due to a direct force there will be a history of a blow. If the injury was *intrinsic* the patient will say that he was running or jumping and felt 'something go' in the front of the thigh which was painful at the time and later he could only walk with a limp. The usual site is just superior to the suprapatellar tendon where a haematoma and area of tenderness will be palpable. Complete separation is possible when a gap in the continuity of the muscle will be palpable. On examination the hip joint will be normal as will the knee joint apart from limitation of flexion and pain felt on resisted extension. With a complete rupture resisted extension will be very weak.

Initially treatment should be the application of an ice pack with a degree of compression to reduce the swelling. The following day deep soft tissue treatment may be commenced and ice packs continued. Ultrasound is also indicated. The patient should adopt a posture with flexion at the hip, and the knee extended to prevent a stretch being placed on the torn fibres. Recurrence is likely if the patient resumes physical activity too soon. Active treatment should continue for a week after the patient is apparently symptom-free and he should not run hard for at least one month after there is no pain. Should the injury be due to a severe blow on the front of the thigh, the possibility of myositis ossificans developing must be remembered as this will require orthopaedic treatment.

Full recovery is when there is full passive flexion of the knee and there is no pain on resisted extension. The mechanics of the joints of the lower extremity (all of them), the pelvis and lumbar spine must be checked out for any resultant defect.

The *hamstrings* are also frequently injured and this injury is all too often recurrent. The lesion may occur at any point in the muscle but mid-thigh is probably the most common. The patient will say that the pain came on as he was running or jumping and he will walk with the knee flexed. There will be a localised area of swelling and tenderness at the site of injury. There will be pain on resisted flexion of the knee and on passive extension – i.e. the straight leg raising test will be positive. There will be no other abnormality found on examination of the knee joint.

Treatment should be as for a quadriceps injury but myositis ossificans does not occur in the hamstrings following a direct blow.

Hamstring injury, especially if recurrent, seems to be frequently associated with mechanical problems in the pelvis where the sacroiliac joints are most often at fault and these must be treated osteopathically before the patient is allowed to start training again after a hamstring injury. It is often useful to advise the patient to rub the old injury well with a rubifacient such as Tiger balm when he resumes activity as this will increase the circulation to the part. Following any muscular injury there will be an area of scar tissue laid down which is less elastic than the original fibres were before injury, so it is essential that the athlete really stretches well before any subsequent activity.

The *popliteus* muscle may be injured, often when the athlete has been training on uneven ground, the balance of muscle power between the hamstrings and quadriceps must be correct. He will complain of pain in the popliteal fossa which is exacerbated when he squats (similar to a lesion of the posterior cruciate ligament). The knee joint will be found to be normal apart from pain felt on passive extension, resisted flexion and resisted medial rotation. (There will be no abnormality found on A–P shift as would be the case if the cruciate were damaged). An area of tenderness within the muscle confirms the diagnosis and the condition responds well to local soft tissue treatment.

The *iliotibial* tract may be strained and this injury seems to be confined to athletes. Typically the patient will say that he felt pain while running, the common site being just above the knee on the lateral aspect. A day or two later the pain had subsided but came on once more when he ran again and was more severe. This picture may well have been repeated until even walking becomes painful. The pain is localised and there is a painful area where the injury has occurred which responds well to soft tissue treatment and ultrasound. Again all relevant mechanics must be checked before normal activity is allowed to be resumed, namely the joints of the lower extremity, the pelvis and the lumbar spine.

| 10.5 | ### Tendon injuries |

Tendons are nearly always traumatised at the tenoperiosteal junction. These are the vulnerable sites around the knee joint.

The *quadriceps* muscle has tendons at the origin and insertion. The straight head of rectus femoris (from the anterior inferior iliac spine) is a common site of injury. As this part of the muscle acts as a flexor of the hip as well as an extensor of the knee both these resisted movements will produce pain. The area may need infiltration if it does not respond to deep soft tissue treatment. Ultrasound may accelerate healing. The injury is particularly common where kicking is involved.

Tendon injury around the *patella* occurs at three sites, namely the suprapatellar tendon, the quadriceps expansion and the infrapatellar tendon (see Fig. 10.7). There will be a history of pain which probably came on during some energetic activity (especially if the athlete did not warm up enough and/or stretch his quadriceps sufficiently). The patient will complain of pain on walking especially upstairs. The site of pain is localised and the area is sensitive to palpation so the diagnosis is clear. Treatment is as for the straight head of rectus femoris. Only occasionally is infiltration necessary. Once the injury has healed it is imperative to make sure that there is no residual shortening of the quadriceps muscle as a whole. Long fibre stretch techniques should be used and the patient advised to stretch the muscle frequently himself until it is completely supple. The correct mechanics of passive movement of the patella on the femur are also essential to avoid the possibility of recurrence.

The patella tendon may be involved and this injury may come about by kneeling on a rough surface. It has to be treated similarly to the quadriceps expansion injury. The injury may be secondary to a patella alta where there is increased stretch placed on the tendon, in which case the quadriceps bellies must be stretched to

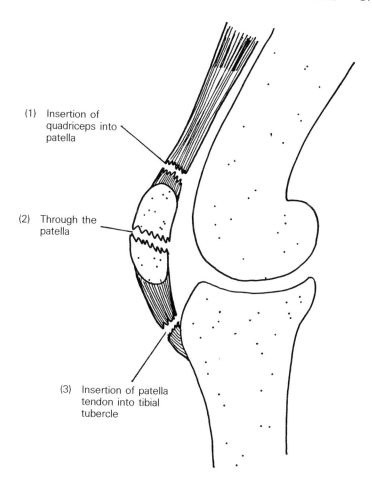

(1) Insertion of
    quadriceps into
    patella

(2) Through the
    patella

(3) Insertion of patella
    tendon into tibial
    tubercle

Fig. 10.7 Common sites of rupture of quadriceps tendon apparatus.

relieve the condition. There may be a bursitis present to complicate the condition − see section 10.13.

The tendons of origin of the *hamstring* muscles especially those from the ischial tuberosity are frequently injured, especially in runners, hurdlers or jumpers. If the injury involves the periosteum it is very difficult to treat satisfactorily, in particular where the injury has been repeated. X-rays may reveal a certain degree of exostosis at the tuberosity and the condition is often complicated by a chronic bursitis. Racing drivers used to be subject to this trouble as the area was repeatedly traumatised by sitting on hard, inflexible seats. Some conditions require surgical 'cleaning up' of the area. It is important to remember that similar symptoms may be present if the patient has an abscess in the ischiorectal fossa but the symptoms will have come on for no apparent reason. In this case there will be a degree of fever and enlargement of the lymph glands in the groin.

The tendons of insertion of the hamstrings are all subject to injury (see Fig. 10.6). There will be localised pain on resisted flexion of the knee and the injured fibres can be palpated and will be tender. All three may be complicated by bursitis. In all these cases it is essential that the injury has healed satisfactorily before full activity is resumed and it is wise to avoid full activity for a month after the lesion has fully resolved during which time stretching and strengthening exercises should be carried out repeatedly. As with any inflammatory condition ice packs help to resolve the condition and the athlete should be advised to apply these. The ideal is six times a day for about five minutes at a time.

The tendons of origin of *gastrocnemius* are often injured especially in runners particularly if the running is in different directions, for example in lawn tennis players. The patient will say that the pain started suddenly as he was diving for a ball. It will be localised to the injured area and will be exacerbated by standing on tiptoes. He will probably walk with the knee slightly bent to prevent stretching the tendon. Plantarflexion of the foot is painful with the knee fully extended but not with the knee flexed to 90° (differential diagnosis of a tear of the soleus muscle). This condition responds well to deep soft tissue treatment but the rule of resumption of activity should be observed. This condition is also often complicated by bursitis. Stretch of the injury can be reduced during healing by raising the height of the heel.

10.6

Musculotendinous injuries

These are also common around the knee joint. The common sites are the quadriceps, hamstrings, popliteus and gastrocnemius. The exact site can be found by palpation and resisted movements will cause pain (as with muscular and tendinous injuries). Recovery is slower than for a muscular injury but quicker than for a tendon. The injury responds well to deep soft tissue treatment and friction and the patient can assist by applying ice packs to the area. The use of a rubifacient to the area is also helpful and should be used as a precaution once normal activity is resumed. The exact location of the musculotendinous junctions around the knee should be checked in an anatomy text book. The history is similar to that of a tendon injury. Muscle injuries occur most often in young athletes and tendon injuries in middle-aged people. Musculotendinous injury can occur at any age.

Musculotendinous injuries around the knee joint are sometimes accompanied by tears of the fascial sheaths especially in the hamstring muscles. The patient will say that the symptoms came on during physical activity, probably running and there will be an area of localised pain. Swelling occurs with use of the muscle concerned which usually subsides quite quickly once the activity ceases, so it may be necessary to observe the athlete immediately after he stops running. This injury usually requires surgical repair as the fascial sheath maintains pressure on the underlying muscle fibres which will, therefore, not be able to function normally if the tear is not repaired. The patient may have noticed a weakness in the muscle since the injury. The exact site is nearly always at the musculotendinous junction.

10.7   Bone injuries

The knee joint is not protected by musculature so the bones are vulnerable to direct trauma. Localised bruising is commonly seen, either alone or with some other condition of the area. Bruising of the periosteum is very painful and obvious to see. Ice packs and rest are the treatment of choice and homeopathic arnica will help resolve the condition. Tincture of arnica may be applied locally *only if the skin is unbroken*. There will be a history of a fall or blow to the area and discolouration is visible. Normal activity can be resumed once the pain has subsided.

Osteoid osteoma are most frequently seen in male patients under the age of 30 and over 50% of these occur in the femur or tibia. The patient will usually complain of pain but may only say that he has noticed a hard lump. Despite the fact that this is a benign tumour, this assumption must never be made without further investigation, so the patient must be referred for an orthopaedic opinion. Once the correct diagnosis is made, surgical excision is carried out and the tumour does not recur.

Fractures around the *knee joint* are not rare. The femur may fracture in the lower part of the shaft, in the supracondylar area, (these are most often seen in elderly people), a condyle may fracture or there may be a fracture-separation of the femoral epiphysis (see Fig. 10.8). Direct violence is usually the cause of a fracture of the femoral shaft or a supracondylar fracture and there will be a history of this. The knee joint will be swollen and very painful, far too painful to move at all. Deformity may be obvious.

Fracture of a *femoral condyle* is caused either by a direct blow or a fall from a height and clinically will resemble the above fractures. Fracture-separation of the femoral epiphysis usually occurs in adolescence, either from a hyperextension or abduction strain and again severe pain, swelling and inability to move the knee are characteristic. All these conditions require expert attention.

The *tibia* is also subject to fracture. The medial condyle is seldom fractured but the lateral is less fortunate. A fall from a height or a direct blow causing a valgus strain drives the condyle upwards into the femoral condyle which remains intact. The shaft of the tibia may fracture either alone or with a fracture of the fibula. In these cases there will be a history of a fall or direct injury, and deformity and extreme pain are present.

A *hyperextension injury* in a child or young adult may not tear

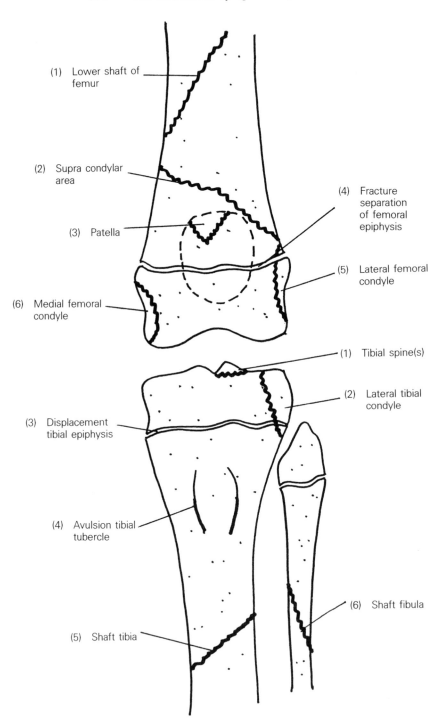

(1) Lower shaft of femur

(2) Supra condylar area

(3) Patella

(4) Fracture separation of femoral epiphysis

(5) Lateral femoral condyle

(6) Medial femoral condyle

(1) Tibial spine(s)

(2) Lateral tibial condyle

(3) Displacement tibial epiphysis

(4) Avulsion tibial tubercle

(5) Shaft tibia

(6) Shaft fibula

Fig. 10.8   Common sites of fracture around the knee joint at the femur, tibia and patella, including sites of epiphysitis and apophysitis.

the anterior cruciate ligament but cause the tibial spine to be avulsed. A lateral X-ray of the knee shows the detachment of the spine from the tibia. Occasionally a resisted extension strain of the knee causes displacement of the tibial epiphysis. In all these fractures there will be a history of injury which should make the osteopath suspicious that a fracture may have occurred. The knee will be too painful to move and swollen and obvious deformity may be seen. All these cases must be referred.

Fracture of the *patella* is not rare. A fall or direct blow onto the bone may fracture it. Resisted extension of the knee may rupture the extensor mechanism. Typically the patient catches his foot and in his attempt to prevent falling contracts his quadriceps violently. The patient is usually middle-aged and surgery to repair the damaged extensor mechanism is essential if he is not to lose the last 10–15° of extension. The direct patella fracture usually resolves itself. In both cases the knee is swollen and held in flexion. Aspiration of an effusion may be necessary and cases should be referred for further advice.

Following the repair of fractures around the knee, there is likely to be a loss of movement and/or power in one or more movements. This is where osteopathic treatment is so useful in restoring normality to the mechanical components. Ligaments may have been stretched or there may be loss of movement especially of the lateral shift of the joint. As this is a safety mechanism of the joint, unless it is restored the joint is likely to suffer from some relatively minor injury. Exercises to restore full muscle power are also essential if the joint is to function fully in the future. The effects of limping or walking with some walking aid may be widespread and any residual inefficiency should be treated.

10.8   Epiphysitis and apophysitis

Epiphysitis may occur at the lower femoral epiphysis or at the upper tibial (or both). It is considered to be an overuse condition of growing bone and excessive physical activity must be reduced. The patient is usually a keen young athlete; he will complain of pain around the inflamed area which is worse after physical activity. Examination reveals an area of tenderness along the epiphyseal line but otherwise the knee joint is normal. X-rays may show widening of the epiphyseal line. Treatment is rest until the symptoms subside. Ice packs will reduce the inflammation and osteopathic treatment to the area is helpful, but normal activity must only be resumed once the inflammation has resolved.

Apophysitis occurs at the tibial tubercle where the patellar tendon is inserted. The condition is often bilateral and is considered to be another overuse condition of growing bone. The typical patient is a young boy aged between 10 and 15 (but it does occur in girls of the same age), who complains of pain felt at the tubercle which is worse after physical activity. The tubercle is swollen and tender to touch. Resisted extension of the knee may cause pain but otherwise the knee joint is normal on examination. The condition resolves in about two years during which time, excess physical activity which involves the quadriceps muscle should be reduced, for example cycling and jumping. X-rays will confirm the diagnosis. Ice packs will help to reduce the inflammation and osteopathic treatment to the knee joint and to the quadriceps muscle is indicated. Kneeling should be avoided while the tibial tubercles are sensitive.

10.9   Ligament injuries

See Fig. 10.9 for diagram of common sites of ligamentous injuries at the knee. The *medial collateral* ligament may be damaged when a valgus strain is imposed on the knee joint. Typically the patient will fall awkwardly, for example while skiing when the knee is flexed and forced into abduction. He may hear a crack and will feel sudden pain. Initially he is able to walk but soon this becomes increasingly painful and he may have to rest the limb completely. The knee has become swollen by this stage. Gradually the pain and swelling subside and the patient resumes use of the knee. Examination reveals a tender area usually across the joint line and there is pain on passive valgus strain of the knee. Strapping to reduce stretch on the damaged fibres is helpful, always avoiding strapping around the limb as this would reduce drainage. Occasionally the ligament ruptures completely rendering the knee joint unstable. Valgus movement will be excessive as will lateral rotation. In athletes such as footballers where the knee has to be stable, surgical repair may be necessary.

The *lateral collateral* ligament is seldom damaged but if it is, varus strain of the joint will be painful and the patient is aware that he has damaged the area. A local tender area confirms the diagnosis and repair usually takes about four weeks. Strapping may be found to give support and relief of pain and ice packs will accelerate healing together with ultrasound and general treatment to the joints and surrounding muscles.

The *coronary* ligaments are frequently strained in sport especially where a rotational strain has been placed on the knee joint, for example in football. There is immediate pain felt at the site of injury which may pass off quite quickly. Some hours later the knee joint will swell up and become painful, and walking the following day may be painful. On examination the knee is inflamed and limited in flexion and extension but most pain is felt on passive rotation of the tibia in 90° of flexion of the knee, and an area of tenderness is found over the affected fibres. There is no pain on valgus or varus strain thus absolving the collateral ligaments. Deep

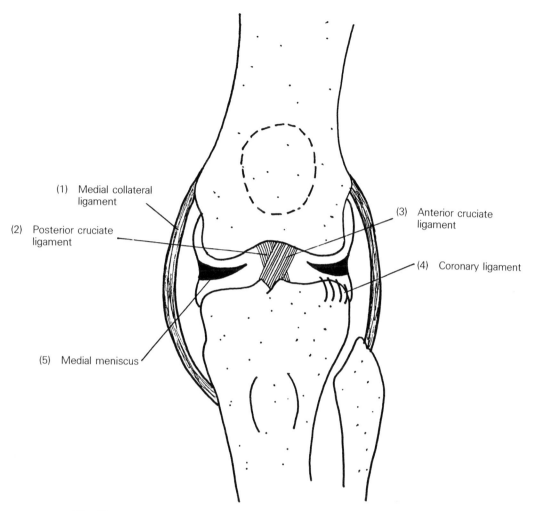

(1) Medial collateral ligament

(2) Posterior cruciate ligament

(3) Anterior cruciate ligament

(4) Coronary ligament

(5) Medial meniscus

Fig. 10.9   Common sites of ligamentous injury at the knee.

friction to the injured fibres and anti-inflammatory treatment to the knee joint together with supporting strapping to the coronary ligament will help and the problem should resolve in about four weeks. A supportive strapping once full activity is resumed is often found to be helpful, if only psychologically.

The *anterior cruciate* ligament can be injured if the tibia is forced backwards on the femur such as may occur in certain martial arts or in football where one player falls on another. Alternatively, if the knee is in hyperextension and a force is applied in the direction of medial rotation, the ligament may suffer. The patient may give a history of such a strain. On examination the joint will be swollen and painful and will have a full range of movement, all extremes causing pain. The ligament cannot be palpated but all others will be pain-free. Valgus and varus strains cause no pain. On A−P movement however, there is pain on anterior shift of the tibia, as this movement stretches the anterior cruciate ligament.

Conversely the *posterior cruciate* ligament will produce pain when the tibia is shifted backwards on the femur. This injury occurs when the knee is subjected to a strain which forces the tibia laterally on the femur with the knee flexed to 90°. Spontaneous recovery is slow and there is often some instability in A−P shift even as long as a year after the initial injury. Stabilisation is desirable but late surgery is often unsuccessful. Vigorous quadriceps exercises are essential and sport may be possible with a brace worn on the joint. If, however, this is unacceptable, surgical repair may be the treatment of choice, but the prognosis of a damaged cruciate ligament is not very good. No osteopathic treatment should be given which will increase the unstable movement of the affected joint.

10.10   **Joint injuries**

Most injuries to the knee joint will involve the synovial membrane and a joint effusion will occur. If the joint swells up over a period of hours, then the effusion is likely to be of synovial fluid. However, if the *swelling* occurs within minutes, the effusion is likely to be blood and a haemarthrosis is present. The former can be treated with ice packs and possible compression whereas the latter must be seen quickly by a medical practitioner as aspiration is probably necessary. The joint effusion may affect a bursa, the commonest one being the suprapatellar bursa, so the swelling may be visible in the lower one-third of the thigh on the anterior aspect. It is often necessary to treat the knee injury as an acute inflammatory synovitis in the early stages as a firm diagnosis cannot always be made for certain, while the knee is acutely inflamed. Ice packs, possible elevation and compression and the use of anti-inflammatory medication are all useful at this stage. Once the acute phase has passed, a complete and thorough examination is possible and a correct diagnosis can be made.

Injury to a *meniscus* is all too often seen in sport. During flexion-extension, the meniscii move with the tibia but when the femur is rotated on the tibia with the knee flexed they move with the femur. Such movement strains the coronary ligaments and the tissue of the meniscii themselves. Hence tearing of a meniscus will occur when there is a strong rotational strain with the knee flexed. This sort of movement occurs in many sports but especially in football. Typically the player feels a click in the joint and sudden agonising pain as he twists the flexed knee. The joint usually gives way and the athlete falls to the ground. When he tries to move his knee he finds that he can bend it but cannot straighten it fully. If he forces it there is a loud click and full extension is restored. For the next few days the knee is painful and swollen and if he twists the joint further it may give way under him and he may fall to the ground once more with the familiar seering pain and the knee locked in flexion again.

The *medial meniscus* is more commonly torn than the lateral as it is attached to the medial collateral ligament of the knee and this restricts its gliding movement somewhat. However, a cyst is not uncommon on the lateral meniscus but extremely rare on the medial. Clinical examination will reveal a degree of synovitis present. Flexion may be full and pain-free but extension will be limited and painful at the extreme. On passive extension there is a classic elastic resistance felt. McMurray's test where rotation is carried out at different levels of flexion is positive. Grinding the meniscii together relaxes the ligaments but causes pain if there is a meniscal injury. Distraction of the joint decompresses the meniscii but puts tension on the ligaments; this causes no pain if the meniscus is damaged but does cause pain if a ligament is injured. It may be possible to replace a small fragment by encouraging extension with the knee under traction but the risk of recurrence must always be taken into account. These patients should be examined by arthroscope.

If there is displacement as well as *rupture* the patient's gait is characteristic. He hops into the surgery with the injured knee flexed, the limb medially rotated and his toes just touching the ground. However much the joint is encouraged to extend there is a persistent springy block felt. No healing of such an injury can occur as the meniscii are devoid of a blood supply and surgery is the treatment of choice.

Other causes of *locking* must be considered. A loose body may be present but is usually demonstrable on X-ray. There is seldom any history of injury and the position of locking usually varies. The patient can usually wiggle the joint free and the locking is only momentary. In adolescents a loose body is usually due to osteochondritis dissecans where a fragment detaches from the femoral condyle. The patient is between the ages of 15 and 20 and there is localised tenderness on one of the femoral condyles. If the knee is flexed to 90° and rotated medially and then gradually straightened, pain is felt which is relieved by lateral rotation. This is known as Wilson's sign. Such fragments need to be removed and osteopathic treatment is only useful during the recuperative period with special emphasis on quadriceps strengthening. Recurrent patellar dislocation may also cause locking. If the patella is pressed laterally with the thumb while flexing the knee slightly, the patient will resist further movement. This is known as the 'apprehension test' and is virtually diagnostic of recurrent patellar dislocation. This condition may be resolved by strengthening the quadriceps muscle especially the vastus medialis. It occurs more frequently in women—

see section 2.4. The last condition which may cause locking of the knee is a fracture of the tibial spine but here there is a history of a hyperextension injury and not of a rotational strain. This fracture should show on an X-ray.

In older patients a *loose body* may result from osteoarthritic change within the knee but there will not be a history of an acute rotational strain.

On occasion the patellar pad of fat becomes *inflamed*. This can mimic a meniscal injury but no locking will occur. There is seldom a history of injury but the area may have been subjected to some direct blow. Treatment is usually unnecessary but local ice packs may accelerate healing. The area is tender to touch and there may be some discomfort felt on strong contraction of the quadriceps. A cyst on a meniscus is invariably palpable when the knee is in full extension and visible when the knee is in full flexion. They are often multiple and are thought to be a result of trauma. If they are obstructive, they need surgical treatment.

Chondromalacia patellae is an inflammatory condition of the articular cartilage of the articular surface of the patella. It is due to friction on the articular surface. Friction may be increased if the patellar tracking is at fault. This may be due to uneven strength in the opposing vasti (medialis and lateralis) and the efficiency of these muscles must be checked and corrected if necessary. Exercises should be given to even out muscular action. Valgus or varus deformity of the knee joint will affect the tracking of the patella and should be detected if present. The effect can be reduced by orthotics. Foot deformities may lead to abnormal tibial rotation which will also affect the patella tracking and should be treated osteopathically if present. The condition of 'patella alta' is probably the commonest cause of chondromalacia patellae. The patella rides high on the femur even when the quadriceps muscle is relaxed. This is often due to a hypertonic condition of the muscle and can be treated very successfully by long fibre stretching and strong corrective articulation of the patella. Activities such as running should be avoided until the patella resumes it's correct position in relation to the femur. Local anti-inflammatory treatment such as ice packs will reduce the inflammation. If it is imperative that the athlete competes while suffering from chondromalacia, a horseshoe strapping placed below the inferior border of the patella thus reducing the movement of the patella during relaxation of the quadriceps will enable him to run without pain, but treatment to correct the defect must be carried out as soon as possible or there is a risk that the patellar tendon may become mechanically stretched if this device is relied upon in the long-term.

10.11   **Facet locking**

A facet lock occurs in any joint in the body if there is loss of mobility of the joint within it's normal range. The prime movements of flexion and extension which are ably assisted mechanically by the presence of the meniscii do not become involved in a facet lock situation although some loss of mobility of either movement may result from the several conditions already described. Rotation however, can be involved in facet locking. There may be a loss of either medial or lateral rotation without any other abnormality being present in the knee. The condition is a result of some force being applied to the joint while it is in a certain position other than the easy normal position of rest. In medial rotation it will be possible to carry the joint further into medial rotation, but lateral rotation will be restricted. Conversely in lateral rotation, further lateral rotation may be possible but medial rotation will be limited. A deviation from normal may be seen in the position of the tibia in relation to the femur at rest. When the leg is relaxed, the anterior border of the tibia lies in line with the apex of the patella. If there is a facet lock in medial rotation the anterior border of the tibia will lie medial to the apex of the patella. Lateral rotation is more often seen, when the anterior border of the tibia lies lateral to the apex of the patella. Correction of this facet lock will lead to full, pain-free rotation in the opposite direction. The hamstrings may be involved as it is these muscles which are the rotators of the knee.

It is not rare to find that the lateral shift is deficient in one or other direction, lateral shift being more commonly reduced than medial shift. Again correction of this loss of mobility will render the knee normally mobile.

The fibula head is usually locked posteriorly, probably because the pull of the biceps is in that direction. Correction of this facet lock will render the area mobile. In all these conditions there will be a low degree of inflammation of which the patient may complain but he is more likely to be aware of some limitation of movement especially at the extreme of one or other prime movements of the knee. The fibula head facet lock may be secondary to some ankle injury while a pelvic problem may be involved where there is loss of the lateral shift.

10.12   **Mobility injury**

Stiffness of the knee joint is frequently associated with shortening or tightness of the hamstring muscles where there may be some loss of flexibility and a history of recurrent problems. Degenerative changes occur fairly commonly in the knee joint as it is a joint which is subjected to tremendous stresses during life. Any sport which stresses the knee will help to precipitate such changes which may well be evident by the age of 40.

Hypermobility is seen, especially where there has been damage to a ligament. The medial collateral ligament may be stretched leading to instability on medial shift and valgus strain, while chronic stretch of the cruciate ligaments will lead to hypermobility in the A–P shift. These joints are best treated with exercises to strengthen the quadriceps and a brace for physical activity to support the weak joint and reduce the probability of further damage.

10.13   **Bursitis**

There is a large number of bursae around the knee joint, any one or more of which may become inflamed either from a direct injury, repeated minor traumata or by virtue of it communicating with the synovial space. The patient who has a bursitis will complain of pain at the site of the bursa which is made worse when it is pressurised. There will be palpable swelling which will be well defined and sensitive to deep pressure. The condition will usually resolve if pressure is kept off it, either by protecting the bursa from direct pressure (for example, no kneeling should be allowed) or by restricting muscle activity if the bursa is one placed under a tendon. Ice packs also help the swelling to go down but if the condition becomes chronic, aspiration or even excision may be necessary. Infiltration will sometimes reduce the bursitis. The details of the peri-articular bursae is given in section 10.1. A Baker's cyst is a protrusion from the synovial joint, posteriorly into the popliteal fossa. These cysts seldom give symptoms unless they are large enough to limit movement. Infiltration is the treatment of choice. See Fig. 10.10.

10.14   **Blood vessel injury**

The main arteries around the knee joint are well protected but veins in the area are superficial. Varicosities are commonly seen, even in young athletes. They are commoner in women than men and seem to be familial in their occurrence. Injury to a varicosity can be extremely serious. If bleeding occurs a pressure pad should be applied and the leg elevated and the patient despatched to hospital immediately. Keen sportsmen who are seen in practice and who have varicosities which are a potential hazard, should be advised to have surgical treatment. Varicose veins can be damaged by sharp objects, falls and blows, for example from a hard ball. Varicose eczema is a complication of varicose veins.

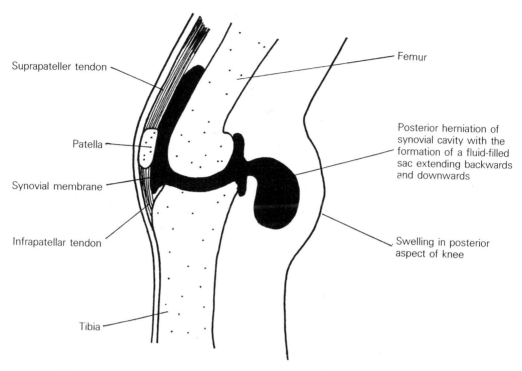

Suprapateller tendon

Patella

Synovial membrane

Infrapatellar tendon

Tibia

Femur

Posterior herniation of synovial cavity with the formation of a fluid-filled sac extending backwards and downwards

Swelling in posterior aspect of knee

Fig. 10.10   Baker's cyst.

10.15

Nerve injury

The lateral popliteal nerve curves around the neck of the fibula where it is liable to direct injury, for example from a blow or as a complication of fracture of this part of the fibula. Mild damage will result in minor symptoms and recovery will be fairly swift. More severe damage can lead to foot drop, loss of sensation over the front and lateral half of the leg and the dorsum of the foot and toes and possible wasting of the peroneal muscles. Recovery takes some months.

10.16

Skin injuries

Grazes around the knee joint are extremely common in athletes. They should be cleaned and dressed with sterile dressings. Cuts are also often seen and may need stitching. Friction burns may occur, especially in runners or footballers on synthetic surfaces. First aid treatment is necessary and referral, if severe injury has occurred.

10.17

Referred pain

Pain may be referred to the knee area from the hip joint, from the sacro-iliac joint and from the lumbar spine. If the pain originates in the hip joint, no abnormality will be found in the knee joint on examination and the hip must be suspected as the cause of pain.

Pain from the sacro-iliac joint is usually felt on the anterior aspect of the thigh and medial aspect of the knee and upper part of the shaft of the tibia (at the insertion of sartorius, gracilis and semitendinosus). The symptoms will be exacerbated by pelvic movement and the knee will be normal on examination. However, there may be a sensitive area at or near the muscular insertions. If the pain is referred from the lumbar spine there will probably be a history of low back pain and/or injury. There may be a reflex change. Examination of the lumbar spine should reveal the source of pain. Treatment to the area of origin of the pain will relieve the symptoms. Treatment may, therefore, have to be aimed and the hip, pelvis and lumbar spine, to both the joints and the soft tissues. Osteopathic treatment is always applied to a widespread area and seldom isolated solely to the apparent site of symptoms.

Chapter 11   The Lower Leg

Anatomical review

Two parallel bones make up the skeletal element of the lower leg. Medially lies the tibia which is much stronger than the fibula which lies laterally. Weight is transmitted through the tibia.

Above and below are joints between the two bones (see Fig. 11.1) The *superior tibiofibular joint* has been dealt with in the Chapter 10. The movement which occurs at this joint is passive and consists of a degree of gliding in the A–P plane. It is a plane synovial joint which has a capsule which is strengthened anteriorly and posteriorly by the anterior and posterior ligaments respectively.

The *inferior tibiofibular joint* is a syndesmosis − that is, a joint in which the opposed bony surfaces are connected by an interosseous membrane. Strong ligaments reinforce the joint anteriorly, posteriorly and inferiorly. The interosseous ligament is continuous with the crural interosseous membrane and consists of many short, strong bands which pass between the adjacent rough surfaces of the bones constituting the chief bond between them. There is a little 'give' between the bones and a small range of passive movement in the A–P plane.

A third joint exists between the tibia and the fibula, namely a *fibrous joint*. The interosseous borders of the two bones are connected by the crural interosseous membrane. This separates the muscles on the front from those on the back of the leg. This membrane consists of fibres which pass obliquely downward and laterally and is continuous inferiorly with the interosseous ligament of the inferior tibiofibular joint. Two openings in the membrane exist; the anterior tibial artery passes to the front of the leg through a large oval opening in the uppermost part of the membrane and the perforating branch of the peroneal artery pierces it inferiorly.

All three joints are only slightly extensible, so that during dorsiflexion of the ankle, slight displacement of the fibula from the tibia is possible. If the movement is reduced, additional stress is placed on the bones, increasing the probability of injury especially during dorsiflexion of the ankle.

Anteriorly there are four muscles (see Fig. 11.2). *Tibialis anterior* lies on the lateral aspect of the tibia. It is a thick fleshy muscle above arising from the upper two-thirds of the lateral surface of the tibia and the adjoining surface of the interosseous membrane. The fibres run downward and end in a tendon which is obvious on

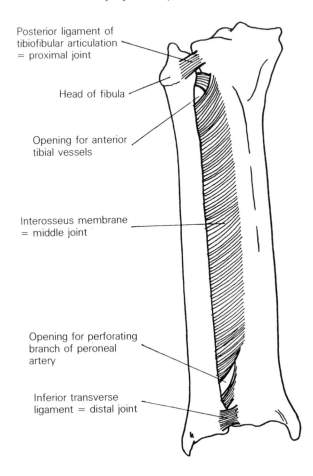

Posterior ligament of
tibiofibular articulation
= proximal joint

Head of fibula

Opening for anterior
tibial vessels

Interosseus membrane
= middle joint

Opening for perforating
branch of peroneal
artery

Inferior transverse
ligament = distal joint

Fig. 11.1 The
tibiofibular
articulations.

the anterior surface of the muscle in the lower one-third of the leg.
The tendon passes through the medial compartment of the superior
and inferior retinacula where it is surrounded by a synovial sheath.
It then passes medially and is inserted into the medial cuneiform
bone and the base of the first metatarsal bone. In the upper part of
the leg the muscle overlaps the anterior tibial vessels and nerve.
There is a bursa between the tendon and the medial cuneiform
bone. Action of this muscle is threefold. When the foot is on the
ground and weight bearing, the muscle raises the longitudinal arch
of the foot and is therefore important in the maintenance of this
arch. When the foot is off the ground the muscle acts as a dorsiflexor of the ankle joint. Thirdly, it acts to draw the leg forward at
the ankle joint thus helping to stabilise posture if there is a
tendency to overbalance backwards. It's nerve supply consists of
the deep peroneal nerve, L4 and L5 (see Fig. 11.2(a)).

Extensor hallucis longus lies between the tibialis anterior and
extensor digitorum longus and is partly hidden by them. It arises
from the medial surface of the fibula in its middle one-half and

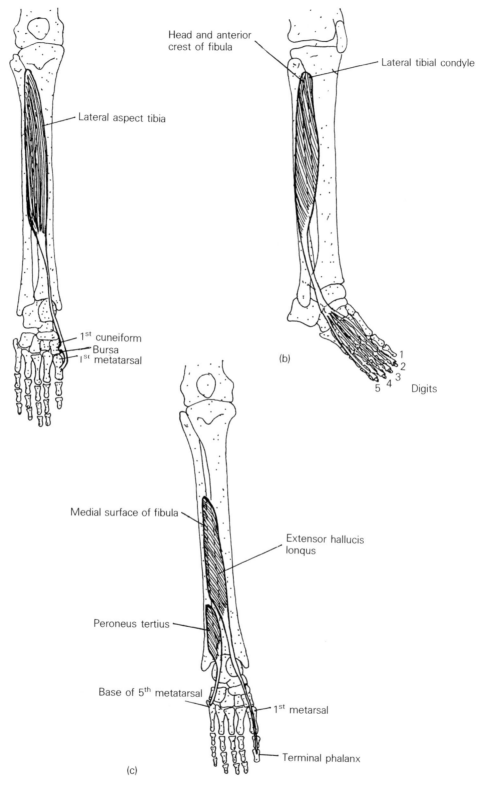

(a)

(b)

(c)

Head and anterior crest of fibula

Lateral tibial condyle

Lateral aspect tibia

1st cuneiform
Bursa
1st metatarsal

1
2
3
4
5 Digits

Medial surface of fibula

Extensor hallucis longus

Peroneus tertius

Base of 5th metatarsal

1st metarsal

Terminal phalanx

Fig. 11.2 (a) Tibialis anterior; (b) extensor digitorum longus; (c) extensor hallucis longus and peroneus tertius.

from the adjacent surface of the interosseous membrane. It forms a tendon which lies in a synovial sheath and passes below the retinacula of the ankle, lies along the first metatarsal and is inserted into the distal phalanx of the great toe. Its action is to extend the hallux and it also acts like tibialis anterior as a stabiliser of the leg. It's nerve supply consists of the deep peroneal nerve L4, L5 and S1. The anterior tibial nerve and vessels lie between this muscle and the tibialis anterior (see Fig. 11.2(c)).

Extensor digitorum longus lies in the lateral part of the front of the leg. It arises from the lateral condyle of the tibia, the upper three-quarters of the shaft of the fibula and the adjacent part of the interosseous membrane and forms a tendon in the lower one-third of the leg. This tendon divides into four parts which have a common synovial sheath as they pass under the retinacula lateral to the tendon of tibialis anterior. The tendons pass over the dorsum of the foot and are inserted into the base of the middle and distal phalanges of the dorsal surface (similar to the extensors of the fingers, see section 8.2). (See Fig. 11.2(b).)

Peroneus tertius is an additional tendon of the extensor digitorum longus which extends to the base of the fifth (and sometimes also the fourth) metatarsal. It is not always present but is considered to be a developing muscle in man. It assists in eversion which will reduce the risk of inversion strains if sufficiently strong. The nerve supply to extensor digitorum longus and peroneus tertius consists of the deep peroneal nerve, L5 and S1 (see Fig. 11.2(c)).

Laterally there are two muscles in the leg (see Fig. 11.3). *Peroneus longus* arises from the head and the upper two-thirds of the lateral surface of the shaft of the fibula and from the anterior and posterior surfaces of the intermuscular septum. Between the fibres of origin from the head and shaft of the fibula there is a gap through which the lateral popliteal nerve passes. The fibres pass vertically down-wards and end in a tendon which runs behind the lateral malleolus with the tendon of peroneus brevis, in a common synovial sheath. The tendons lie in a groove behind the lateral malleolus which is converted into a tunnel by the superior peroneal retinaculum. The tendon then passes forwards under the peroneal tubercle of the calcaneum covered there by the inferior peroneal retinaculum. It then crosses the lateral side of the cuboid bone in a groove which is converted into a canal by the long plantar ligament of the foot, crosses the sole of the foot obliquely and is finally inserted into the lateral side of the first metatarsal and the lateral side of the medial cuneiform bones. Below the lateral malleolus, the tendon is protected by a sesamoid fibrocartilage (sometimes bone). Within the canal on the sole of the foot the tendons are situated within another synovial sheath. The nerve supply consists of the superficial peroneal nerve, L5 and S1 (see Fig. 11.3(a)).

Peroneus brevis arises from the lower two-thirds of the lateral

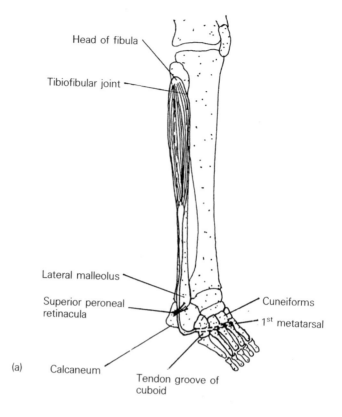

(a)

Head of fibula

Tibiofibular joint

Lateral malleolus

Superior peroneal retinacula

Calcaneum

Cuneiforms

1st metatarsal

Tendon groove of cuboid

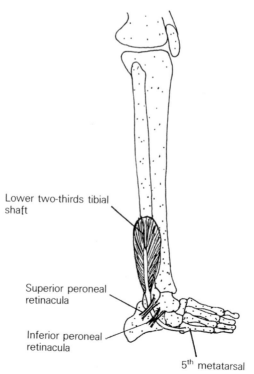

Lower two-thirds tibial shaft

Superior peroneal retinacula

Inferior peroneal retinacula

5th metatarsal

Fig. 11.3 (a) Peroneus longus; (b) peroneus brevis.

(b)

surface of the shaft of the tibia in front of peroneus longus. The tendon runs with that of peroneus longus and in front of that tendon but it passes above the peroneal tubercle of the calcaneum (peroneus longus lies below the tubercle) and is finally inserted into the tubercle on the base of the fifth metatarsal on its lateral side. It's nerve supply consists of the superficial peroneal nerve, L5 and S1 (see Fig. 11.3(b)).

The peroneal muscles both act as everters of the foot when the foot is off the ground. When weight bearing they act as muscles which brace the transverse arch of the foot. When standing on one leg only, the muscles help to steady the leg on the foot, for in this position there is a tendency for the body weight to throw the leg medially.

Posteriorly the muscles of the leg are divided into a superficial and a deep group (see Fig. 11.4). The superficial muscles are gastrocnemius, soleus and plantaris. *Gastrocnemius* forms the bulk of the calf. It arises by two tendons, one from each condyle of the femur. Under the medial head there is a bursa and under the lateral head there is a fibrocartilagenous sesamoid. Approximately halfway down the calf, the fibres of this muscle blend with those of the soleus muscle on its deep surface and the two muscles are inserted into the calcaneum on the posterior surface by the *tendo calcaneus*.

The nerve supply consists of the medial popliteal nerve, S1 and S2.

Soleus arises from the head and the upper one-quarter of the posterior aspect of the shaft of the fibula, from the soleal line and the middle one-third of the medial border of the tibia and from the fibrous band which arches over the popliteal vessels and medial popliteal nerve. The fibres end in a tendon which blends with that of gastrocnemius to form the tendo calcaneus. The nerve supply consists of the medial popliteal nerve, S1 and S2 and the posterior tibial nerve, L5 and S1.

The *tendo calcaneus* is the thickest and strongest tendon in the body. It begins at the middle of the leg and receives fleshy fibres from the soleus muscle from there down to its lower end and from gastrocnemius on its posterior surface. Together with *plantaris* (see section 10.1) this mechanism is known as the *triceps surae*. Its action is to lift the weight of the body both in standing and walking and provides the propelling force in most sports. The tremendous strength of these superficial muscles of the calf is directly related to the upright posture in man. The tendo calcaneus is inserted into the posterior aspect of the calcaneum and separated from the bone by a bursa. There is no synovial sheath.

There are four deep muscles (see Figs. 11.5 and 11.6). *Popliteus* forms the floor of the lower part of the popliteal fossa, see section 10.1.

Tibialis posterior arises from the upper two-thirds of the lateral

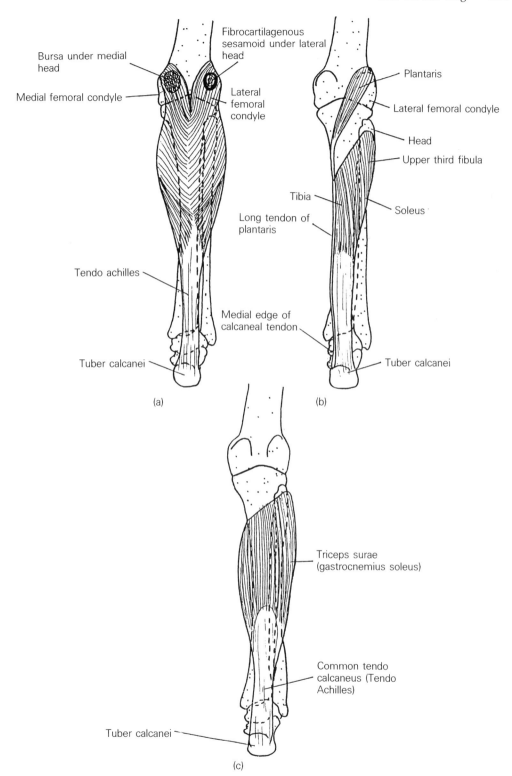

Fig. 11.4 (a) Gastrocnemius; (b) plantaris and soleus; (c) triceps surae.

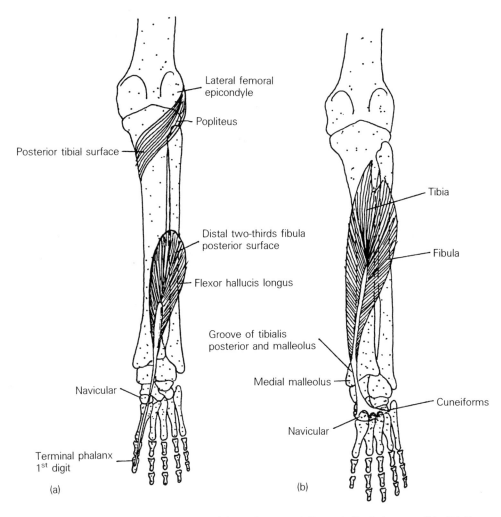

Lateral femoral
epicondyle

Popliteus

Posterior tibial surface

Distal two-thirds fibula
posterior surface

Flexor hallucis longus

Groove of tibialis
posterior and malleolus

Medial malleolus

Navicular

Terminal phalanx
1ˢᵗ digit

(a)

Tibia

Fibula

Cuneiforms

Navicular

(b)

Fig. 11.5   Posterior aspect (a) popliteus and flexor hallucis longus; (b) tibialis posterior.

portion of the posterior surface of the shaft of the tibia, the upper two-thirds of the medial part of the shaft of the fibula and from the intervening interosseous membrane. It is the deepest of the posterior muscles of the leg. The tendon passes in a groove behind the medial malleolus, deep to the tendon of flexor digitorum longus where it is enclosed in its own synovial sheath. It then passes behind the flexor retinaculum and superficial to the deltoid ligament of the ankle joint, then below the plantar calcaneonavicular ligament from which it is protected by a fibrocartilagenous sesamoid. It is inserted into the tuberosity of the navicular bone. Slips also pass to the sustentaculum tali (on the calcaneum) and to the three cuneiform bones, the bases of the second, third, fourth and sometimes fifth metatarsals. The nerve supply consists of the posterior tibial nerve,

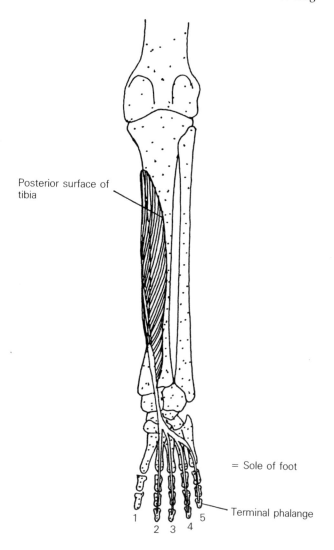

Posterior surface of tibia

= Sole of foot

Fig. 11.6 Flexor digitorum longus, posterior aspect.

Terminal phalange

1 2 3 4 5

L4 and L5. In the non-weight bearing leg, tibialis posterior acts as a plantar flexor and supinator of the foot. In the weight bearing leg it acts as a stabiliser, approximating the heel to the calf of the leg. Occasionally this muscle is absent, when there is likely to be a loss of normal stability of the leg especially when weight bearing (see Fig. 11.5(b)).

Flexor hallucis longus arises from the distal two-thirds of the posterior surface of the fibula, the adjacent interosseous membrane and the intermuscular septum, overlapping tibialis posterior. It terminates in a tendon which occupies nearly the whole length of the posterior surface of the muscle. It lies in a groove which crosses the lower end of the tibia, posteriorly, the posterior surface of the talus and the under surface of the sustentaculum tali of the calcaneum where it is invested in a synovial sheath. It passes beneath the flexor retinaculum to the sole of the foot and is inserted into the base of the distal phalanx of the great toe on the inferior surface. Distal to the sustentaculum tali this tendon is crossed superficially by the tendon of flexor digitorum longus. It's nerve supply consists of the posterior tibial nerve, L5, S1 and S2. The muscle flexes the great toe but it is important as it supports the longitudinal arch of the foot and will therefore help prevent the development of pes planus (see Fig. 11.5(a)).

Flexor digitorum longus lies on the tibial side of the leg (see Fig. 11.6). It arises from the posterior surface of the shaft of the tibia from just below the soleal line to within 10 cm of the lower end of the bone. The fibres end in a tendon which runs nearly the whole length of the posterior surface of the muscle. This tendon crosses the posterior tibialis tendon and passes behind the medial malleolus in a groove common to it and the tibialis posterior but separated from it by a fibrous septum. Each tendon lies within its own synovial sheath. Having passed into the sole of the foot, it crosses superficial to the tendon of flexor hallucis longus and divides into four separate tendons, one to be inserted into the distal phalanx of each of the four lateral toes. At the level of the middle phalanx these tendons penetrate the tendons of the flexor digitorum brevis. The nerve supply consists of the posterior tibial nerve, L5, S1 and S2. In the non-weight bearing leg, the muscle flexes the toes. In the weight bearing leg it acts to support the longitudinal arch of the foot.

Between the superficial and deep muscles of the posterior aspect of the leg lie the posterior tibial vessels and nerve which can be compressed by hypertonic conditions of these muscles.

11.2   Muscle injuries

The *dorsiflexor* muscles may be subject to direct injury, for example a blow on the front of the leg. There will be a history of such injury, and swelling and possible bruising will be evident. The initial treatment is ice, compression and elevation, followed the next day by soft tissue treatment as soon as possible and active stretching by the patient and gentle but increasing use of the muscle, to the point of discomfort but never to the point of pain. Ice packs should be continued until the swelling has completely subsided. The normal activity may not be resumed until resisted movement and passive stretching are no longer painful.

Pain which originates in these muscles is elicited by testing active and resisted dorsiflexion of the ankle, hallux and toes. Weakness will be elicited commonly in lumbar disc lesions, lower motor neuron conditions such as poliomyelitis and possibly as an early sign of an upper motor neuron lesion all of which could present in an athlete.

The *tibialis anterior* is subject to myosynovitis when there is pain felt above the front of the ankle on use of the muscle. The tendon is unaffected and is not sensitive to palpation. However the fibres of the muscle are sensitive, usually at the junction of the middle and lower one-third of the tibia and occasionally crepitus can be elicited at that point. The condition seems to develop in sports which involve the use of stiff boots, especially skiing, but is also seen in runners and in those who have been skipping or jumping repetitively.

The *extensor hallucis longus* may develop ischaemis contracture following a fracture of the tibia at its midpoint. In such a case each time the foot is plantarflexed, the big toe extends. It will then be forced against the upper of the shoe and become sore and discoloured.

In cases of *pes planus* there is shortening of the dorsiflexor muscles and eventually this will result in clawing of the toes and possible irritation of the extensor tendons by shoe pressure.

Shin splints is a condition of these muscles which is considered to be a form of cramp. When an athlete runs, especially on hard surfaces and if he has not done so for a while, the muscles fatigue and build up an oxygen debt when they may accumulate large amounts of lactic acid. At a certain point the muscle fibres go into spasm, the area involved being generally small but the problem is recurrent with use of the muscle. Examination will reveal pain on resisted movement and there will be one or more areas of hypertonia and sensitivity. The hypertonic state pressurises the veins thus further engorging the muscle fibres, so relaxation of the area is essential. Treatment to relax the fibres is effective.

Shin splints may also affect the periosteum or even the bone structure, see section 11.5. Symptoms resembling intermittent claudication occur in the dorsiflexor muscles, resulting from a tightness in the fascial compartment of these muscles. In minor cases the athlete will say that after walking possibly for about a mile, he finds difficulty in actively dorsiflexing his foot but experiences no pain. After a short rest the muscle recovers. In severe cases the athlete complains of pain at the front of the mid leg after exertion. Oedema and redness are seen over the lesioned part of the tibialis muscle. This may respond to soft tissue treatment but if it does not, the fascial sheath has to be divided or ischaemic necrosis may result and the efficiency of the muscle may be permanently impaired. Mild cases respond well to soft tissue treatment. Older patients may have a thrombus or even an embolus in the anterior tibial artery which can produce similar symptoms but in such a case the arterial pulse will be defective and there may be swelling of the limb below the arterial problem. This will require expert treatment and should be referred if there appears to be a possibility of such a case presenting.

Anterior skin splints are characterised by pain, tenderness, and tightness along the distal one-third of the medial aspect of the tibia and along its lateral border. Sprinting, uphill running, stiff footwear and hard surfaces are causative factors. Most cases occur when unaccustomed activity is undertaken but some cases seem to develop from overuse. Pain on resisted dorsiflexion is always present and the condition is invariably recurrent before the athlete seeks advice.

Bone scans of the area are helpful in the differential diagnosis of shin splints, compartment syndrome (fascial sheath tightness) and fracture. Shin splints will probably appear normal on a scan, compartment syndromes will show increased uptake but not as much as will be seen in the case of a fracture. These require expert interpretation. Where the conditions respond to soft tissue treatment the mechanical efficiency of all the surrounding joints must be fully checked for complete mobility before the athlete is allowed to return to normal activity. This must include examination and treatment if necessary, of any pelvic and lumbar spine condition.

The *peroneal* muscles are not often injured within the muscle belly. Any injury is more likely to affect the tendons − see section 11.3. However, there may be trauma to the muscles in cases of severe inversion strains of the ankle joint when the peronei may be stretched and thus traumatised. If the muscles are damaged, there will be pain localised to the injured area and there will be a palpable area of tenderness at the site of injury. Resisted eversion of the foot will also cause pain and passive stretching of the muscles may cause pain too. In each case the pain will be localised to the area of injury. As with other muscle fibre injuries the treatment is deep soft tissue treatment and in this case, as the muscles are long and thin, the treatment is more effective if given along the length of the muscle rather than cross fibre. The fascial sheath of the peronei is sometimes irritated, invariably in cases of overuse. If severe, the common peroneal nerve may be compressed, leading to weakness or even paralysis of dorsiflexion of the foot. Surgical release is the treatment of choice. Before normal activity can be resumed the mechanical integrity of both the superior and inferior tibiofibular joints together with the joints of the foot and leg, must be checked. There may well be some contributory mechanical dysfunction in the pelvis and lumbar spine which must be treated if necessary.

Injury to the *triceps surae* is common. One of the basic problems of design is that muscle fibres of gastrocnemius and soleus blend together in the mid calf and this is the commonest site of injury. In general, anywhere where fibres blend is weaker than where fibres are continuous. Typically the patient will complain of pain in the calf which will have come on suddenly as he made a sudden movement. He may well report that he thought something had hit him in the calf and he looked round to see what it was. He will present walking on tiptoe on the affected side. When asked to stand on tiptoe the pain is worse. Resisted plantarflexion causes pain and there will be an area of sensitivity and swelling in the calf. There may be local bruising. With the patient prone, resisted plantarflexion is tested first with the knee fully extended and then with the knee flexed to a right angle. Bending the knee relaxes the femoral extremity of the gastrocnemius muscle but does not alter the strain on soleus. Hence abolition of pain caused by resisted plantarflexion when the knee is flexed, incriminates the gastrocnemius muscle. If both are painful, then the injury has occurred to both gastrocnemius and soleus. This condition is sometimes called 'tennis leg' as it is common in tennis players who make sudden movements when playing. As the injured fibres are in spasm the muscle is shortened as a whole. A raised heel will help to relieve the need for the athlete to stretch the injured fibres, or the area may be strapped from below the heel to just above the torn area thus supporting the muscle. Never strap around the limb as this will impede venous drainage. On the day of injury the leg should be rested, elevated and ice packs applied. The patient should be encouraged to gently keep the ankle plantar- and dorsi-flexed to the point of discomfort but not to the point of pain. The following day deep soft tissue treatment can be started and continued until healing has occurred. Muscle tears are more likely to occur in this area if the muscles are inherently short — i.e. if they have not been sufficiently stretched before use. In cold weather when the legs are not covered by clothing the circulation is reduced superficially and injury is more likely. So, prevention will include thorough stretching, adequate clothing in cold weather and as a further protection the area should be well rubbed with a rubifacient such as Tiger balm before use, especially for a while after the injury. With adequate treatment the athlete should return to his sport in about two weeks. Without, the injury may last several weeks or even months. In chronic cases there will be a palpable area of scar tissue which should be broken down by deep soft tissue treatment and ultrasound. Where there is a palpable gap within the muscle, any exercise on tiptoe while weight bearing should be avoided for about a month, or until the gap is no longer palpable.

The invertors of the foot are the *tibiales anterior* and *posterior*, so if there is pain on resisted inversion, one or other of these is at fault. If dorsiflexion is also painful, the tibialis anterior is at fault; conversely if inversion is painful and dorsiflexion is not, then tibialis posterior is at fault.

Injury within the *flexor hallucis longus* and the *flexor digitorum longus* occurs less frequently. If involved, either resisted flexion of the great toe or one or other of the lateral toes will cause pain and the area of injury is palpable in the leg. Soft tissue treatment is indicated and full recovery should be achieved before the athlete is allowed to resume normal activity.

11.3   Tendon injury

There are many tendons around the lower leg area, all of them part of a muscle which produces movement in a weight bearing part of the body. Hence injury of a tendon here is common. The tendo calcaneus or tendo Achilles is the most commonly injured.

Tendinitis is an inflammatory condition which may result from overuse or from direct injury, possibly from ill-fitting footwear or from a direct blow. The history may be helpful, therefore. The patient complains of pain in the area of the problem in all cases. The pain will be made worse by active and resisted plantarflexion and by passive dorsiflexion when the tendon is stretched. There will be an area of palpable tenderness and possible swelling but this is not always very apparent especially in chronic cases. The symptoms will probably have come on after some unaccustomed activity possibly barefoot (when the tendon will have been stretched more than is usual). Standing on tiptoe also exacerbates the symptoms. Tendinitis may occur on either the posterior or anterior aspect of the tendon, the latter being far more common then the former, so careful palpation is essential. Fibres of the tendon are usually involved on either or both sides and some visible swelling may be seen on the affected side of the tendon. A soft tissue X-ray may reveal some discontinuity of the tendon but not always. Where there is discontinuity of the fibres the prognosis is not as good as where this is not so, as in the former cases there seems to be an increased likelihood of recurrence. The condition responds well to deep friction given transversely so it is of prime importance to locate the problem accurately and give the treatment exactly where it is needed, particular emphasis being required in the diagnosis of the anterior tendinitis. If the acute case is not treated correctly it may well become chronic with resultant thickening of the tendon and resultant loss of elasticity, predisposing it to further injury. It is thought that infiltration of the tendon also predisposes to further trouble and many athletes refuse such treatment.

Rupture of the tendo Achilles may be complete or partial (see Fig. 11.7). Total rupture occurs with some sudden movement where the tendon is suddenly stretched. The patient will say that at the time he experienced sudden pain and his foot gave way and he could not continue playing. Plantarflexion is not lost as the other flexor muscles are still intact but it is extremely weak as will be seen when resisted plantarflexion is tested. If the rupture is complete, the foot will not plantarflex when the belly of gastrocnemius is firmly squeezed in the calf. The defect in the tendon is easy to palpate and is usually located about the middle of the tendon.

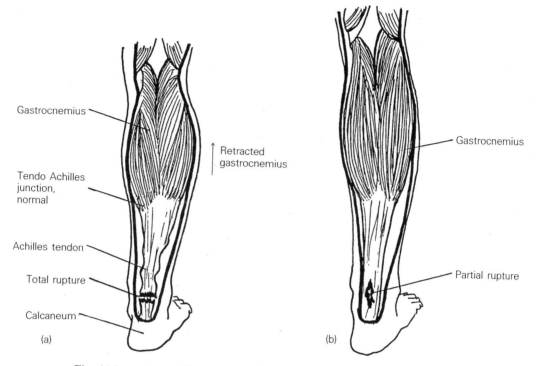

Gastrocnemius

Retracted gastrocnemius

Tendo Achilles junction, normal

Achilles tendon

Total rupture

Calcaneum

(a)

Gastrocnemius

Partial rupture

(b)

Fig. 11.7   The achilles tendon. (a) A total rupture; (b) a partial rupture.

Surgical repair is the treatment of choice in complete rupture cases and should be done before contracture of the calf muscle occurs – i.e. as soon as possible and at the longest within a few days of injury. The result is then better. Postoperatively the patient is not allowed to rise on tiptoe for several weeks. Partial rupture will repair if the foot is strapped or plastered in plantarflexion, the treatment depending on the degree of injury. During the repair period the heel will need to be raised, possibly with a surgical lift. Following repair, osteopathic treatment will be needed to mobilise the joints which will have been kept immobile and to stretch and strengthen all the surrounding muscles which will have been shortened and weakened. Repair takes at least eight weeks. The patient is likely to be aged 40 or more.

The *peroneal* muscles are subject to problems within the tendons. The patient will complain of pain at the site of injury and swelling may be present and palpable. Active eversion will cause pain and passive inversion may also. Resisted eversion is painful too. The site of tendinitis may be anywhere along the course of the tendons – i.e. anywhere between the lower part of the fibula to the cuboid and base of the fifth metatarsal bone. This condition is a common complication of a sprained ankle and may be persistent. It responds well to soft tissue treatment especially if given transversely and supporting strapping to minimise eversion helps during the recovery phase. The peroneal tendons may loosen within their groove on the posterior surface of the fibula and slip forward over the lateral malleolus, causing what is known as a 'snapping ankle'. Seldom does this cause pain or disability but may give concern to the athlete who will say 'it feels odd'. The tendons slip back behind the malleolus when the foot is plantarflexed. If the condition causes weakness and/or disability, surgical intervention is necessary. Post-operative osteopathic treatment to assist rehabilitation of the surrounding joints and strengthening of the peronei is helpful to the athlete who should be able to resume full training. The peroneal tendons are subject to ganglion formation. Ganglia, generally are not rare around the ankle. Some can be dispersed by deep pressure or by infiltration but some are resistant to these measures and will require surgical removal. It should be remembered that some ganglia disappear as quickly as they came without any treatment.

Tenosynovitis is common around the ankle joint as there are many tendon sheaths in the area (see Figs. 11.8 and 11.9). The patient will complain of pain at the site of the problem which is made worse when the muscle concerned is actively used. There will be thickening at the site of injury and crepitus will be palpable on movement of the muscle. The principle of treatment is to restore friction-free movement between the tendon and it's sheath. Some cases respond well to deep soft tissue treatment. Some respond

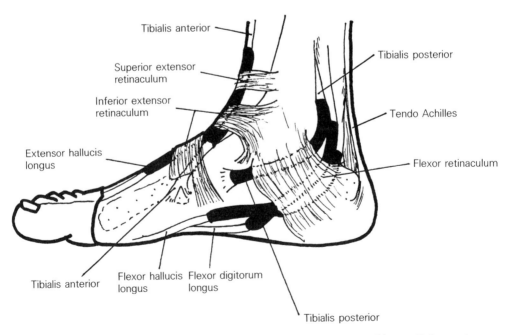

Fig. 11.8   Synovial sheaths of the tendons at the right ankle, medial aspect.

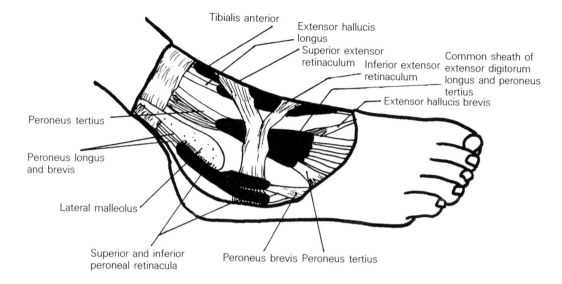

Tibialis anterior
Extensor hallucis longus
Superior extensor retinaculum
Inferior extensor retinaculum
Common sheath of extensor digitorum longus and peroneus tertius
Extensor hallucis brevis
Peroneus tertius
Peroneus longus and brevis
Lateral malleolus
Superior and inferior peroneal retinacula
Peroneus brevis   Peroneus tertius

Fig. 11.9   Synovial sheaths of the tendons at the right ankle, lateral aspect.

to immobilisation, for example by strapping, to minimise active movement of the affected muscle, but some require infiltration between the tendon and it's sheath. If all these measures fail to relieve the condition, the tendon sheath has to be surgically opened. Until recovery has taken place, all activities which cause pain have to be avoided; exercises, therefore are contraindicated.

Between the tendo Achilles and it's point of insertion into the calcaneum lies a bursa which may become inflamed (see Fig. 5.22). It is usually caused by shoe pressure and is seen most often in athletes who have high arched feet when the calcaneum is particularly prominent. Others who are more likely to suffer are those who have a very narrow heel as the movement which causes the condition is one of side to side movement of the calcaneum inside the shoe. Initially, there is probably an area of redness or blister formation at the back of the heel but after sufficient friction the bursa itself becomes inflamed. The athlete will complain of pain in the back of the heel. Differentiation from the diagnosis of tendinitis is made by the fact that the athlete with bursitis can run, jump and hop barefoot, without pain, whereas if he had a tendinitis the pain would be similar with and without shoes. The bursa is usually palpable and will be painful if squeezed, deep to the tendon. To be sure that the pain is not caused by the presence of an os trigonum, which may have become inflamed, an X-ray should be taken to exclude the presence of one. Treatment is to rest the inflamed bursa and prevent further shoe pressure. Infiltration is often helpful. Correct shoes must be advised if the condition is not to recur.

A bursitis may also occur under the medial head of gastrocnemius at it's origin. If present, the athlete will complain of pain at that site on use of the muscle − i.e. plantarflexion. Palpation deep to the medial head of the muscle will reveal the enlarged and painful bursa; again, rest and possible infiltration will resolve the problem.

11.4

Musculotendinous injury

These are not as common around the ankle as one might expect. Most injuries seem to occur within the tendon rather than the musculotendinous junction. However, they do occur and are diagnosed by locating the exact site of pain which will be felt on active movement, passive stretch and resisted movement of the muscle concerned. Treatment consists of deep soft tissue treatment, increasing the blood supply by any means, for example by the use of Tiger balm and massage with ice, the latter two by the athlete himself, frequently (at least six times a day). Once healing has taken place the osteopath should decide why the injury occurred in the first place. Any predisposing mechanical faults must be resolved before full activity is resumed.

A wobble board is helpful in the rehabilitation of all muscular, tendinous and musculotendinous injuries around the lower leg and ankle, and advice as to which particular movements needs emphasis will help full recovery to be obtained as quickly as possible.

11.5

Bone injury

Periostitis is a common injury in the leg because there is little protection to the tibia which may well be subjected to direct injury, for example by a kick or being struck by a hard ball. The area will be painful and swollen but there will be no loss of active movement. Treatment consists of the application of an ice pack as soon as possible following the injury to minimise the swelling, and elevation of the limb will be helpful to assist drainage. Seldom is the condition serious and recovery is swift. Active plantarflexion/dorsiflexion will also assist drainage.

Shin splints may well involve the periosteum. This is a condition of the dorsiflexors of the foot especially the tibialis anterior muscle. This muscle arises from the periosteum of the shaft of the tibia in a fleshy form so the periosteal tissue may be involved in cases of increased tension of the muscle. The diagnosis is made by eliciting the exact site of pain; if this is along the shaft of the tibia, then the periosteum is involved. As described in section 11.2, treatment to the muscle is usually effective but it is essential to make certain that there is no abnormal stress placed on the muscle due to immobility or incorrect alignment of the joints on which the muscle acts. The application of ice to the affected area helps to reduce the inflammation. Full use should be avoided until complete recovery has taken place.

In severe cases where the pain is particularly persistent and does not seem to respond readily to treatment, X-rays may reveal small *stress fractures* at the site of pain. In such cases treatment should continue as described but the area must be rested from athletic activity until these fractures are no longer evident. Non-weight bearing activity is advisable, for example swimming, and no activity on hard surfaces is allowed until recovery is complete.

Fractures are fairly commonly seen in this area as a result of sporting activities. Most involve both bones of the leg and are usually due to direct violence. However, a twisting force applied to the foot may cause a spiral fracture here, usually in the midshaft and the tibia may well pierce the skin. The other common cause of a fracture in this area is when one player falls on another across the leg — i.e. an angulation force. The history will reveal the cause and the athlete must receive expert orthopaedic treatment. Following bony union there may be a residual shortening of the limb, and the ankle, foot and knee may have been injured by the damaging force. Osteopathic treatment to all these areas is then necessary to restore full mobility, and exercises have to be prescribed to restore full strength and muscular balance. Where there is residual shortening the athlete may be able to compensate fully for this. In some cases, however, the alteration of weight bearing may affect the spine and/or pelvis and osteopathic treatment aimed at assisting the body to overcome these difficulties is invaluable. Some athletes may require a heel lift to assist them and reduce the apparent shortening. Again it is impossible to predict accurately whether this measure will need to be permanent or temporary and advice to the athlete will depend on how he accomodates to the shortening over a period of time.

Fractures of the *fibula* may occur without bony injury to the tibia. This is a common complication of a sprained ankle or a knee injury. The bone may also be fractured by a direct force when the fracture is usually transverse. There is pain and local tenderness but the athlete can weight-bear and there may be normal movement of both ankle and knee. These fractures resolve without any special treatment but there may well be residual problems in the adjacent joints following the injury which will require osteopathic treatment.

Fracture of the *tibia* alone is seen occasionally in children, following a twisting injury to the leg and is usually of the spiral type so may be missed on X-ray but will be evident after a few days once the callus has started to form. An athlete of any age may have a fracture of the tibia alone following a direct blow such as a kick, so X-rays should be taken to eliminate the possibility of such injury if a severe blow has occurred. These cases require referral for orthopaedic treatment but osteopathic treatment following union is advisable to ensure full mobility of the surrounding joints.

11.6   **Epiphysitis**

This is not a common problem around the lower leg but is often seen in the upper part – see section 10.8. If present, the young athlete will complain of pain in the lower part of the tibia and/or fibula which is made worse following any weight bearing athletic activity, especially on hard ground. As it is an overuse condition of growing bone, rest and any anti-inflammatory treatment such as ice packs is indicated and the patient should be encouraged to reduce weight bearing activity and increase non-weight bearing activity such as swimming, which will not aggravate the condition. At the worst, the condition will resolve when growth is complete.

11.7   **Mobility injury**

Stiffness of the muscles of the leg is a common complaint of athletes. It is invariably due to insufficient warming down following athletic activity, when there is insufficient removal of the products of muscular activity, see section 3.2. The patient will complain of pain in the affected muscle which is made worse by use and will feel stiff when placed on full stretch. The condition responds well to soft tissue treatment and full recovery should be achieved before full activity is resumed. To prevent recurrence, the athlete should be advised on a warm down programme and made to realise the importance of doing this regularly following activity.

Cramp also occurs frequently, especially in the plantarflexors but may occur in the dorsiflexor muscles. It is a condition where the muscle goes into a state of involuntary contraction and can be very painful. The precipitating factor may be fatigue of the muscle during use, for example during extended running but there seems to be an underlying factor, namely reduced circulation to the muscle. In the case of the plantarflexor muscles, the arterial supply is via the posterior popliteal artery which lies between soleus and tibialis posterior together with the posterior popliteal vein. Any hypertonic state of these muscles can therefore cause direct pressure on the vessels and this may well be a contributory factor in many cases. If this is so, the circulation can be improved by relaxing the muscle fibres and this can be done by osteopathic treatment. Stretching of the muscle is also useful. Cramp can also be caused by hyperventilation (not uncommon in some runners) or by salt deprivation which is likely to occur where excessive perspiration, for example in hot climates when the athlete is not accustomed to heat, is produced. An increased salt intake in such conditions will resolve the problem. Some cases seem to be associated with a past attack of nerve root problems especially of the sciatic nerve. All cases therefore should be examined not only locally but in the spine too, and any osteopathic faults rectified.

11.8   **Blood vessel injury**

Direct injury to blood vessels may occur as a complication of fracture. In such cases bleeding must be stopped by pressure application while the patient is awaiting transfer to hospital. Claudication is sometimes seen in osteopathic practice in older athletes. The patient will complain that he has pain in the plantarflexors after a certain amount of activity, for example he may say that he is alright up to a certain green on the golf course but the pain comes on at the next. The patient is invariably an older man (seldom a woman). The pain is relieved by rest after which he is able to walk the same distance again before the pain recurs. On examination all movements are normal and pain-free, but if the patient is asked to plantarflex and dorsiflex his foot quickly, the familiar pain comes on. This is a circulatory disorder and usually requires medical treatment although relaxing the muscle fibres concerned may help at least temporarily. The condition is particularly prevalent in the gastrocnemius due to the fact that the arterial supply is via two arteries which follow it's length and do not anastamose (unlike the supply to soleus).

The veins of the leg are subject to great pressure as the venous return is impeded by gravity. The one way flow is maintained by virtue of valves which may break down under pressure causing varicosities to occur. The veins will enlarge and so are more likely to receive direct damage. In such cases the patient will complain of pain along the affected part of the vein and engorgement will be seen. Complications include ulceration and eczema and all cases of varicosity should be advised to have expert treatment preferably before complications result. The pain is made worse when the limb is dependent and immobile, e.g. when standing still.

The possibility of a deep vein *thrombosis* must always be considered. The patient will complain of pain in the affected area, usually in the mid-calf which is not affected by using the limb (unlike an injury to a muscle). There will be some swelling of the limb below the site of the thrombus and there may be some discolouration. Palpation will reveal an area of sensitivity in the viscinity of the thrombus. All active movements will be normal and there will not be additional pain felt on resisted movements. These cases require referral.

Phlebitis is a similar condition where the vein is inflamed but no thrombus has formed. Palpation will reveal tenderness along the affected vessel and there will be considerable pain and swelling. This condition is also serious as it often precedes thrombus formation and any suspicion of its being present must lead to the immediate referral of the patient.

11.9   **Skin injury**

This may occur alone or as a result of a deeper injury, for example a fracture. There will be a history of direct injury. Grazes should be cleaned and dressed but more serious wounds may need stitching and should be referred to hospital. To minimise the possibility of infection all athletes should keep their antitetanus treatment up to date.

Skin conditions as a result of varicosities also need specialist treatment and should be referred for the same.

Chapter 12   The Ankle

12.1   **The inferior tibiofibular joint**

This is dealt with in section 11.1.

12.2   **The tibiotaloid joint**

This joint is the articulation between the lower end of the tibia and the articular surface on the upper part of the talus (see Figs 12.1 and 12.2). The two malleoli are included in the joint and give bony support to the two sides of the joint. The joint is of the hinge type. The articular surface of the talus is concave from side to side and convex from in front backwards and is wider in front than behind. The medial malleolus articulates with the talus on the upper part of it's medial surface and the lateral malleolus articulates with the talus laterally. This mortise formation renders the ankle joint extremely stable which is vital as the talus transmits all the body weight from the leg to the foot.

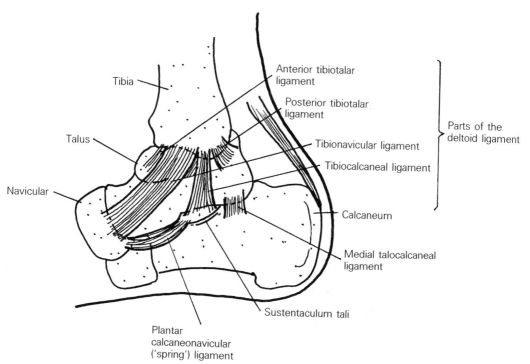

Fig. 12.1   The tibiotalar and subtalar joints, medial aspect.

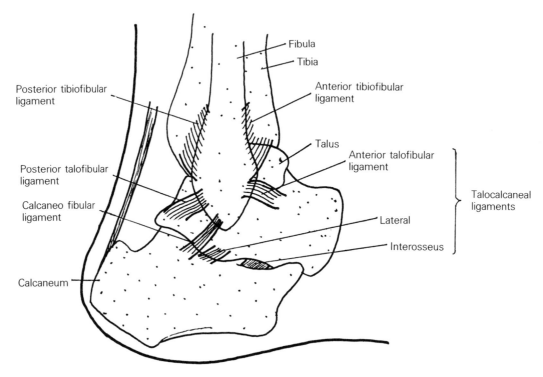

Fig. 12.2   The tibiotalar and subtalar joints, lateral aspect.

The *capsule* is attached to the margins of the articular surfaces and is synovial lined. It is reinforced by ligaments, the largest and strongest being the deltoid ligament which is attached above to the medial malleolus. The superficial fibres of this ligament pass (a) to the tuberosity of the navicular bone, these form the tibionavicular ligament; (b) to the sustentaculum tali of the calcaneum, these form the calcaneotibial ligament and (c) to the medial side of the talus, these form the posterior talotibial ligament. Deep fibres pass to the medial surface of the talus.

The *lateral ligament* consists of three separate bands. The anterior part runs from the anterior margin of the lateral malleolus forward and medially to become attached to the lateral aspect of the neck of the talus. The posterior talofibular fibres run from the lower part of the malleolus to the tubercle of the talus. These fibres are extremely strong and run almost horizontally. The calcaneofibular fibres run from the front of the malleolus, pass downward and posteriorly to become attached to the tubercle on the lateral surface of the calcaneum. These are the fibres which are frequently damaged in sprains of the ankle joint. The peroneal tendons cross these fibres.

The *anterior ligament* runs from the anterior margin of the lower end of the tibia to the talus below. These fibres are irritated by the formation of exostoses on the anterior surface of the ankle joint.

The movements which occur are plantarflexion and dorsiflexion. *Plantarflexion* is brought about by the contraction of gastrocnemius and soleus and these muscles are assisted by flexor hallucis longus, flexor digitorum longus and tibialis posterior. The movement is limited by tension in the opposing muscles and by tension in the anterior fibres of the deltoid ligament. For a description of these muscles see section 11.1.

Dorsiflexion is brought about by the contraction of tibialis anterior assisted by extensor hallucis longus and extensor digitorum longus. The movement is limited by tension of the tendo Achilles and tension in the posterior fibres of the deltoid ligament. As the articular surface of the talus is broader in front than behind, an increased space is needed between the malleoli during dorsiflexion. This comes about as a result of the movement which can occur at the inferior tibiofibular joint and some movement must also take place at the superior tibiofibular joint. The movement is of a gliding type and must always be checked by the examining osteopath in conditions of the ankle joint and foot. Locking at either of these joints will interfere with the normal mechanics of the ankle joint. Conversely hypermobility at either joint will lead to instability especially in dorsiflexion of the ankle.

12.3

The talocalcaneal joint

This is the articulation between the inferior surface of the talus and the calcaneum below (see Fig. 12.3). There are two such joints, the posterior and the talocalcaneonavicular (anterior) joint.

The posterior joint is of the plane type and is formed by the posterior facet on the superior surface of the calcaneum and the corresponding facet on the inferior surface of the talus – i.e. the posterior facet. The capsule is attached around the articular margins and is synovial lined and does not connect with any other joint. Posteriorly it is reinforced by a strong ligament, the interosseous talocalcanean ligament, the lateral part of which is especially strong and becomes taut during inversion of the foot thus limiting that movement from becoming excessive.

The anterior talocalcaneal joint is a complex articulation, namely between the anterior articular facet on the superior surface of the calcaneum, the facet on the posterior surface of the navicular, the upper surface of the plantar calcaneonavicular ligament and the rounded head of the talus above. The capsule is thickened posteriorly and the joint is reinforced by the plantar calcaneonavicular ligament below – the so-called spring ligament which is so important in the stability of the foot (see Fig. 12.4). The movements which occur are inversion and eversion while in addition there is

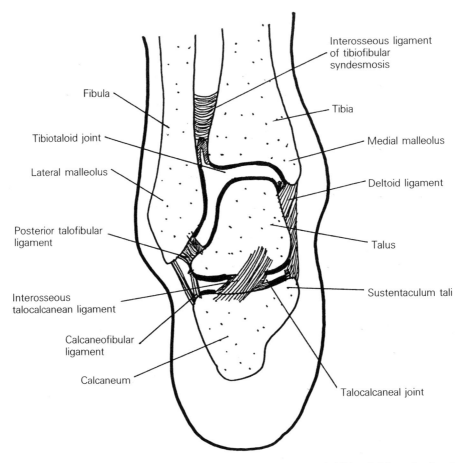

Fig. 12.3   Coronal section through the left talocrural (tibiotaloid) and talocalcaneal joints.

considerable gliding during movements of the foot. These passive movements are important to the mechanical integrity of the foot and ankle and will always need to be checked for full integrity in foot problems. Inversion is brought about by the action of tibialis anterior and posterior and eversion by the action of the peroneal muscles. Inversion is limited by tension in the peronei and in the talocalcaneal ligament and eversion by tension in the tibialis muscles and in the deltoid ligament. The anatomy of the muscles concerned is described in section 11.1.

The tibiotaloid joint and the talocalcaneal joints move together in active sport. The ankle is a hinge and the subtalar joints are of the plane and ball-and-socket types, so movement occurs in a wide range yet the joints are very strong and resist considerable stresses especially during activities such as running, jumping and hopping on one foot. Inversion is the movement which elevates the medial

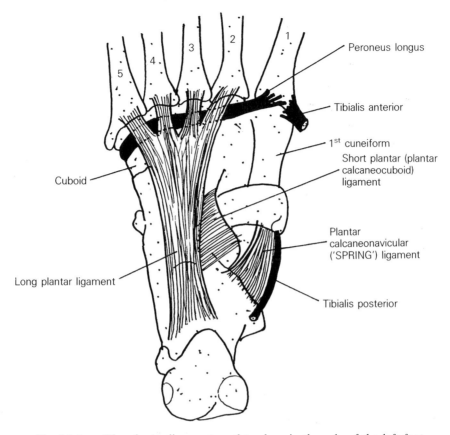

Peroneus longus

Tibialis anterior

1st cuneiform

Short plantar (plantar calcaneocuboid) ligament

Cuboid

Plantar calcaneonavicular ('SPRING') ligament

Long plantar ligament

Tibialis posterior

Fig. 12.4   The plantar ligaments and tendons in the sole of the left foot.

edge of the foot and is often known as supination, while eversion elevates the lateral side of the foot and is known as pronation. These two terms are used when describing the gait of an athlete, a pronated gait being the commoner fault seen.

Muscular injuries are described in Chapter 11.

12.4   **Tendon injury**

These have also been described in the Chapter 11. As a reminder the common tendons to be injured around the ankle are the tendo Achilles and the peroneal tendons which may recurrently dislocate. Tenosynovitis is also frequently seen and has already been described. See Fig. 5.10.

12.5   **Bone injury**

Periostitis is seen around the ankle joint either as a result of direct trauma such as a blow from a hard ball, or at the lateral aspect of the joint resulting from jumping. In this case the athlete has forced his foot into eversion and dorsiflexion as he took off to jump thus forcing the superolateral margin of the calcaneum against the antero-inferior surface of the fibula. Examination of the joints reveals nothing as there is no injury to muscle or ligament. Pain can only be elicited by superimposing dorsiflexion on the fully everted foot, passively, when the inflamed periosteum on the antero-inferior aspect of the fibula will be pressed against the calcaneum. Palpation will then reveal localised tenderness on the fibula but no corresponding tenderness on the calcaneum. The athlete will report that he only feels the pain as he takes off to jump. The swiftest way to relieve the pain is to infiltrate the area and give it rest until the tenderness has subsided. If the periostitis has been caused by a direct blow there will be a history of such an event. Ice and elevation are indicated and arnica can be applied *if the skin is not broken*. Occasionally there is a residual bony exostosis following a severe periosteal injury but it is usually of no consequence. The malleoli are the most vulnerable sites and if there is any possibility of a fracture, this must be excluded by X-ray.

Fracture of the *talus* is rare and will usually be caused by a severe injury rather than a sports injury, for example a road traffic accident. Some, however, do occur as a result of a fall from a height so it is possible to see one of these in such sports as gymnastics or pole vaulting or even equestrian events. There will be extreme pain and usually gross deformity and the patient should be transferred to a specialist unit at least to have the possibility of such a fracture excluded.

Fracture of the *calcaneum* is not so rare. It is usually caused by a fall from a height onto the heel such as might happen in high jump or even in basketball, netball or vaulting. Pain is felt in the heel, especially on weight bearing. As this fracture is so often missed it is wise to X-ray all athletes who have fallen onto the heel from a height and have pain in the area of the calcaneum. Treatment is required from a specialist. The common complication of this fracture is immobility in the subtalar joints and restoration of this movement is essential if full foot mobility is to be restored. Some patients have a residual periostitis in the lateral malleolus as described above.

The development of an *exostosis* in this area is not rare (see Fig. 12.5). Repeated friction may cause an exostosis which will usually develop on the posterior aspect of the calcaneum. It is usually due to ill-fitting footwear and has already been mentioned. On the inferior aspect of the calcaneum a bony spur may develop which may or may not cause pain. If it does, the patient will complain of pain which is made worse by any springing movement of the foot. The lesion is probably caused by repeated injury to the calcaneal attachment of the plantar fascia during which the peri-

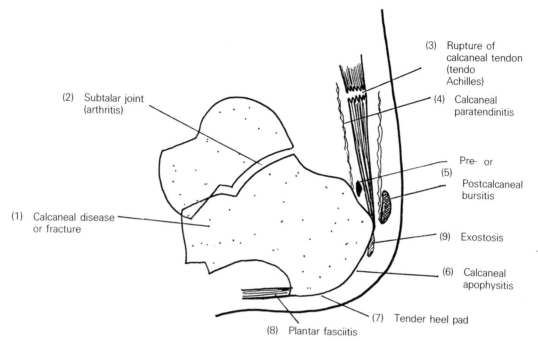

Fig. 12.5   Causes of a painful heel.

osteum has been repeatedly damaged. If the spur is giving symptoms, a pad with a hole in it which will cover the spur and therefore prevent weight being transferred through it, will alleviate the pain. Usually a period of rest from weight bearing will deal with the problem and recurrence is found to be rare.

A generalised periostitis of the calcaneum is also sometimes seen. The patient complains of pain on weight bearing which covers a wide area of the bone. Palpation reveals tenderness often of the posterior as well as the inferior surfaces of the bone and some swelling may also palpable. The cause of this is uncertain but it may well be an overuse condition. It is often seen in middle-aged men. Soft footwear and anti-inflammatory treatment is the most successful way of dealing with the problem.

Exostoses may form on the anterior margins of both of the ankle joint bones usually from sports such as football where it is thought to result from repetitive kicking strains with the foot in plantar-flexion imposed on the joint. All active and passive movements may cause pain but resisted movements will not. Articulation of the joint with compression will increase the pain. In early cases the symptoms may be relieved by increasing the range of movement of the joint but in more severe cases surgery may be necessary to remove the exostoses after which full mobilisation of all joints in the area will be needed before full activity is resumed.

In cases of *anterior spur formation* the pain is caused by the irritation of the anterior ligament of the joint.

All these injuries predispose to the early development of *degenerative change* within the joint. The probability seems to be increased when the mechanics of the area are left in a faulty state after injury. Treatment to restore normal mechanics seems to minimise the risk of degeneration occurring prematurely, so every effort to correct faults has to be of great importance to athletes. Pathologies are not rare in the calcaneum. Any persistent pain which is resistant to treatment should give rise to the possible presence of a pathology. Paget's disease may affect the calcaneum; this will give rise to a deep-seated pain which does not respond to osteopathic treatment. An infective abscess is occasionally present; in this case there will be lymphatic involvement and the athlete will not feel 'well' and may have a fluctuating body temperature. The possibility of pain referred from the lumbar spine and /or the pelvis must always be considered in cases of pain felt in the region of the heel and examination of these areas must always be carried out thoroughly. It is often possible to recreate the symptoms by certain movements of the upper area if it is at fault and there is often a linear type of pain involved. There may or may not be a reflex change or a positive straight leg raising test. Osteopathic examination is never complete unless the centrally related area of the body is fully examined and treated as and when necessary.

12.6 **Epiphysitis and apophysitis**

Epiphysitis of the inferior end of the tibia is not commonly seen and has been mentioned in section 11.6.

Apophysitis is usually seen in boys aged about 10 and is known as Sever's disease which is a misnomer as the condition is not a disease but a mild traction injury of the calcaneal apophysis. The young athlete will complain of pain in the posterior aspect of the calcaneum which is made worse on activity, especially when the dorsiflexor muscles are used strongly. There is tenderness and some swelling in the area of the insertion of the tendo Achilles. X-rays are helpful in confirming the diagnosis when the apophysis will appear to have increased density and possible fragmentation, but the other calcaneum may well appear similar, yet is symptom-free. A slightly raised heel and rest from weight bearing activity together with osteopathic treatment to the foot, lower leg and spinally associated areas is helpful and the condition usually resolves in a few weeks when full activity can be resumed. Swimming is a useful form of exercise during the recovery phase as it is a non-weight bearing activity and will therefore not stress the apophysis. Occasionally the apophysis may detach due to an excessive strain being placed on the dorsiflexors and will require specialist attention and regulated exercises following repair. There may be some residual bony protrusion following an apophysitis but is usually of no importance unless it is subjected to friction thereafter.

Joint and ligament injury

Shortening of the posterior calf muscles will render the ankle joint limited in dorsiflexion and this will be the only abnormal finding on clinical examination. It may well give rise to strains of the midtarsus. If severe the condition is obvious as the athlete walks into the surgery when he will be seen to have a lateral rotation of the lower extremity. The condition is usually bilateral. Treatment consists of stretching the gastrocnemius and soleus muscles out separately — the former by straight knee stretching and the latter by knee flexion with the heel on the ground. Passive osteopathic stretching is also essential as well as these exercises. As there is bound to be an associated loss of joint mobility this has to be treated too. In severe cases in adults, the tendo Achilles may have to be lengthened surgically after which osteopathic treatment to all the associated areas is indicated. A wobble board is useful to help stretch out the affected muscles.

Osteoarthritis is commonly seen in older athletes especially when their chosen sport has repeatedly traumatised the joints, for example runners. The patient will complain of a diffuse pain in the joint which is worse following weight bearing activity. Examination will reveal a loss of mobility in all ranges which may be accompanied by discomfort or pain. Resisted movements will not cause pain. Osteopathic treatment to increase the range of movement in all ranges is extremely helpful but may have to be repeated at regular intervals as the condition is progressive. Non-weight bearing exercises are also useful to help maintain mobility.

A *loose body* in the ankle joint will produce a classic symptom picture. The athlete will complain of severe momentary pain in the joint usually on plantarflexion, for example when descending a step. His reaction is to shake the foot when the pain ceases and he can again bear weight. This episode is likely to be repeated. Examination of the joint appears normal. X-rays will also reveal nothing abnormal as the loose body is likely to be cartilagenous. If this diagnosis is suspected, an arthroscopic examination may well be the immediate treatment of choice.

A *sprain* of the ankle is the most commonly seen condition in the treatment of sports injuries. It may be a simple strain of one ligament of the joint or may involve injury to more than one. It may also involve a disturbance of the mechanics of the joint, temporarily or permanently. The commonest injury is an inversion strain which traumatises the lateral ligament and may also involve one or more muscles, for example the peronei, or the long flexors if the ankle was in plantarflexion at the time of injury.

The athlete will be aware of the diagnosis himself. He will complain of pain especially when he attempts to bear weight which he feels mostly on the lateral aspect of the joint. There may be considerable swelling and bruising may be severe. If the swelling appeared within minutes of the injury a haemarthrosis must be suspected and expert attention is needed as aspiration may be required. Most cases take hours rather than minutes for the swelling to become gross. This swelling may well impede the examination of the joint making an accurate diagnosis impossible. Severe bruising which appears quickly may suggest a complete tear of the lateral ligament whereas bruising which appears a day or so after the injury suggests a partial tear. Active movement may be impossible due to pain. Passive inversion will always increase the pain and plantarflexion may do so also. Passive inversion will only be excessive if there is a complete tear of the ligament; in partial tears the range is normal (or limited by swelling and/or pain). The exact site of injury should be determined by careful palpation, the commonest being the fibular attachment of the lateral ligament. Should the inferior aspect of the fibula be sensitive to pressure, the possibility of a fracture of the lateral malleolus should be excluded by X-ray.

Treatment in the acute phase has to be aimed at reducing the swelling and the application of ice is indicated. The limb should be elevated (above the level of the heart) and plantarflexion and dorsiflexion carried out regularly and repeatedly in this position to assist drainage. Ice packs need to be used at least six times a day for about five minutes at a time. In less severe cases, a horseshoe strapping should be applied which is put on from the inner aspect of the ankle, under the heel to the outer aspect thus pulling the ankle into eversion and approximating the damaged fibres. This will help to minimise lengthening of the ligament during healing and the athlete will be able to walk comparatively comfortably. It will also not impede drainage of the area. In this way inversion will be supported and plantarflexion and dorsiflexion will not be restricted. Friction to the damaged fibres is also helpful. Any damage to muscle, tendon or tendon sheath will also not be aggravated and friction to these injuries will help them to heal. Once the athlete can walk with less pain, the mechanics of the tibiotaloid joint must be assessed. Almost always there is found to be a forward shift of the talus and associated limitation of movement. This has to be corrected which is easily done if the foot is put into full dorsiflexion and a traction-gapping of the joint achieved when the movement will be improved, if not completely normalised immediately − the technique may have to be repeated if the joint is resistant to total correction. A wobble board is useful to normalise any muscular insufficiency and helps to keep the joint mobile. All such injuries will resolve more quickly if the ankle is actively used. If it is not, adhesions are likely to result. These can be satisfactorily dealt with by osteopathic treatment but are better avoided.

If the lateral ligament has a complete *tear*, there will be excessive inversion at the joint; the talus will tilt unduly on inversion and this can be seen on a mobility X-ray by comparison with the unaffected side. Surgical repair is then needed but osteopathic treatment to the immobile areas is indicated after repair of the ligament. In these cases it may take several weeks for full mobility to be restored but it can invariably be achieved and will render the athlete less liable to further injury.

Instability in the ankle renders the joint liable to recurrent sprains. The athlete will complain that his ankle 'turns over easily' and may swell and ache after physical activity. The peroneal muscles may be weak in which case strengthening can be achieved by using a wobble board. If, however, the lateral ligament is chronically stretched, the athlete should reinforce the unstable ankle by using a support during activity to prevent progressive weakening.

Eversion sprains of the ankle are rare. They can occur when the foot is trapped in a certain position, for example in a stirrup as the rider falls off or in a skiing injury when the ski does not release. Pain will be felt on the medial aspect of the joint and will be made worse by active and passive eversion of the foot. There may be involvement of the posterior tibialis tendon. Friction to the injured fibres and attention to any abnormality in the associated mechanics will accelerate healing. This condition may be associated with pronation of gait when the tibionavicular and tibiocalcaneal ligaments become chronically stretched. Some cases will respond well to strengthening of the tibialis anterior and posterior muscles but chronic cases may need orthotics to reduce the strain on the medial aspect of the ankle.

An *os trigonum* may be irritated by repeated plantarflexion of the ankle if one is present. Pain felt in the posterior aspect of the ankle with tenderness deep to the tendo Achilles without pain on partial plantarflexion (i.e. use of the dorsiflexor muscles) should alert the osteopath to the possibility of one being present. If it has become inflamed, rest from forced or repetitive plantarflexion usually results in the inflammation subsiding; seldom is surgical removal needed (see Fig. 4.1).

12.8   Facet locking

The *tibiotaloid joint* may be facet locked when active and passive plantarflexion and/or dorsiflexion will be limited. Resisted movements will be normal. The injury usually results from jumping down onto the heel with insufficient flexion of the knee. As the joint is of the mortise type, the two articulatory surfaces are forcibly approximated. This type of injury is seen in high and long jump, netball and in certain bad landings in gymnastics. The athlete will complain of discomfort in the ankle especially after physical activity when there may be a little swelling. Examination reveals some loss of active and passive plantarflexion and/or dorsiflexion and there will be a palpably reduced sulcus on the anterior aspect of the tibiotaloid joint which is easily discerned when the affected ankle is compared with the other side. Corrective gapping of the joint will help the condition subside and full mobility is restored.

Facet locking of the *talocalcaneal joints* will result in loss of the full range of inversion and/or eversion. With sprains of the ankle, one or other of these movements is reduced but not both. The athlete will complain of discomfort in the area of the joints especially after activity. Palpation will reveal little or no tenderness in the region of the periosteum but the joint line may be tender. Osteopathic correction will render the mechanics normal and the symptoms will subside. All the associated joints may need treatment as the effect of this condition is likely to become widespread by the time the athlete seeks advice.

Facet locking of these joints may be as a result of an ankle sprain where insufficient emphasis has been placed on restoration of full mobility both active and passive.

12.9   Mobility injury

Both the tibiotaloid and talocalcaneal joints may be stiff, probably following a fracture or a severe sprain. This may be due to shortening of the surrounding ligaments and not to facet locking, but both are possible. In the latter there will be a reduction of passive movements whereas in a case of ligamentous shortening the passive movements are likely to be normal. The shortened ligaments will respond well to stretching/articulatory techniques and normal movements can be restored this way, but it may take some time in chronic cases.

Sudeck's atrophy occasionally affects the foot, following a comparatively minor injury. Pain and stiffness come on a few weeks after injury for no apparent reason. The ankle and foot become swollen and there is patchy discolouration of the area. There is often hypersensitivity and the skin may be unusually moist. The condition responds well to gentle osteopathic treatment and full mobility is restored, but it may take several months to resolve fully.

Hypermobility is seen in the ankle usually following a sprain or a series of repeated sprains. Usually there is increased inversion and laxity of the lateral ligament. Exercise to strengthen the peroneal muscles is helpful and correction of any defective mechanics in any surrounding joint, but the athlete may have to wear an ankle support for further athletics to minimise the chance of further strain. Many athletes apply a protective strapping to the ankle routinely, which may be a wise move.

Bursitis

On the posterior aspect of the calcaneum a bursa may become inflamed either subcutaneously or deep to the tendo Achilles. If the bursitis is subcutaneous it will be seen as a swelling on the back of the heel and will have been caused by pressure or friction. The athlete will complain of pain and swelling and will prefer to walk barefoot. Protection from pressure and the application of ice packs will encourage the bursa to subside, but attention to correct footwear is essential to prevent further trouble. A bursitis deep to the tendo Achilles will also produce pain but this will be felt more deeply by the athlete and will be made worse by contraction of the plantarflexor muscles. When present this is usually palpable deep to the tendon. Rest from active plantarflexion and possible infiltration of the bursa will resolve the problem and only occasionally is excision needed. A protective pad helps to reduce pressure from footwear, in both cases.

Skin injuries

As the heel is subjected to weight bearing during most athletic activities, attention to skin conditions may be necessary. It is important to remember that the condition of the skin on the heel may indicate some abnormality of gait, for example there may be a great deal of hard skin on the outer aspect of the heel by comparison with the inner aspect, where the body weight is not taken evenly on the area. This could be secondary to a postural problem in the foot, leg, or even spine or pelvis and may need attention and correction even though it may not be producing symptoms other then uneven distribution of body weight on the heel.

Blisters are common in the area of the heel and are caused by friction from footwear. The fluid may be released by using a sterilised needle but the epidermal layer must never be cut away. The area should then be covered with a sterile dressing. Prevention is better than cure! Two pairs of socks which are made of a natural fibre and correctly fitting shoes should stop recurrence and the skin can be made tougher by bathing the feet in surgical spirit regularly.

Hard skin is a frequent problem to athletes especially when it cracks open and the advice of a State Registered Chiropodist is to be recommended.

A *verruca* is often seen in this area and if persistently troublesome the athlete should take the advice of a chiropodist. The condition seldom requires surgical treatment and responds well to a homeopathic remedy. These conditions are important to recognise as they may cause the athlete to walk and run in some peculiar manner, thus disturbing his normal mechanics and even causing pain or disability elsewhere in the body.

Chapter 13   The Foot

The midfoot and forefoot

The part of the foot described in Chapter 12 comprises what is known as the hind foot. The *mid foot* is made up of the tarsal bones namely the navicular, medial intermediate and lateral cuneiform bones and the cuboid which is placed on the lateral aspect of the foot. Joints exist between these bones which are best illustrated by diagram, see Fig. 13.1. Note that there is no joint between the calcaneum and the navicular but these bones are connected by means of the extremely strong lateral calcaneonavicular ligament and the plantar calcaneonavicular ligament or 'spring ligament'. The movement which occurs between these bones is of a gliding

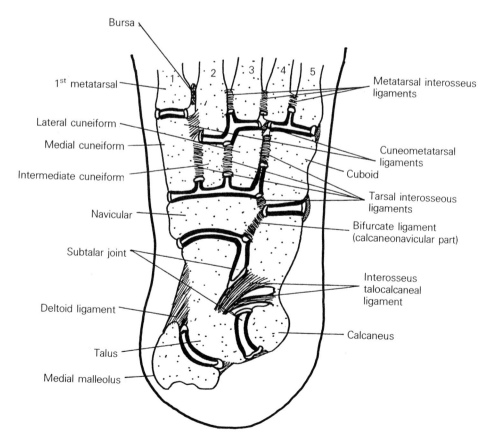

Fig. 13.1   Intertarsal joints of the right foot, oblique section.

type and of small range. No such movement can be carried out voluntarily when the foot is raised from the ground. All movement occurs when the body weight is placed on the anterior part of the foot as when starting to run or jump. The joints serve to increase the flexibility and suppleness of the foot and allow alteration in the arches of the foot during weight bearing activities. Osteopathic examination therefore, will include palpation of the passive movement at each and every one of these joints which must be fully analysed for it's full integrity in all foot problems which are met in practice.

The ligaments which support these joints are shown in Figs 13.2, 13.3 and 13.4. By virtue of their tissue construction, they cannot fatigue but if they become overstretched they are unable to return to their original length. These are supported in turn by muscles which can fatigue and have less resistance to stress than ligaments. The bone arches are supported by ligaments which are in turn supported by muscles; it is therefore evident that muscular strength is imperative if the ligaments are not to become stretched and the integrity of the arches maintained.

The *forefoot* comprises the metatarsals and the phalanges and there is an important arch present between the metatarsal heads. When the foot is weight bearing on the ground, it rests on

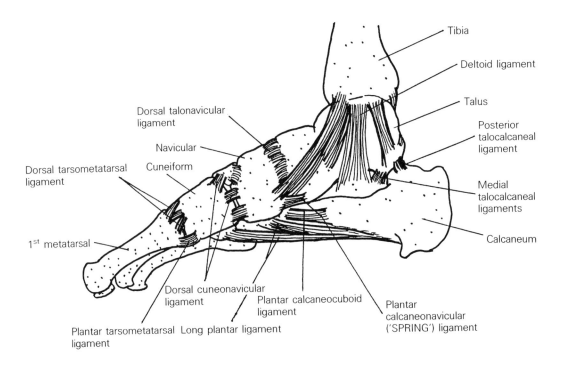

Fig. 13.2   Ligaments of the right foot, medial aspect.

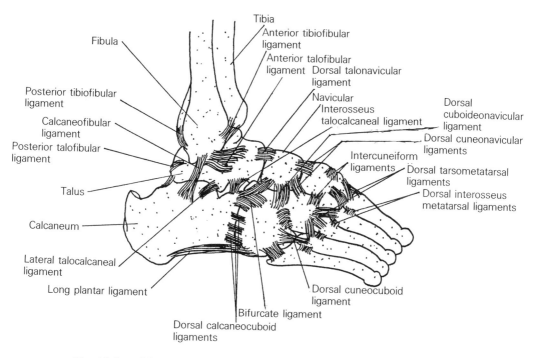

Fig. 13.3   Ligaments of the right foot, lateral aspect.

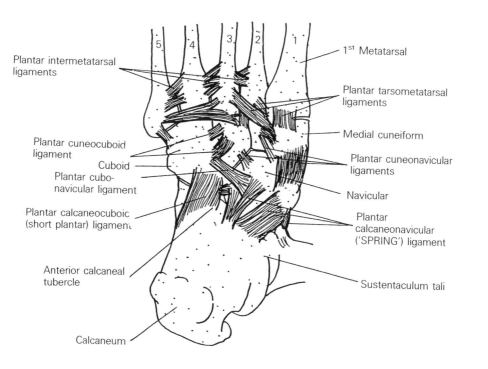

Fig. 13.4   Ligaments of the right foot, plantar aspect (long plantar ligament removed).

the ground in three places, namely the calcaneum posteriorly, the head of the first metatarsal anteromedially and the head of the fifth metatarsal anterolaterally. These points form a triangle, see Fig. 13.5.

The medial arch lies between the calcaneum and the first metatarsal head and comprises five bones, namely the calcaneum, the talus, the navicular, the medial cuneiform and the first metatarsal head (see Fig. 13.6). The plantar ligaments which support this arch are the talocalcaneal ligament, the plantar calcaneonavicular ligament (the spring ligament and the most important of all), the cuneonavicular ligament and the the cuneometatarsal ligament. These serve to resist violent shortlasting stresses. Sustained stresses are withstood by the muscles which support the arch, namely the tibialis posterior, the peroneus longus, flexor hallucis longus, flexor digitorum longus and the abductor hallucis longus. The antagonists are the extensor hallucis longus and the tibialis anterior, both of which are inserted into the convexity of the arch and therefore can reduce it's curvature.

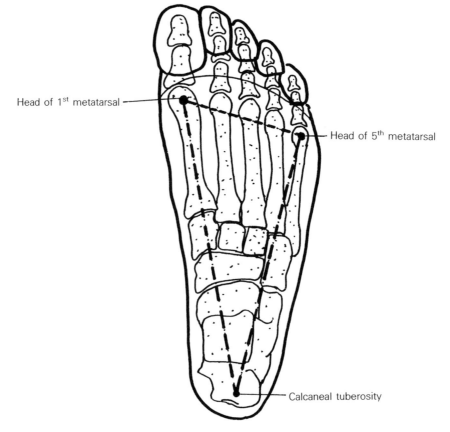

Head of 1st metatarsal

Head of 5th metatarsal

Calcaneal tuberosity

Fig. 13.5   Weight bearing points of the foot, plantar arch, inferior aspect.

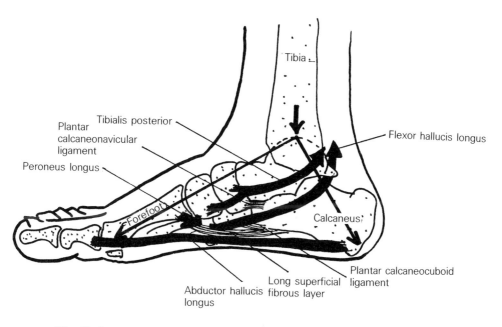

Fibularis label text within figure:

Tibia

Tibialis posterior

Plantar
calcaneonavicular
ligament

Peroneus longus

Flexor hallucis longus

Forefoot

Calcaneus

Abductor hallucis
longus

Long superficial
fibrous layer

Plantar calcaneocuboid
ligament

Fig. 13.6   Weight bearing points of the foot, medial arch.

The lateral arch spans the area from the calcaneum to the fifth metatarsal head and includes three bones, namely the calcaneum, the cuboid and the fifth metatarsal (see Fig. 13.7). It is not as high as the medial arch and is less flexible. The long plantar ligament runs from the plantar surface of the calcaneum to the plantar surface of the cuboid and some superficial fibres run further anteriorly to be attached to the plantar surface of the second, third and fourth metatarsals. It is an extremely strong ligament and inferiorly lies the short plantar ligament which runs from the inferior surface of the calcaneum to the adjacent surface of the cuboid. Together these ligaments resist sudden stresses on the lateral arch of the foot. The muscles which maintain the lateral arch are the peroneus longus, the peroneus brevis and the abductor digiti minimi and the antagonists are the peroneus tertius and the extensor digitorum longus muscles. Contraction of the plantarflexors of the ankle also tends to reduce the concavity of the lateral arch.

The anterior transverse arch of the foot lies between the head of the first metatarsal and the head of the fifth metatarsal bone (see Fig. 13.8). The apex of this arch is the head of the second metatarsal which is why metatarsal arch problems are usually seen clinically affecting this bone. The arch is relatively flat but it's integrity is of prime importance as the heads of the second, third and fourth metatarsals are not adapted to direct weight bearing. The arch is supported on the plantar surface by the relatively weak intermetatarsal ligaments with muscular support from the transverse head of

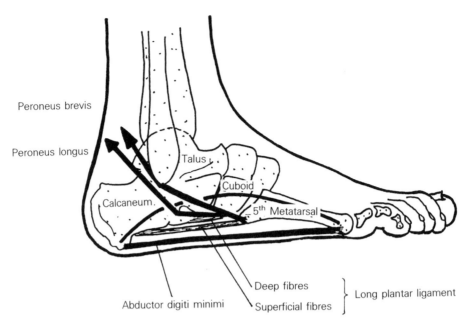

Peroneus brevis

Peroneus longus

Talus

Cuboid

Calcaneum

5th Metatarsal

Abductor digiti minimi

Deep fibres

Superficial fibres

Long plantar ligament

Fig. 13.7   Weight bearing points of the foot, lateral arch.

the abductor hallucis muscle which is also relatively weak. That is why the arch is frequently flattened and then callouses forms under the metatarsal heads and the heads themselves may even be forced to weight bear, causing pain. The lumbrical and interosseous muscles help to stabilise the metatarsals and are often found to be weak in cases of dropped metatarsal arch. The posterior transverse arch extends in the tarsal area from the navicular medially to the cuboid laterally and is supported by the interosseous ligaments and especially by the plantar expansion of the tibialis posterior muscle assisted by the adductor hallucis and the peroneus longus muscles.

It is evident that the integrity of the various arches of the foot depends largely on the muscular strength and balance of the long muscles of the foot which arise in the leg, aided by the intrinsic muscles of the foot. Many foot problems arise from weakness in these muscles.

On the dorsum of the foot there is only one intrinsic muscle, namely the extensor digitorum brevis which arises from the upper lateral surface of the calcaneum and runs obliquely forwards across the dorsum of the foot and divides into four tendons. The medial one is often referred to as the extensor hallucis muscle and is inserted into the dorsal surface of the base of the proximal phalanx of the great toe. The other three tendons are inserted into the sides of the tendons of the extensor digitorum longus of the second, third and fourth toes. It acts as an extensor of the toes and is often

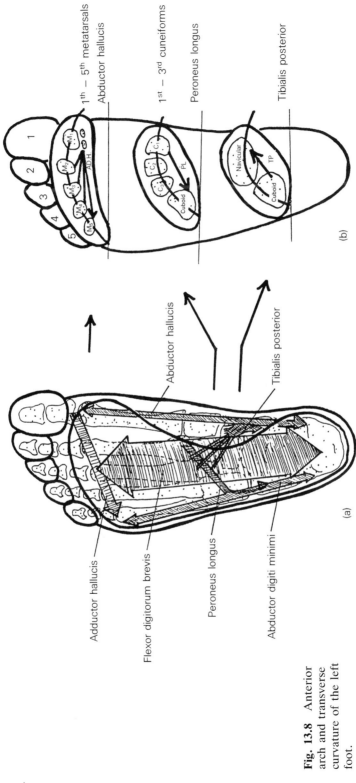

1th – 5th metatarsals
Abductor hallucis

1st – 3rd cuneiforms

Peroneus longus

Tibialis posterior

(b)

Adductor hallucis

Abductor hallucis

Flexor digitorum brevis

Peroneus longus

Tibialis posterior

Abductor digiti minimi

(a)

Fig. 13.8 Anterior arch and transverse curvature of the left foot.

overdeveloped in rowers who use the muscle to stabilise the foot while rowing. Its nerve supply consists of the deep peroneal nerve, S1 and S2.

The plantar surface of the foot has three groups of intrinsic muscles. Superficial to these lies the plantar aponeurosis which is thick and strong and arises from the calcaneum and radiates anteriorly into each of the five toes. Transverse fibres interconnect the longitudinal fibrous bundles, the spaces between them being filled with fat which acts as a protective pad in the sole of the foot, see Fig. 13.9.

The muscles of the great toe

The *abductor hallucis* lies along the medial border of the foot. It arises from the medial tubercle of the calcaneum, the flexor retinaculum and the plantar aponeurosis and ends in a tendon which is inserted with the medial tendon of the flexor hallucis brevis into the medial side of the base of the proximal phalanx of the great

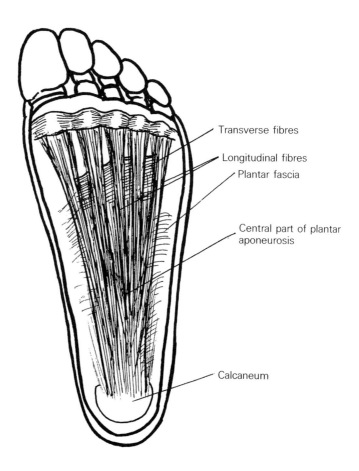

Transverse fibres

Longitudinal fibres

Plantar fascia

Central part of plantar aponeurosis

Calcaneum

Fig. 13.9 Plantar aponeurosis of the left foot.

toe. Its nerve supply consists of the medial plantar nerve, S2 and S3.

The *flexor hallucis brevis* lies deeper; it arises from the planar surface of the cuboid and adjacent surface of the lateral cuneiform and from the tendon of the tibialis posterior. It divides into a medial and lateral portion each having a tendinous insertion. The medial head combines with the abductor hallucis to be inserted into the medial side of the base of the proximal phalanx of the great toe and there is a sesamoid bone in the tendon of insertion. The lateral head blends with the adductor hallucis to be inserted into the lateral side of the base of the proximal phalanx where there is also a sesamoid present in the tendon of insertion. The nerve supply consists of the medial plantar nerve, S2 and S3. This is an important plantarflexor of the hallux and is especially developed in athletes.

The *adductor hallucis* has two heads of origin. The stronger oblique head arises from the bases of 2−4 metatarsals and the tendon sheath of peroneus longus. The weaker transverse head arises from the plantar metatarsophalangeal ligaments of the third, fourth, and fifth toes and the deep transvere metatarsal ligaments. The tendon of insertion blends with that of the lateral head of the flexor hallucis brevis to be inserted into the lateral side of the base of the proximal phalanx of the great toe where there is a sesamoid in the tendon of insertion. The nerve supply consists of the lateral plantar nerve, S1 and S2. The transverse head is important in maintaining the anterior transverse arch of the foot. See Fig. 13.10.

The muscles of the little toe

The *flexor digiti minimi* arises from the plantar surface of the base of the fifth metatarsal bone, the long plantar ligament and from the tendon sheath of the peroneus longus muscle. It's tendon of insertion is attached to the lateral side of the proximal phalanx of the fifth toe at it's base. Sometimes a few deep fibres are inserted into the lateral part of the distal half of the fifth metatarsal and are known as the opponens digiti minimi but they are by no means always present. The nerve supply consists of the lateral plantar nerve, S2 and S3.

The *abductor digiti minimi* lies along the lateral border of the foot and is the largest and longest muscle of the fifth toe. It arises from the lateral and inferior surfaces of the calcaneum, the tuberosity of the fifth metatarsal and from the plantar aponeurosis and is inserted with the flexor digiti minimi into the lateral side of the base of the proximal phalanx of the little toe.

The nerve supply consists of the lateral plantar nerve, S2 and S3. See Fig. 13.10.

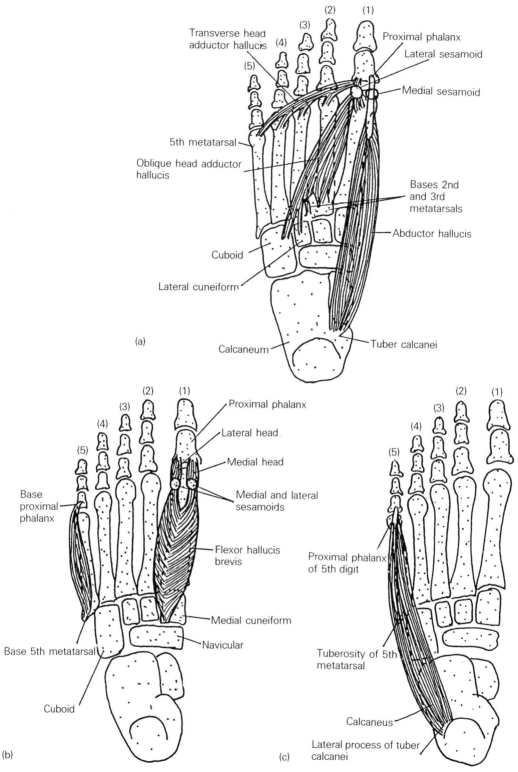

Fig. 13.10 Small muscles of the big and little digit. (a) Abductor hallucis and adductor hallucis; (b) flexor hallucis brevis and flexor digiti minimi; (c) abductor digiti minimi.

Muscles in the centre of the sole of the foot

The *quadratus plantae* (also known as the *flexor digitorum access-orius*) arises by two slips from the medial and lateral margins of the plantar surface of the calcaneum which unite to form a fleshy belly. It is inserted into the tendon of the superior surface and lateral margin of the tendon of flexor digitorum longus. Its nerve supply consists of the lateral plantar nerve, S2 and S3.

The *lumbricals* are four small muscles which arise from the tendons of the *flexor digitorum longus*. The medial muscle arises from only the medial border of the first tendon but the lateral three arise from the adjacent borders of the tendons; they are inserted via tendons into the medial margins of the proximal phalanges of the second, third, fourth and fifth toes and radiate into the dorsal digital expansion. The nerve supply for the medial muscle is the medial plantar nerve, L5 and S1 and the others are supplied by the lateral plantar nerve S1 and S2. These muscles are not always present. They help to reinforce the plantar arch. See Fig. 13.11.

The *interossei* are dorsal and plantar. The dorsal interossei are four in number and arise from the opposing surfaces of all the metatarsals. They are attached to the bases of the proximal phalanges of the second, third and fourth digits. They act as abductors of the toes moving them away from the second toe which is the axis of the foot. There are three plantar interossei, each arising from a single head from the medial side of the third, fourth and fifth metatarsal bone. They are inserted into the medial side of the base of the proximal phalanx of the third, fourth and fifth toe. They act as adductors. The nerve supply consists of the lateral plantar nerve, S1 and S2. See Fig. 13.11.

The metatarsophalangeal and interphalangeal joints of the toes are of the hinge type and flexion and extension are the active movements which take place. In addition, there is a passive lateral shift and a passive A−P shift. Passive movement also occurs between the adjacent metatarsal heads which are joined by ligaments.

There are several tendon sheaths in the sole of the foot (see Fig. 13.12). A tendon sheath surrounds the tendon of the peroneus longus, deep, as it passes to insert into the first metatarsal and medial cuneiform bones. The tendons of the flexor digitorum longus and the tibialis posterior muscles are also enclosed in a synovial sheath. In addition, there is a separate synovial sheath for each digit inferior to the phalanges.

To sum up the flexors of the toes are flexor hallucis longus, flexor hallucis brevis, flexor digitorum longus, flexor digitorum brevis, quadratus plantae and flexor digiti minimi.

Extensors of the toes are the extensor hallucis longus, extensor

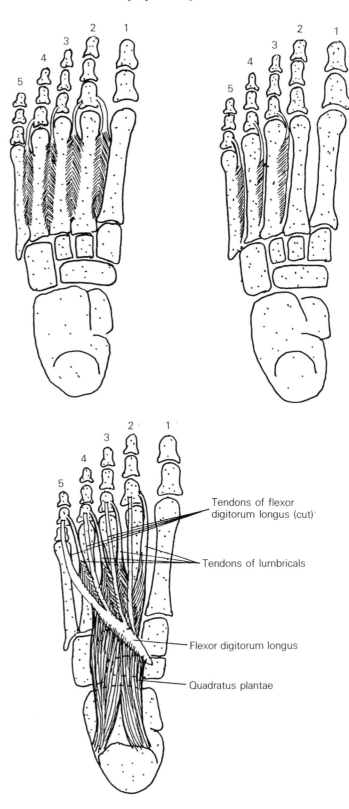

Fig. 13.11 (a) Dorsal interossei; (b) plantar interossei; (c) lumbricals and quadratus plantae.

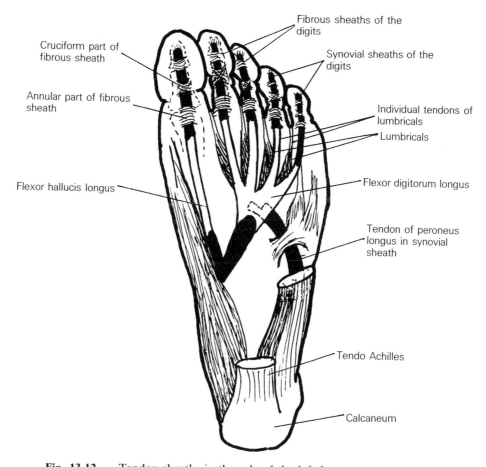

Fibrous sheaths of the digits

Cruciform part of fibrous sheath

Synovial sheaths of the digits

Annular part of fibrous sheath

Individual tendons of lumbricals

Lumbricals

Flexor hallucis longus

Flexor digitorum longus

Tendon of peroneus longus in synovial sheath

Tendo Achilles

Calcaneum

Fig. 13.12   Tendon sheaths in the sole of the left foot.

hallucis brevis, extensor digitorum longus, extensor digitorum brevis.

Abductors are the abductor hallucis, the dorsal interossei and abductor digiti minimi. Adduction depends on the action of the adductor hallucis and the plantar interossei.

Maintenance of the arches of the foot depends on the interaction of the various muscles which support the arches and the action of the antagonists. When these muscles are not sufficiently strong, stress is placed on the very strong supporting ligaments which will become irreversibly stretched in time. They are designed to withstand sudden acute stress and not longstanding strain.

13.2   Muscle and tendon injuries

The short intrinsic muscles of the foot are seldom injured. The long muscles which arise from the leg are more likely to be strained than the short ones. Similarly the tendons of the long muscles are more likely to be damaged than the short muscles which are comparatively protected by virtue of their position within the foot. In the midtarsal area the tendons of tibialis anterior may become damaged at or near it's insertion into the medial cuneiform bone or the bursa which lies under the tendon may become inflamed either from direct pressure, for example from ill-fitting footwear or from a direct blow onto that part of the foot. In the sole of the foot the tendons of flexor hallucis longus, flexor digitorum longus and tibialis posterior are sometimes damaged, usually from a direct cause, either a blow or possibly treading on a sharp object with insufficient protection to the foot. In the latter case there will probably be obvious bruising as well as pain. Typically there is crepitus felt within the tendon sheath when the muscle is actively used and careful palpation of the area should enable a correct diagnosis to be made. It is helpful to refer to the exact anatomical arrangement when assessing the possibility of a tenosynovitis around the foot.

13.3   **Abnormalities of the arches of the foot**

Pes planus or 'flatfoot' is the commonest abnormality seen. The normal footprint shows that the weight distribution is mainly on the medial aspect of the calcaneum and the head of the first metatarsal bone with clear impressions of the five digits; there is some impression from the lateral border of the foot. In cases of flatfoot there is a wide flattened impression of the whole of the sole of the foot (see Fig. 13.13). This condition does not always cause pain but if it does it must be treated. The athlete will probably be a young male in his mid-teens and will complain of pain felt under the medial arch particularly at or near the navicular which is made worse after a period of exercise. There may also be pain in the leg. Both feet are usually affected. The calcaneonavicular ligament becomes painful, stretched and tender on palpation and is often prominent. The midtarsal ligaments and the plantar fascia become stretched and painful too. The condition would not have come about had the supporting muscles been strong enough to support the arch, so treatment has to be aimed at strengthening these, namely tibialis posterior, flexor hallucis longus, flexor digitorum longus and the small muscles of the sole of the foot. Clinical examination will reveal that the tuberosity of the navicular is prominent, the tendo Achilles is bowed, concave laterally and the heels are in the valgus position when the athlete is standing (see Fig. 13.14(a)). There will also be distortion of the shoes. Passive movements of the ankle are normal but those of the subtalar and midtarsal joints are limited and may cause pain. Osteopathic treatment to the restricted joints is essential together with exercises to

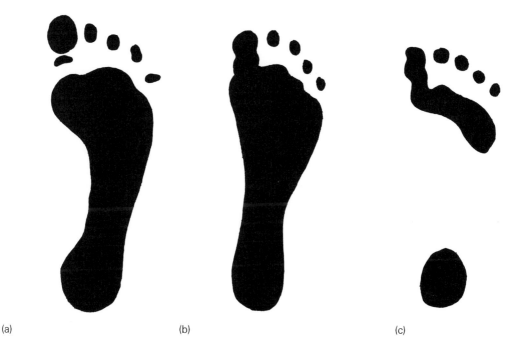

(a)   (b)   (c)

Fig. 13.13   (a) Normal foot (pes rectus); (b) flatfoot (pes planus); (c) pes cavus.

strengthen the muscles. Full recovery is to be expected within about three months if the athlete is willing to play his part fully.

Pes cavus is the opposite condition. The foot print will show that the body weight is transmitted on the lateral side of the calcaneum and across the metatarsal heads. The lateral border of the foot does not touch the ground (see Fig. 13.13(c)). There is often a family history of the condition. The athlete may complain of a general ache in the foot and calf after exercise or be subject to recurrent sprained ankles. Standing examination reveals that the subtalar joint is held in inversion and the tendo Achilles is seen to be concave medially (see Fig. 13.14(b)). The midtarsal area is prominent on the dorsum of the foot. The metatarsophalangeal joints are held in extension and the interphalangeal joints in flexion. Callous formation is present under the metatarsal heads which may cause pain. As the condition is due to weakness of the lumbricals and interosseous muscles, exercises to strengthen these must be prescribed. The long muscles on the dorsum of the foot will have become shortened and the tendons may be prominent. This can lead to pressure problems on these tendons, so stretching of the muscles is also imperative. Corrective articulation of the joints of the foot, osteopathically, is also essential and improvement but seldom complete correction is expected within a few months. The aim has to be to correct the foot sufficiently for the requirements

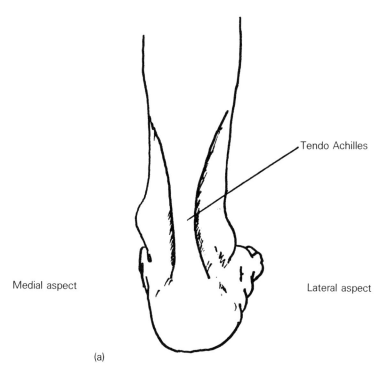

Tendo Achilles

Medial aspect

Lateral aspect

(a)

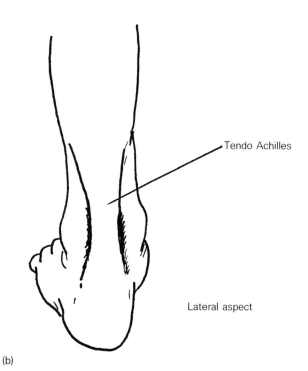

Tendo Achilles

Medial aspect

Lateral aspect

Fig. 13.14 (a) Pes planus tendo Achilles; (b) pes cavus tendo Achilles.

(b)

of the athlete and not to expect perfection. The callouses should be dealt with by a chiropodist.

Advice on suitable footwear in both cases of pes planus and pes cavus should emphasise the need for adequate support in the heel of the shoe. Cases of pes cavus are often seen wearing shoes which are too short. There may be an exostosis developing on the first metatarsal due to the cavus deformity and shoe pressure, and this should be padded to relieve the pressure if necessary.

The pronated gait is seen as a result of pes planus. There is eversion at the subtalar joint on weight bearing. There may be prominence of the navicular which can be subjected to pressure from footwear and a localised periostitis or the development of an adventitious bursa may result. The mechanics of sport, especially running, will be abnormal and can result in all sorts of clinical pictures, so it is imperative to examine the athlete completely, both weight bearing and non-weight bearing, to obtain a complete picture of his locomotive mechanism. In postural disorders it is often helpful to seek the assistance of other disciplines such as a physiotherapist or chiropodist who is conversant with orthotics.

The spring ligament may become stretched and painful. The athlete will complain of localised pain which is made worse by activities such as running. The pain will usually continue for some time after the activity ceases. It is particularly likely to occur in athletes who have a higher than average medial arch and/or short calf muscles. Clinically there will be pain on the extreme of passive movement at the midtarsal joint which will probably be limited in it's range of movement. Osteopathic correction of the range of movement and attention to the intrinsic muscles of the foot and to those of the calf will render the athlete symptom-free.

Plantar fasciitis is one of the commonest problems seen in long distance runners due to overuse, running on hard surfaces, inadequate footwear and possible inherent structural problems within the foot or leg. A runner with a high arch is the most likely to develop plantar fasciitis. The athlete complains of pain under the posterior part of the long arch of the foot which is made worse by running, standing or walking. A frequent complaint is pain felt immediately on adopting the upright position from sitting. The pain is immediately relieved by avoiding weight bearing. The pain may well have started some time ago and have been getting progressively worse. Continued strain of the fascia may result in periosteal damage to the calcaneum where the fascia is attached, and possible *spur* formation. Examination will reveal an area of tenderness under the calcaneum; usually the middle fibres of the fascia are affected as these are the thinnest. All movements of the joints of the ankle and foot are normal. Treatment consists of deep friction to the damaged fibres and correction of any predisposing conditions, for example attention to the pes cavus if present. A heel lift to take some of the strain off the fascia is useful. Recovery is often slow and may take several months.

Early *degenerative change* in the midtarsal area is a common condition. It may be secondary to some previous bony damage or it may come on for no apparent reason. The athlete most likely to suffer is the middle-aged person who has taken up long distance running late in life. Clinically there is loss of the full range of movement in the midtarsus and the symptoms will be relieved by strong articulation of the area and re-education of the muscles of the leg and foot to strengthen them sufficiently for the athlete's new requirements. Pain will be felt in the affected joints especially when running although the gentler pastime of walking may not produce symptoms. X-rays may show some degree of degeneration. Bony injury in the midtarsal area is not likely to be seen as a result of sport, the only possible exception being a direct injury such as a blow from a hard ball or one player falling on another. The possibility of a chip fracture must then be considered if the symptoms of fracture are present. X-rays will exclude such an injury and should be taken if any doubt exists in the osteopath's mind.

Pain in the region of the navicular bone in children may be due to osteochondritis, so called *Kohler's disease*. The young athlete is likely to be aged about 10, probably a boy and will complain of pain in the navicular region especially on athletic activity. All movements of the foot will be normal but the navicular may be tender and inflamed. Treatment consists of rest from athletics and possible strapping for a few weeks when the pain will subside and full activity can be resumed. There may be slight enlargement of the bone thereafter which occasionally gets pressurised by footwear. Padding can be advised to relieve this problem.

Facet locking may occur at any of the midtarsal joints; it may be due to some irregularity of gait, a sudden strain, some unaccustomed activity, ill-fitting footwear or even from some extrinsic force. The athlete will complain of pain especially on one or more movements and may know the cause of the problem. Correction of the mechanical fault is needed and any advice on footwear or corrective exercises should be given and seen to be carried out. It is wise to get an athlete to return for a checkup in about a month to make sure he has been carrying out the instructions he was given and to check that he is doing his part of the treatment correctly. This is both practical and psychologically useful as he feels that the osteopath still retains an interest in his case.

13.4   Metatarsal injuries

The joint between the medial cuneiform and the first metatarsal bone may be subjected to an acute inflammatory change. The athlete will usually be a young girl of about 15 who complains of pain on the dorsal aspect of the joint which has come on for no apparent reason. The pain is made worse by any pressure on the dorsal surface of the joint, for example from wearing lace up shoes. The condition may be bilateral. The severe pain lasts for about a week after which there is a bony protrusion present which may in turn give pain if pressurised and may need to be protected by a felt ring. The condition usually subsides spontaneously. An exostosis in men may appear at the same site and is usually caused by lacing shoes too tightly. Sports shoes should be laced such that there is no pressure over the exostosis yet they are still firmly fixed which is easily done by varying the holes through which the laces are passed possibly missing one out. Alternatively a ring pad may be prescribed or even two strips of chiropody felt, one on either side of the exostosis to take the pressure off.

Sudden twinges of acute pain may occur in athletes when running, especially sprinting. The pain is disabling and occurs regularly in every sprint but soon wears off afterwards. The athlete may describe the pain as similar to locking. Examination may not reveal any apparent abnormality and joint mobility may not be impaired. The condition resolves with traction-release techniques which suggests that there may have been some internal derangement.

The metatarsal bones are commonly *fractured*. There may be a history of an extrinsic force, stubbing the toe under the foot or there maybe nothing obvious. The fracture can occur at the base, the shaft, the neck or the head. Stress fractures can occur in any bone which is subjected to continuous trauma, so the metatarsals are likely candidates and the second and fourth are the most vulnerable. The athlete will complain of pain which is made worse by weight bearing and even worse if he tries to run or jump. There will be some swelling and usually an area of hyperaemia on the sole of the foot beneath the fracture. X-rays may not reveal the fracture if it is of the stress type until a few days after it has occurred when the callus starts to form. Treatment consists of supporting the foot with strapping and walking should then be possible even if somewhat uncomfortable. Union takes about six weeks. If the fracture is in the head of the metatarsal, a pad can be fitted to take some of the weight bearing strain off the lesion. The foot and leg should be checked for any residual mechanical problem after healing has occurred and before the athlete is advised to resume full activity. Frequently there is residual pain in the interosseous muscles which will have been traumatised; these respond well to deep soft tissue treatment.

Avulsion fractures are sometimes seen in the metatarsals. The commonest site is the tubercle of the fifth metatarsal due to the muscular pull of the peronei especially in severe ankle sprains. The long flexor and extensor tendons of the hallux may also occasionally cause an avulsion at their point of attachment to the toe. These can be seen on X-ray examination. Metatarsal fractures heal well but avulsions can cause problems and may need orthopaedic attention in athletes.

Pain may occur at the base of the fourth metatarsal bone where it is found to be slightly elevated on palpation and there is restriction of movement at the joint between it and the cuboid. This is caused by some compressive force applied along the line of the fourth metatarsal from it's distal part. It is common in athletes who do not wear footwear, for example certain martial artists and is seen in dancers and gymnasts. The condition is easily treated osteopathically by reducing what is in fact, a facet lock.

Osteochondritis may occur, usually in the second metatarsal head (but sometimes in the third). The athlete is aged about 14, usually a girl and she will complain of pain in the area on weight bearing especially if she puts her foot into full dorsiflexion, thus throwing the weight onto the metatarsal heads. The head of the bone will be enlarged and is palpably so, and tender. Pain may be felt on passive movements of the second metatarsophalangeal joint. X-rays show the head to be wider than normal and the neck of the bone thickened. The condition subsides without active treatment and rest is indicative. As the metatarsal head remains enlarged the condition predisposes to Morton's metatarsalgia but this may occur without osteochondritis, or Freiberg's disease as it is known, having occurred previously.

Morton's metatarsalgia is associated with a neuroma on one of the interdigital nerves. The condition is most frequently seen in women of middle age. Pain is felt at the site of the neuroma and distally from it, where there may also be paraesthesia. It can be severe. The pain is only felt when wearing shoes; clinically it can be reproduced by pressing the adjacent metatarsal heads together strongly. Some cases can be rendered symptom-free by placing a pad beneath the adjacent metatarsal heads thus holding them relatively apart but if this is not so, the neuroma will need surgical removal. This condition may well come on as a result of some unaccustomed physical activity, for example a middle-aged lady who starts running and may not have done so before. She may be aiming at marathons. Following surgery she will need to be given exercises to strengthen the intrinsic muscles of her foot and osteopathic treatment to mobilise the joints fully. Her posture may also need attention.

13.5   **Metatarsophalangeal injuries**

Metatarsalgia or pain felt under the metatarsal heads and in the metatarsophalangeal joints is very commonly seen in athletes. The commonest cause is a dropped metatarsal arch when the supporting ligaments become weight bearing and inflamed as may the metatarsal heads themselves. Dislocation of one or more of the meta-tarsal heads can also occur. The athlete has probably taken up some new running activity without due consideration of the mech-anical efficiency of the feet beforehand but he may have atonic feet which are a potential hazard to any athlete. Osteopathic treatment will need to include the athlete as a whole, with attention to posture, muscular strength and balance and joint mobility especially of the feet. Correction of a dropped metatarsal head should be followed by a supportive strapping while strengthening exercises are carried out, or the condition is liable to recur.

The first metatarsophalangeal joint suffers from two particular problems, namely hallux valgus and hallux rigidus. *Hallux valgus* is the condition where the first metatarsal approximates the lateral four toes. It is not normally painful unless complicated by the development of an adventitious bursa subcutaneously, or if there is shoe pressure on the deformity. Treatment is aimed at reducing the deformity by strengthening the abductor hallucis muscle and preventing shoe pressure by correct fitting and possible padding.

Hallux rigidus is more of a problem to athletes. It is usually a result of an acute idiopathic inflammation which occurs at the joint in adolescence or as a result of direct injury such as that experienced by repeated compression of the joint. This type of repeated com-pression can be caused by certain martial arts or by kicking balls when unsuitable footwear is worn. The joint becomes progressively more inflexible and is marginally inflamed and often tender to touch, especially on it's upper surface. The real problem arises when there is less than 15° of extension at the joint as this range is needed for walking; 25° is needed for running. If this range is reduced below these figures, the joint becomes strained with every step and an acute joint strain presents clinically. In some cases the range can be increased sufficiently for the athlete's needs and this movement must be encouraged daily by the athlete himself. Some cases, however, will require surgical treatment but it is always worth trying physical means first. Untreated the condition is progressive.

Fractures of the phalanges are sometimes seen in athletes when the foot has been subjected to a compression strain. The injured toe is strapped to its neighbour and healing takes about six weeks.

Dislocation of these joints occurs when the foot is subjected to a violent twist, or the dislocation may happen at the tarsometatarsal articulation. The first metatarsal is the most commonly dislocated and this may be associated with a fracture. The condition is serious as it may endanger the circulation of the foot and expert treatment is always necessary. Diagnosis is confirmed by X-ray examination.

Under the first metatarsophalangeal joint are two sesamoid bones which may become *inflamed* in athletes. The cause is invariably due to insufficient padding or protection on the sole of the foot from shoe or boot. Footwear is commonly worn out for this condition to occur. Pain is felt as the inflamed sesamoid is forced to take weight. Sometimes there is an associated rotation of the first metatarsal which will need correction but treatment is aimed at taking weight off the bone by means of padding until the inflammation subsides. A ring pad cut from thick chiropody felt suffices.

A *hammer toe* may cause problems to an athlete as it is subjected to shoe pressure. It is a deformity of fixed flexion at the proximal interphalangeal joint with hyperextension at the distal joint. Surgical correction may be needed if protective padding is not sufficient to stop shoe pressure.

The first metatarsophalangeal joint may be subject to attacks of *gout*, a condition far more commonly seen than is sometimes realised. The patient will complain of pain which is acute and the attack will have come on for no apparent reason. The joint swells and is warm to touch and the surrounding skin becomes reddened. The athlete is often middle-aged, but not always. Diagnosis depends on blood tests and treatment is medical.

A similar appearance of the joint may occur with *rheumatoid arthritis* but this condition is likely to affect more than one of the small joints of the body. Rheumatological investigation and treatment are required, so the athlete should be referred for further investigation. Whereas gout is more likely to affect men, rheumatoid arthritis is more often seen in female athletes, and possibly in a younger age group.

13.6

Skin injuries

The skin of the foot of the athlete is subjected to enormous pressures and athletes are notoriously negligent about routinely caring for their feet. Friction from ill-fitting footwear will produce *blisters* as could a spike pushing through from below. Spenco second skin is invaluable in treating these. See also section 12.11. Continuous pressure will eventually produce a *corn*; these should be treated by a chiropodist as should *verrucae*, also mentioned in section 12.11.

A foreign body may become *embedded* in the foot causing pain. Some are easily removed but others are difficult to locate exactly and should receive expert attention. Callouses form where there is undue pressure and should be treated by a chiropodist. The reason for the formation of a callus should be decided and the cause treated, for example a callus under the metatarsal heads in a case of pes cavus where the pes cavus needs treating osteopathically.

Areas of *hard skin* on the sole of the foot will demonstrate where the body weight is being distributed and can be helpful in weight bearing problems but the skin condition needs chiropody treatment. The so-called 'tennis toe' is seen in many athletes and can cause considerable discomfort. The condition is caused by sudden stops, quick changes of direction and moving sharply forwards, thus ramming the toes against the front of the inside of the shoe and small haemhorrages result under the toe nails, usually the big toe nail. This can cause pain, swelling and discolouration. If really acute, the haemhorrage may have to be released by puncturing the nail with a sterile needle. More commonly the condition is chronic.

Ingrowing toe nails are often a problem with athletes who invariably make the condition worse by cutting the nail away at the side. They are best treated by a chiropodist.

Most of these conditions are caused by incorrect footwear and sensible advice can be given to the athlete once the cause of the problem has been determined.

13.7

Shoes

Examination of the shoe is part of the examination of the foot of any athlete. The sole of the shoe will show any undue wear or uneven distribution of weight during the sporting activity. Examination of the inside of the shoe will reveal where pressure or friction has been put on the foot, for there will be areas of undue wear which can be felt. Most athletes are aware of the need for the correct footwear for the particular sport but it is still amazing that some people will wear the wrong type of shoe. As so much research has been put into footwear by manufacturers in recent years there is no excuse for athletes wearing incorrect shoes, and causing foot problems for themselves.

Chapter 14   The Head and Neck

14.1 **Introduction**

Before we consider this region of the body we should review the function of the cranium and vertebral column as a whole.

(1) This forms the central axis of the body, transmitting weight from the trunk to the pelvis and lower extremities.
(2) It provides a support for the head.
(3) It provides protection for the central nervous system.
(4) It has sufficient flexibility to enable movement to occur by means of a series of joints between each pair of adjacent vertebrae. The movement depends on muscular action.
(5) It has sufficient rigidity to provide the necessary support. The rigidity depends on bony strength and ligamentous support.
(6) It must have elasticity to withstand the various shocks which are imposed upon it especially during activities such as jumping and twisting. This elasticity is largely provided by the inter-vertebral discs and the A−P curves.

Normally the spine is straight in the vertical plane. If viewed from the side, the cervical spine is seen to curve forward, the thoracic backwards, the lumbar forwards and the sacral backwards. The cervical and lumbar curves are developmental and the others are primary (i.e. present at birth). See Figs. 4.10 and 4.11. There are variations within the 'normal' range of these curves and spinal function will be partially dependent on their integrity. In some athletes the spine curves from side to side when viewed from the back, a condition known as scoliosis. This may be generalised throughout the spine or localised to one region, for example in an athlete who partakes of a one-sided sport such as lawn tennis. In general, movement will be of a greater range when the concavity is exaggerated than when the convexity is exaggerated by active or passive movement. In addition the spine has to bend sideways when the whole of the body weight is taken on one leg as the pelvis tilts to the opposite side; the lumbar spine becomes concave on the side of the weight bearing leg and the reverse occurs in the thoracic area. The equality of this movement can be seen on standing examination and is important in the equalisation of the weight bearing strains during athletic activity.

A typical vertebra is made up of two parts, the body and the arch (see Fig. 14.1). The *body* is more or less cylindrical and

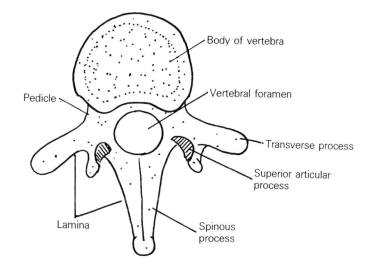

(a)

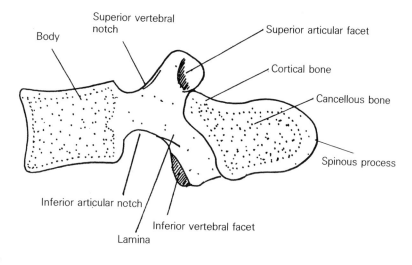

Fig. 14.1 A typical vertebra. (a) Superior aspect; (b) lateral aspect.

(b)

increases in size from the head down to the pelvis. The opposed surfaces of the bodies of adjoining vertebrae are firmly attached to the intervening intervertebral disc. The *arch* is composed of a pedicle on either side, which projects backwards. The lamina is a broad plate of bone which passes backwards and medially from the pedicle; the two laminae fuse to form the spinous process. Articular processes, two upper and two lower arise from the junction of the pedicle and lamina on each side. The transverse processes project laterally from the junction of the pedicle and lamina and serve for ligamentous and muscular attachment. In addition, in the thoracic region the transverse processes articulate with the ribs. The articular processes form the articular surfaces of the adjacent apophyseal joints.

Various ligaments connect the vertebrae (see Fig. 14.2). The *anterior longitudinal ligament* stretches from the basi-occiput above, to the sacrum below, on the anterior aspect of the spine and is attached to the bodies and the intervertebral discs. Similarly the *posterior longitudinal ligament* runs on the posterior aspect of the bodies and discs (i.e. it lies within the vertebral canal, anterior to the spinal cord). The *ligamentum flavum* is very strong and thick and connects adjacent laminae. The *interspinous ligament* connects adjacent spinous processes and is continuous posteriorly with the *supraspinous ligament* which is very strong in the cervical region.

The *intertransverse ligaments* connect adjacent transverse processes. Each apophyseal joint has a capsule which is reinforced by anterior and posterior ligaments. These ligaments form a strong link between the vertebrae throughout the vertebral column.

Each intervertebral disc consists of an outer fibrous 'annulus' and an inner soft pulpy 'nucleus'. Damage to the annulus can render a protrusion of the nuclear material. See Fig. 14.3.

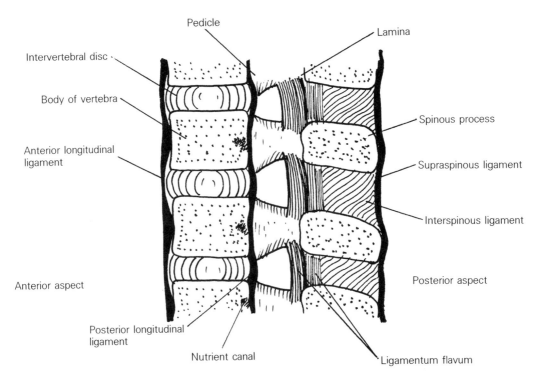

Fig. 14.2   Ligaments of the vertebral column: sagittal section.

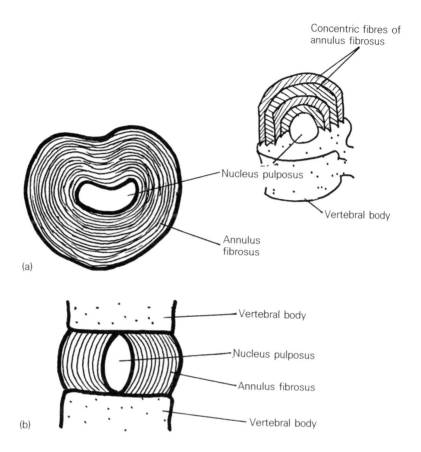

Fig. 14.3 An intervertebral disc. (a) Superior aspect; (b) median sagittal section.

Between each pair of vertebrae there is a foramen through which a segmental nerve passes. Every part of the skin and all muscles and joints are supplied by these nerves.

The sympathetic trunks are two gangliated nerve cords which extend from the base of the skull to the coccyx. In the neck, each trunk lies in front of the transverse processes of the cervical vertebrae, in the thoracic region on the heads of the ribs and in the lumbar region on the anterolateral aspect of the bodies of the lumbar vertebrae. There is ample evidence according to the work of Professor Korr that mechanical disturbances of the vertebral mechanics can influence the function of the sympathetic nervous system. In all sporting activities, especially when competition in undertaken, the sympathetic nervous system becomes vitally important − it is the 'flight and fright' system of the body. In addition there are several important ganglia in the chain, the most important being the three cervical ganglia. The superior cervical ganglion lies at the level of the second and third cervical vertebrae and supplies branches to the larynx, heart and cardiac plexus. The middle cervical ganglion lies at the level of the sixth cervical vertebra; branches run to the thyroid gland, the heart and the cardiac plexus. The inferior cervical plexus lies between the transverse process of the seventh cervical vertebra and the neck of the first rib and sends a branch to the heart and one which links with the vagus nerve (the tenth cranial nerve).

The movements which occur are flexion, extension, lateral flexion or side bending to both right and left and rotation to right and left.

The overall range of *flexion* of an 'average' athlete is greatest in the cervical and lumbar areas, as is extension, which is particularly marked in the lower cervical joints and lumbar joints. This degree of mobility lays these joints open to overstrain injuries more often than the less mobile joints of the spine. Flexion is brought about by the action of the anterior muscles and limited by tension in the posterior muscles and intervertebral ligaments.

Extension occurs due to the muscular action of the posterior muscles and is limited largely by tension in the anterior longitudinal ligament.

Lateral flexion is greatest in the thoracic area and approximately equal in the cervical and lumbar areas and is limited by tension in the antagonistic muscles and intervertebral ligaments. It is brought about by the unilateral action of the lateral spinal muscles.

Rotation is greatest in the thoracic region and only slight in the lumbar spine which lays this area open to rotational strains.

The range of movement is dictated by the plane of the facets of the apophyseal joints in general, and surrounding structures such as the ribs in the thoracic area which obstruct a wide range of lateral flexion in that region. Generally there is little individual movement between adjacent vertebrae but the summation of movement gives a relatively wide range throughout the column as a whole.

When assessing the spinal movements both actively and passively it is essential to note the quantity and quality of each, not only throughout the column but at each intervertebral level as well. This gives the osteopath a clinical picture of the spinal mechanics which can be related to the athlete's particular activity; some sports require a greater range of movement than others and some require flexibility in particular areas of the spine whereas other sports require less flexibility and more strength of muscle.

Head injuries

Injury to the head in sport is all too common especially in body contact sports or where a hard ball is used. A direct blow on the head or a fall which strikes the head on the ground or possibly a wall such as in enclosed court racket games may lead to bruising only, but this must never be assumed without further investigation to eliminate the possibility of fracture of the skull (or neck). A fracture to the base of the skull is usually caused by a severe blow on the mandible or a fall on the feet or coccyx, when the force is transmitted to the base of the skull. The history may be helpful but if the casualty is unconscious this may have to be elicited from another player. Unconsciousness occurs when there is injury to the brain. The casualty's eye may appear bloodshot or there may be blood or cerebrospinal fluid discharged from the ear, or blood from the nose or mouth. All such cases need urgent hospitalisation.

There are several causes of unconsciousness according to the St John Ambulance Association. Those which may occur at any time to an athlete are:

(1) Head injury
(2) Fainting
(3) Heart attack
(4) Epilepsy
(5) Hypoglycemia

Poisoning and a cerebrovascular accident are not likely to affect an athlete.

The association also gives guidelines for assessing the level of consciousness of an injured person and the level should be recorded at intervals of no more than five minutes, more often if this seems necessary. Carefully recording this level will show whether the athlete is recovering from his head injury or is getting worse which could imply that he may have a serious head injury.

The levels of responsiveness are:

(1) The patient may respond normally to both questions and conversation.
(2) The casualty may answer only direct questions.
(3) The casualty may respond only vaguely to questions.
(4) The casualty may obey direct commands.
(5) The casualty may respond to pain.
(6) The casualty may not respond at all.

Even mild cases of concussion should be treated seriously and the ten second rule should apply in all sports. The possibility of a complication such as a subdural haematoma must never be overlooked.

Other common sites of fracture are the mandible, zygoma and nose, again usually caused by a direct blow and in either case the patient may be suffering from some degree of unconsciousness.

Other injuries include damage to the teeth, ear or eye. Wearing adequate headgear or mouth guards will reduce the possibility of such an injury but will not eliminate it. Such protection is commonly used in boxing, cricket and American football but not in sports such as lacrosse or golf where there is a possibility of such an

injury from the ball. The commonest injury to the ear is the so-
called 'cauliflower ear' where there is a severe haematoma usually
due to direct injury. The possibility of an underlying fracture must
always be considered. All injuries to the eye should be considered
as serious and specialist treatment is always needed initially. Because
the eye is protected within the orbit, injury to the eye itself is not
too frequent. Foreign bodies may get into the eye in sports such as
football, horse riding or from sand bunkers on golf courses.
Abrasions of the cornea occur in sports such as water polo or
wrestling where there is the possibility of a finger getting into the
eye because of the close physical contact in the sport. The eye
becomes sore, red and waters a great deal and gets progressively
more painful. Injury to the orbit can occur from any small ball
moving at high velocity, such as in racketball or from a sharp
object such as a broken racket or string. There is immediate very
sharp pain and loss of vision, and haemorrhages or retinal tears
can be caused this way. All such injuries need expert attention as
soon as possible.

Following head injury there may be some residual problems
within the cranium, producing symptoms such as head pain, vertigo
etc. These cases respond well to osteopathic cranial treatment and
there is usually some disturbance of the cervical structures as well,
which will require osteopathic attention.

The *temperomandibular joint* warrants special mention as it is
sometimes damaged in sports, especially of the body contact type,
boxing in particular (see Fig. 14.4). Anatomically the joint is
divided into two parts by the articular disc which forms a mobile
socket for the head of the mandible. Inferiorly the disc is made up
of very thick, dense fibrous tissue and is attached to the posterior
margin of the head of the mandible. The superior portion is
fibro-elastic and is attached to the posterior wall of the mandibular
fossa of the temporal bone. The capsule is thin and loose, as the
range of movement of the joint is extensive. Medially the joint is
strengthened by the sphenomandibular ligament which is a flat
band running from the spine of the sphenoid bone to the lingula of
the mandibular foramen. Laterally the temperomandibular ligament
is attached above to the zygomatic process of the temporal bone
and below to the lateral surface and posterior portion of the neck
of the mandible. The parotid gland lies superficial to this ligament.
The stylomandibular ligament runs from the styloid process of the
temporal bone to the posterior border of the ramus of the mandible
(see Fig. 14.5).

Dislocation is not uncommon and can be reduced safely by
applying pressure to the lower back molar teeth and at the same
time raising the chin; this action overcomes the spasm in the
muscles of mastication. The joint becomes more vulnerable in the
absence of teeth. In close relationship to this joint lies the tympanic

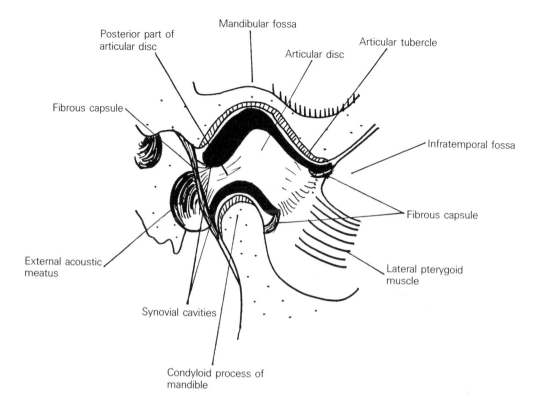

Fig. 14.4   Right temperomandibular joint, lateral aspect.

cavity which may be involved in damage to this area and inflammatory conditions of the joint may extend to the auditory mechanism. Dislocation may be unilateral or bilateral.

Sprain of the temperomandibular joint is not uncommon in sporting activity, especially where the skull is subjected to direct force of an extrinsic nature. The history will be clear; active movement may be painful and limited and there will be some swelling around the joint. Passive and resisted movements may also cause pain and the former may be limited by the intra-articular swelling. Treatment is aimed at reducing the swelling initially, by anti-inflammatories and/or ice packs. Localised treatment to the capsule, stylomandibular ligament and the surrounding muscles helps the condition to resolve; deep soft tissue treatment to the injured fibres is indicated and the condition usually resolves within a few weeks as healing is assisted by the rich blood supply to the area. Isometric exercises to the surrounding muscles are also helpful and active use of the joint can be encouraged by chewing gum.

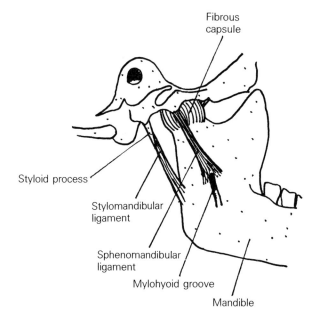

(a)

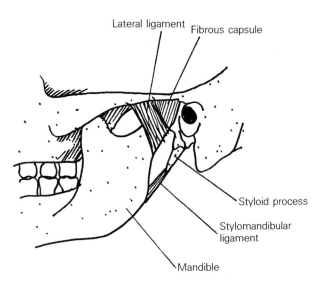

Fig. 14.5 The left temperomandibular joint and its ligaments. (a) Medial aspect; (b) lateral aspect.

(b)

14.2   **The neck**

Seven cervical vertebrae comprise the cervical spine (see Fig. 14.6). The first, the atlas (see Fig. 14.7), the second, the axis (see Fig. 14.8), and the seventh, the vertebra prominans (see Fig. 14.9) differ from the remaining four vertebrae which are similar to one another in structure. The cervical vertebrae are characterised by the presence of the foramen transversarium in each transverse process which transmits the vertebral artery and veins and a branch from the inferior cervical ganglion of the sympathetic trunk.

The first cervical vertebra, the *atlas*, has no body, as this part of

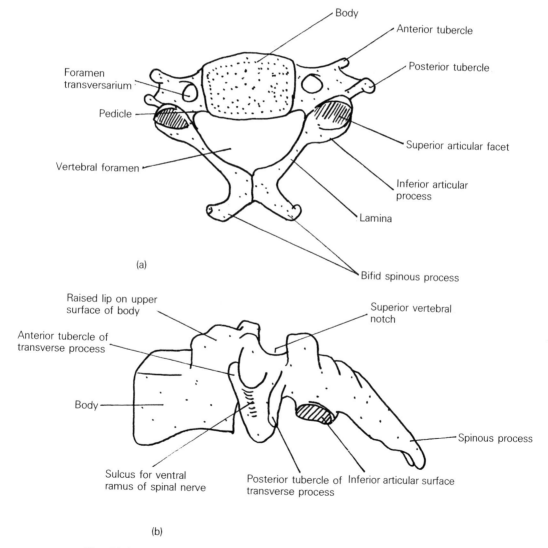

(a)

(b)

Fig. 14.6   A typical cervical vertebra. (a) Superior aspect; (b) left lateral aspect.

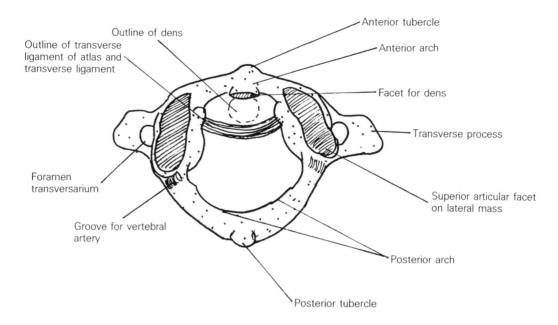

Outline of dens

Outline of transverse
ligament of atlas and
transverse ligament

Anterior tubercle

Anterior arch

Facet for dens

Transverse process

Foramen
transversarium

Groove for vertebral
artery

Superior articular facet
on lateral mass

Posterior arch

Posterior tubercle

Fig. 14.7 The atlas, first cervical vertebra, superior aspect.

the bone has fused to the second cervical vertebra, the axis. The atlas has no spine; it consists of two lateral masses connected by an anterior and a posterior arch. The transverse processes are long, providing adequate leverage for the rotational movements of the head. This is easily palpable between the mastoid process and the angle of the mandible.

The *axis* is characterised by the odontoid process which projects upwards from the body of the vertebra. It articulates with the facet on the posterior surface of the anterior arch of the atlas. The spine is large but the transverse processes are small. The spine provides attachment for muscles which extend the neck and for those which retract and rotate the head.

The *seventh cervical vertebra* is characterised by it's long spine which provides attachment for many muscles. The transverse processes are large and the anterior part of the transverse process may remain as a separate entity − a cervical rib − which will then articulate with the vertebra. Cervical ribs are more often present on the left than the right but may be bilateral. The occipito-atlantal joints are the articulations between the condyles of the occiput and the superior articular facets of the lateral mass of the atlas on each side (see Fig. 14.10). These joints often communicate with the median atlanto-axial joint which is the articulation between the odontoid process of the axis and the ring formed by the transverse ligament of the atlas and the anterior arch of that bone. In addition, there is a lateral atlanto-axial joint on each side, being

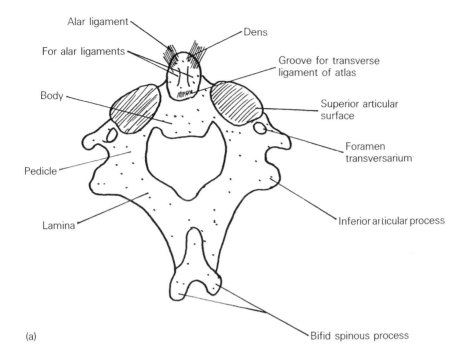

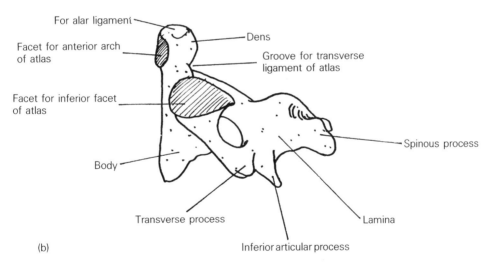

Fig. 14.8   The axis, second cervical vertebra. (a) Posterosuperior aspect; (b) left lateral aspect.

the joint between the inferior facet on the lateral mass of the atlas and the superior facet of the axis. Several ligaments reinforce the thin, loose capsules of these joints. They are:

(1) The apical ligament which runs from the tip of the odontoid process to the anterior margin of the foramen magnum.

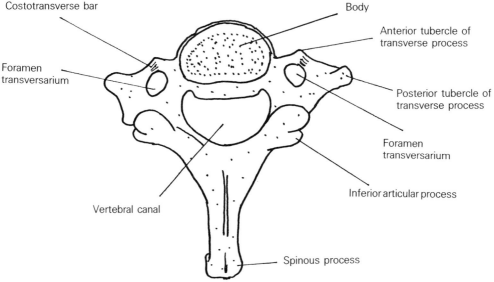

Costotransverse bar

Body

Anterior tubercle of
transverse process

Foramen
transversarium

Posterior tubercle of
transverse process

Foramen
transversarium

Inferior articular process

Vertebral canal

Spinous process

Fig. 14.9   Seventh cervical vertebra, superior aspect.

(2) The transverse ligament of the atlas which runs between the
    lateral masses of the atlas, posterior to the odontoid process
    and supporting and stabilising it. This is strengthened by the
    longitudinal bands which run upward to the anterior margin
    of the foramen magnum and downward to the posterior surface
    of the body of the axis.
(3) The cruciform ligament of the atlas, which is formed from the
    transverse ligament and the longitudinal bands.
(4) The alar ligaments, paired, which run from the odontoid
    process to the lateral margin of the foramen magnum on each
    side.
(5) The tectorial membrane which lies within the spinal canal; it
    is a prolongation of the posterior longitudinal ligament, fixed
    to the posterior surface of the body of the axis below, and
    above it is attached to the basilar part of the occiput where it
    blends with the cranial dura mater, a point of great importance
    in the art of treating patients by cranial osteopathic techniques.
(6) The anterior longitudinal ligament − see section 14.1.
(7) The posterior longitudinal ligament − see section 14.1.
(8) The ligamentum flava − see this section 14.1.
(9) The ligamentum nuchae which is very strong and is a continu-
    ation of the supraspinous ligaments of the thoracic area. It
    forms a septum between the muscles on either side of the
    neck.
(10) The interspinous ligaments which are not well developed in
    the neck.

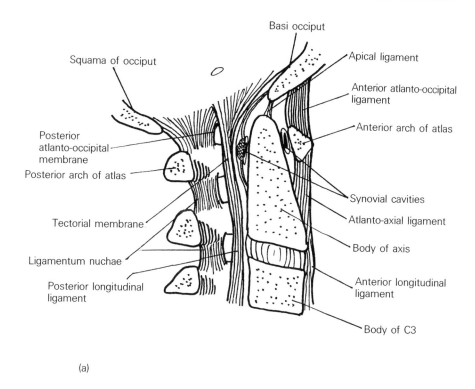

(a)

(b)

Fig. 14.10   (a) Atlanto- occipital joint, median sagittal section; (b) atlanto-axial joint, posterior aspect.

(11) The intertransverse ligaments which are also poorly defined in the neck.

In addition there are the *'uncovertebral' joints* of the cervical region (see Fig. 14.11). As the intervertebral disc does not reach the lateral margin of the vertebrae, a small synovial joint may develop on each side. This process occurs between the age of five and ten and is more or less complete by ten years of age. Initially this will add to the general flexibility of the cervical area but it is thought that it may predispose to cervical disc conditions later in life.

Flexion of the neck takes place at each vertebral level. The overall range is limited by the apposition of the mandible on the anterior thoracic wall. Flexion is brought about by the action of the anterior cervical muscles; unilateral contraction of these muscles also causes lateral flexion and/or rotation to occur (see Fig. 14.12). The deepest of these muscles is the *longus cervicis*, also known as the *longus colli* which consists of three groups of fibres. The superior oblique fibres arise from the anterior tubercles of the transverse processes of C5 to C2 inclusive and are inserted into the anterior tubercle of the atlas. The inferior oblique fibres arise from the bodies of T1 to T3 inclusive and are inserted into the anterior tubercle of the transverse process of C6. The medial fibres, deeper

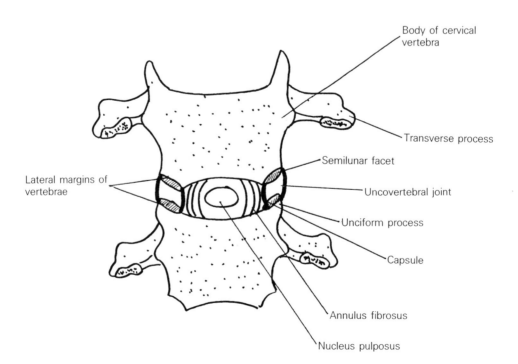

Fig. 14.11   An uncovertebral joint, frontal section.

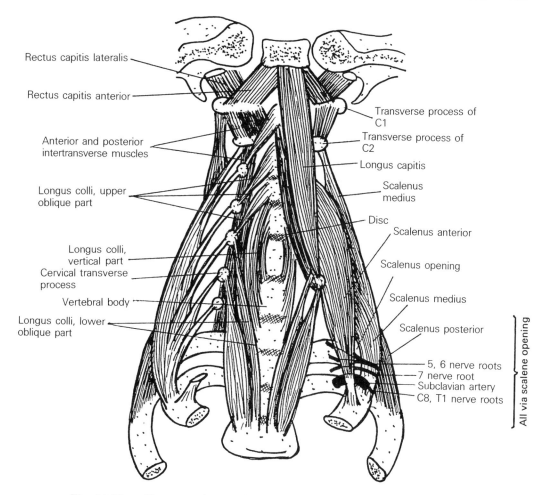

Rectus capitis lateralis

Rectus capitis anterior

Anterior and posterior
intertransverse muscles

Longus colli, upper
oblique part

Longus colli,
vertical part
Cervical transverse
process

Vertebral body

Longus colli, lower
oblique part

Transverse process of
C1
Transverse process of
C2
Longus capitis

Scalenus
medius

Disc
Scalenus anterior

Scalenus opening

Scalenus medius

Scalenus posterior

5, 6 nerve roots
7 nerve root
Subclavian artery
C8, T1 nerve roots

All via scalene opening

Fig. 14.12   Deep anterior cervical muscles with scalenus opening.

than the previous ones, run from the front of the bodies of T3 to
C5 inclusive and are inserted into the front of the bodies of C2 to
C4 inclusive. The nerve supply consists of the anterior primary
rami of C2 to C8.

This muscle is important in the maintenance of the cervical
posture. Bilateral contraction causes flexion of the cervical column
and unilateral contraction, forward and lateral flexion. When both
sides contract simultaneously they reduce the cervical curve.

Longus capitis arises from the anterior tubercles of the transverse
processes of C3 to C6 and is inserted into the inferior surface of
the basilar part of the occiput. It's nerve supply consists of the
anterior primary rami of C1 to C4. Bilateral contraction flexes the
head and unilateral contraction tilts the head sideways.

The *rectus capitis anterior* arises from the lateral mass of the
atlas and is inserted into the basilar part of the occiput. It's action

is to flex the head. It's nerve supply consists of the anterior primary rami of C1 and C2.

The *hyoid bone* lies anterior to the above group of muscles. Four muscles run from the skull to the hyoid, all of which are associated with swallowing, mastication and speech and none of which is directly involved in sport (see Fig. 14.13). The four muscles which arise from the hyoid and are inserted below the bone are weak flexors of the neck and the omohyoid muscle is involved in prolonged inspirational efforts, as in sport.

The *omohyoid* consists of an inferior and a superior belly which are connected by an intervening tendon. The superior belly arises from the body of the hyoid bone and the fibres pass obliquely downwards ending in the aforementioned intermediate tendon. The inferior belly passes from this tendon downwards and laterally to become attached to the scapula just medial to the suprascapular notch. The intermediate tendon lies on the internal jugular vein

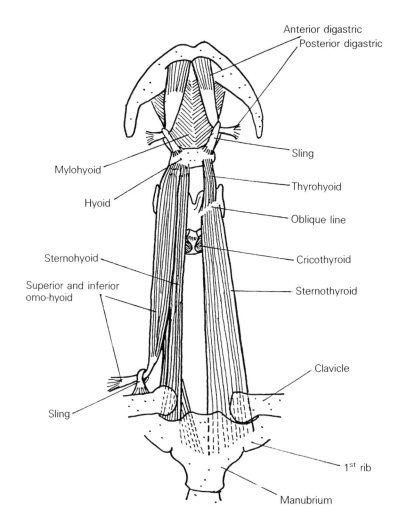

Fig. 14.13 The infrahyoid muscles.

where it is held in position by a band of the deep cervical fascia which is in turn attached to the clavicle and first rib. The nerve supply consists of the hypoglossal nerve. The *sternohyoid muscle* arises from the posterior surface of the manubrium (of the sternum) and from the sternoclavicular joint. It is inserted into the upper margin of the posterior surface of the hyoid. It's nerve supply consists of the hypoglossal nerve. The *sternothyroid muscle* closely invests the thyroid gland. It arises from the posterior surface of the manubrium and is inserted into the thyroid cartilage. It's nerve supply consists of the hypoglossal nerve. The *thyrohyoid* is a continuation of the sternothyroid muscle, arising from the thyroid cartilage and is inserted into the posterior surface of the hyoid bone. It's nerve supply consists of the hypoglossal nerve.

All these four muscles are responsible for lowering the hyoid bone and for stabilising the laryngeal cartilages. Their efficiency is partly dependent on the correct mobility of the hyoid and the balance of the action of the supra- and infrahyoid muscles.

Together with the omohyoid, the trapezius, sternocleidomastoid and levator scapulae muscles attach the neck to the shoulder girdle (see Fig. 14.14). *Trapezius* is a flat triangular muscle covering the back of the neck and shoulder. The descending part arises from the superior nuchal line, the external occipital protuberance and the ligamentum nuchae and is inserted into the lateral one-third of the clavicle. The transverse part, or horizontal fibres, arises from the spinous processes of C7 to T3 and from the supraspinous ligaments and is inserted into the acromial tip of the clavicle, the acromion process and the superior lip of the spine of the scapula. The ascending portion of the muscle arises from the spines of T2 to T12 inclusive and from the supraspinous ligaments and is inserted into the spinal trigone and the adjacent part of the spine of the scapula. It's nerve supply consists of the accessory nerve and C2, C3 and C4. The primary function of trapezius is to stabilise the shoulder girdle (in association with other muscles) and so it is important in the postural maintenance of the shoulder, especially in all active use of the arm. It is frequently unilaterally overdeveloped in athletes who partake of one-sided sports. When the shoulder is fixed, trapezius extends the neck; it elevates the scapula and point of the shoulder when acting with levator scapulae; acting with serratus anterior it rotates the scapula forward so that the arm can be raised above the head, while in conjunction with the rhomboids it rotates the scapula posteriorly and braces the shoulder backwards. See section 6.10.

Sternocleidomastoideus forms a prominent visible landmark across the side of the neck. The sternal head arises from the upper part of the anterior surface of the manubrium sterni. The clavicular head arises from the anterior surface of the middle one-third of the clavicle. As the two heads ascend, the clavicular head blends with

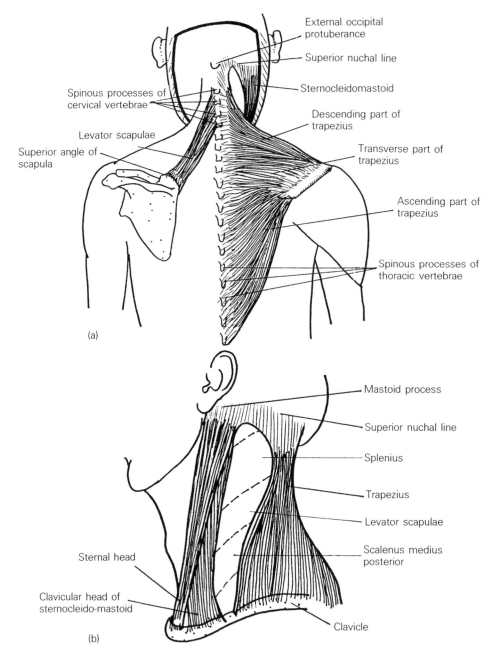

Fig. 14.14   The trapezius, levator scapulae and sternocleidomastoid muscles. (a) posterior aspect; (b) left lateral aspect.

the deep surface of the sternal head and the muscle is inserted by means of a strong tendon into the lateral surface of the mastoid process and the superior nuchal line of the occiput. It's nerve supply consists of the accessory nerve and C1 and C2 from the cervical plexus. Unilateral action of the muscle rotates the head to the opposite side and bilateral contraction lifts the head. The condition known as 'wry neck' is due to contraction of the muscle as a result of direct irritation of the fibres or of the nerve supply. Spasm of the muscle is commonly seen, especially with a similar condition of the trapezius.

The *levator scapulae muscle* lies at the back and side of the neck. It arises from the transverse processes of C1 to C4 inclusive. It passes downward to be inserted into the medial border of the scapula close to the medial end of the spine of that bone. It's nerve supply consists of C3, C4 and C5. If the shoulder is fixed, this muscle acts as a side bender of the neck. Acting with trapezius, when the cervical spine is fixed it will elevate the shoulder and assist in the action of carrying a weight on the shoulder.

The *scalene muscles* lie on the lateral aspect of the neck. The *scalenus anterior* lies deep, behind sternomastoideus. It arises from the transverse processes of C3 to C6 inclusive, descends almost vertically and is inserted by means of a tendon into the scalene tubercle of the first rib. It's nerve supply consists of the anterior primary rami of C4, C5 and C6. Acting from below, this muscle flexes the neck while acting from above, it elevates the first rib. Unilaterally it rotates the neck towards the opposite side.

The *scalenus medius* is the largest and longest of the scalenes. It arises from the posterior tubercles of the transverse processes of C2 to C7 inclusive. It is inserted into the first rib behind the groove for the subclavian artery. It's nerve supply consists of the anterior primary rami of C4 to C8. Acting from above, this muscle acts as a neck flexor, from below it raises the first rib and unilaterally it acts to side bend the neck to the same side.

The *scalenus posterior* is the smallest and deepest of the scalenes. It arises from the posterior tubercles of the transverse processes of C4, C5 and C6 and is inserted by a thin tendon into the outer surface of the second rib. It's nerve supply consists of the anterior primary rami of C6–C8. It acts as a flexor of the lower part of the neck; acting from below it helps to elevate the second rib and unilaterally it acts to side bend the neck when the second rib is fixed.

The scalene opening lies between the scalenus anterior and the scalenus medius. Passing through this opening are the subclavian vessels and the brachial plexus which can be pressurised by conditions of these muscles. Retroversion of the arm may also occlude the vessels and/or irritate the nerves.

On the posterior aspect of the neck, under cover of the trapezius, lies the *splenius capitis* muscle. It arises from the spinous processes of C4 to T3 and the adjacent part of the ligamentum nuchae, and is inserted into the mastoid process. The splenius cervicis is longer and larger. It arises from the spinous processes of T3 to T6 and is inserted into the transverse processes of C1 and C2. It's nerve supply consists of the dorsal rami C1 to C8. The two splenius muscles act together as supporting muscles of the erect posture. Bilateral contraction will produce cervical extension and unilaterally, rotation to the same side. See Fig. 14.15.

Lying between the transverse processes in this area are two muscles. The *longissimus capitis* arises from the transverse processes of C5 to T5 and is inserted into the mastoid process. The *longissimus cervicis* arises from the upper six thoracic transverse processes and is inserted into the posterior tubercles of the transverse processes

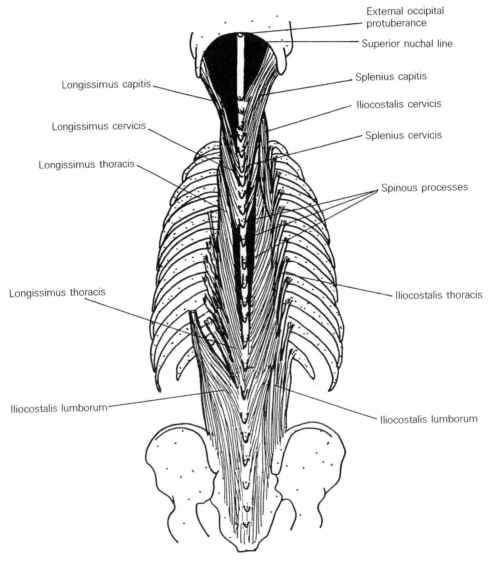

Fig. 14.15   Intrinsic muscles of the back (lateral tract).

of C2 to C5. The nerve supply to both muscles is from the dorsal rami of C2 to T5. These, too, are largely postural muscles but in addition, act as extensors of the neck. See Fig. 14.15.

The *interspinales* are arranged intersegmentally between the adjacent spinous processes and are especially well developed in the neck. The intertransversarii are similarly segmentally arranged between the transverse processes and are well developed between C2 and C7. The nerve supply is segmental from the dorsal rami. These muscles act largely in maintaining the postural integrity, but can also assist in cervical extension.

The *rotatores* are poorly defined in the neck; each is segmentally arranged running from the transverse process of one vertebra to the adjacent or next but one spinous process. The *multifides* are also small segmental muscles which arise from the articular processes of the lower four cervical vertebrae and pass upward to be inserted into the spinous process of two to four vertebrae above.

The *semispinalis cervicis* arises from the transverse processes of the upper five or six thoracic vertebrae and the fibres are inserted into the spinous processes of the upper five cervical vertebrae (see Fig. 14.16). The *semispinalis capitis* is one of the strongest muscles of the neck; it arises from the tips of the transverse processes of the upper six or seven thoracic vertebrae and the lower four cervical vertebrae and is inserted into the occiput between the superior and inferior nuchal lines. It's nerve supply consists of the dorsal rami. The semispinalis muscles are strong extensors of the neck when acting together and side benders when acting unilaterally. The rotatores and multifides act as rotators.

The *suboccipital muscles* act on the head joints (see Fig. 14.17). Bilateral contraction causes cervical extension and unilateral contraction causes side bending to occur. The *rectus capitis posterior major* runs from the spine of the axis to the lateral part of the inferior nuchal line of the occiput. Unilaterally it acts as a rotator of the head to the same side. The *rectus capitis posterior minor* arises from the tubercle on the posterior arch of the atlas and is inserted into the medial part of the inferior nuchal line of the occiput. It acts solely as an extensor of the head. The *oblique capitis inferior* arises from the lateral surface of the spine of the axis and is inserted into the lower part of the transverse process of the atlas. It acts as a rotator of the head and has a good mechanical advantage due to the length of the transverse process of the atlas. The *oblique capitis superior* runs from the upper surface of the transverse process of the atlas to be inserted into the occiput between the two nuchal lines. The nerve supply of all the suboccipital muscles is dorsal ramus of C1.

Rectus capitis lateralis runs from the transverse process of the atlas to the occiput and acts to side bend the head. It's nerve supply is C1.

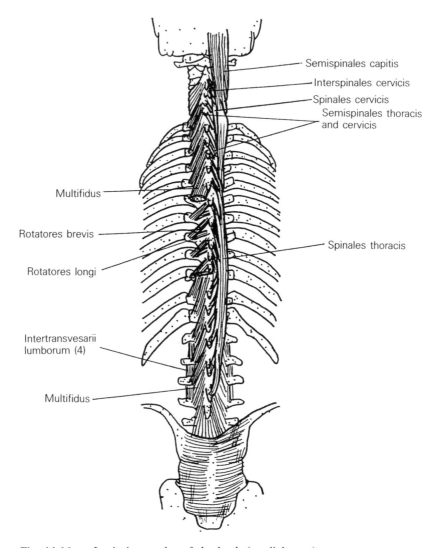

Fig. 14.16   Intrinsic muscles of the back (medial tract).

The *anterior intertransversarii cervicis* are small bundles of muscle which run between the anterior protuberances of the transverse processes of the cervical vertebrae and act as stabilisers of the neck.

The *posterior serratus superior* arises from the lower two cervical vertebrae from their spinous processes and is inserted into the second to fifth ribs, acting as an elevator of these ribs. It's nerve supply consists of the intercostal nerves, T1 to T4.

To sum up, flexion is brought about by the contraction of the anterior cervical muscles and is limited by the apposition of the mandible on the anterior chest wall. Segmentally the movement is limited by tension in the posterior ligaments and muscles. Extension

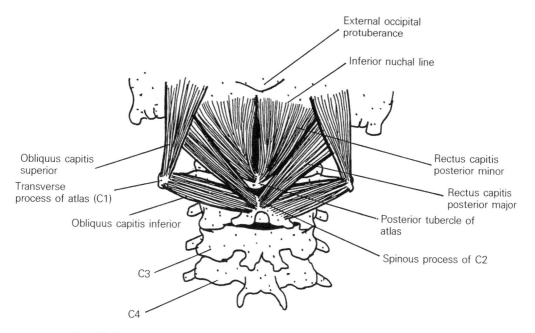

Fig. 14.17   The suboccipital muscles.

is brought about by the bilateral contraction of the posterior muscles and is limited by tension in the anterior structures. The range increases in the lower cervical segments and hypermobility is not unusual in C6/7 and C5/6. The exact range of movement at each joint can be assessed by palpation and from mobility X-rays. Side bending is brought about by the unilateral action of the lateral muscles and is limited by tension in the opposing muscles and in the ligaments, as is rotation. It must be appreciated that side bending is always accompanied by rotation and vice versa, as neither movement is pure in the neck due to the anatomical conformity of the joints. Most of the short muscles are principally postural whereas the long muscles are prime movers. It is the long muscles which are most often traumatised in sport, thus limiting the range of movement which is possible.

14.3   **Muscle injury**

The majority of muscle injuries in the neck are complications of joint injury or are accompanied by some joint involvement. Anterior muscle injury is unusual but can occur as a result of direct injury. Insidious posterior muscle injury is often accompanied by poor development of the anterior musculature so that the cervical curve becomes accentuated and injury is more likely. Many amateur athletes spend time strengthening the posterior muscles without

Table 14.1 Muscles
of the neck supplied
by the cervical nerves

	Anterior primary rami	Posterior primary rami
C1	Rectus capitis anterior Longissimus capitis Infrahyoid muscles	Rectus capitis posterior Oblique inferior Semispinalis capitis
C2	Longissimus capitis Longissimus cervicis Sternocleidomastoideus Infrahyoid muscles	Oblique inferior Semispinalis capitis Longissimus capitis
C3	Longissimus capitis Longissimus cervicis Scalenus medius Infrahyoid muscles Levator scapulae Trapezius	Semispinalis capitis Splenii and deep muscles of back of neck
C4	Longissimus capitis Longissimus cervicis Scalenus medius Levator scapulae Diaphragm	Semispinalis capitis Splenii and deep muscles of back of neck
C5	Longissimus cervicis Scalenes	Deep muscles of back of neck
C6	Longissimus cervicis Scalenus medius Scalenus posterior	Deep muscles of back of neck
C7	Scalenus medius	Deep muscles of back of neck
C8		Deep muscles of back of neck

the necessary attention being paid to the anterior muscles of the
neck. This development of the posterior muscles also tends to
shorten them and some time should be spent on stretching, in
order to lengthen them.

Because of the complexity of the muscular arrangement in the
neck, muscular problems invariably affect more than one muscle at
a time.

Trapezius is the most superficial muscle, posteriorly, and covers
a large area. It is often seen in spasm; the athlete will complain of
pain in the area of the muscle and active use of the arm may be
painful as well as cervical extension. The area which is causing
symptoms is easily palpated, most often the horizontal fibres. The
muscle responds well to soft tissue treatment especially if this is
given cross-fibre (remembering the different directions of the fibres).
The use of a rubifacient is also helpful but ice treatment may be
indicated if there is joint involvement. Rest from all active sports
which involve use of the arm is necessary until the problem has
resolved. Osteopathic examination and treatment of all the cervical

joints and all those of the thoracic spine which need attention is also necessary, together with the shoulder joint and the acromio-clavicular and sternoclavicular joints. This muscle seems to be particularly sensitive to exposure to cold and may be irritated in sports played in cold weather, more particularly if it is windy and the athlete has insufficient clothing. In sports such as golf which is not as active as sports such as football, a pure silk scarf will protect the player from the elements.

Lying on the side of the neck is the *sternocleidomastoid muscle* which is also involved (with trapezius) in the stability of the shoulder girdle and clavicle. It is a strong rotator of the neck, an activity which is necessary in most sports. It is, therefore, fairly commonly injured. The athlete may say that he awoke with the problem, probably the day after some sporting activity. He will complain of pain especially when rotating the neck − in fact he may be unable to do so. Rest and warmth are indicated, initially, and deep soft tissue treatment, again cross-fibre. The mechanics of the clavicle are often overlooked as a contributory or causative factor and must be corrected if necessary. The neck joints must also be checked out, especially the occipito-atlantal and atlantoaxial areas. Like problems affecting trapezius, this muscle is often injured by overuse of the arm, not only neck rotation.

Similarly, *levator scapulae* is often injured by overuse of the arm. Like the previous muscles it can be easily palpated, especially at its point of insertion into the scapula. Treatment is as for the two previous muscles and in this case must include correction of any restriction of scapular rotation. All these muscles are commonly injured when the athlete has been using weights, probably without adequate guidance. This group of muscles is also involved in sports which include throwing and any which involves the use of the arm above the head − i.e. many ball games.

The *scalene muscles* lie on the side of the neck and are attached below to the first and second ribs. They are, therefore, accessory muscles of respiration and assist movement of these ribs during full inspiration. Strong use of the arm above the horizontal will cause these ribs to be elevated, for example in volleying at tennis. The muscles are frequently strained. The athlete will complain of pain, aggravated by neck flexion and rotation to the opposite side from the injury. Palpation may reveal that the first and/or second ribs are elevated (facet locked) and the rib(s) will not depress during full expiration. Usually all three scalenes are involved. As the brachial plexus and subclavian vessels pass through the scalene opening between scalenus anterior and scalenus medius, the athlete may well complain of symptoms of pressure on these structures. Nerve irritation to the whole of the plexus is the commonest complaint and in fact this is the site where such irritation to the *whole* plexus most commonly occurs. It is, therefore vital to take a very careful history and obtain a clear clinical picture so that this condition is not confused with a possible foraminal irritation or even a carpal tunnel syndrome. The former will give symptoms indicative of *one* nerve root being irritated and the latter of the median nerve − *not* the whole plexus. Treatment will be aimed at the joints of the neck, upper thoracic area and upper ribs as well as local soft tissue treatment to the muscle(s). All use of the arm above the horizontal level is contraindicated until the condition has been successfully treated. The patient can assist recovery by passively stretching the muscle(s) himself, to the point of discomfort but not to the point of pain.

The *posterior serratus superior* lies more posteriorly than the scalene muscles but it too is involved in respiration as it helps elevation of the second to fifth ribs inclusive. It is a deep muscle and also acts as an extensor of the neck, so may be injured in forced flexion strains, for example in body contact sports. The athlete will complain of a deep pain in the lower cervical and upper thoracic areas which may be aggravated by full inspiration. Rest, deep soft tissue treatment and correction of any joint problems will assist recovery.

Deep to the trapezius lie the *splenii*. These are also often involved in neck problems and the athlete will complain of pain on extension and rotation of the neck to the same side as the injured muscle(s).

The *longissimi* may be injured with other extensor muscles of the neck; it is virtually impossible to differentiate exactly which of these deep extensor muscles is injured and in fact, invariably more than one will be injured at any one time, again probably from forced flexion in body contact sports.

Similarly the *semispinales*, being strong muscles, may be injured. As the semispinalis arises from as low down as the seventh thoracic vertebra it is essential in all posterior muscle conditions of the neck to check the joint integrity as far as T7. Injury to the semispinales will also give pain on side bending.

The *suboccipital muscles* are at risk in compression injuries of the neck, for example when heading a ball in football or following a fall onto the head or a direct blow to it. The upper cervical area will usually be held in extension or possibly rotation and will be painful. The increased tone of the muscles involved is easy to palpate. Soft tissue treatment can be given but this may be difficult, in which case gentle occipital springing will help to relieve the spasm. The underlying joints must be checked for their mobility and corrected as necessary.

The *infrahyoid muscles* may be hypertonic; this is usually due to hypermobility of the hyoid which should be articulated as necessary to relieve the condition. If these muscles are involved in a neck condition they are unlikely to be a primary injury but secondary to other muscles being traumatised.

Severe spasm of the *cervical muscles* occurs not uncommonly; it can be extremely painful in which case a collar, muscle relaxants and anti-inflammatories may be needed to relieve the condition. A collar can be improvised with tubigrip and foam rubber.

14.4 **Bone injury**

Fortunately bony injuries of the neck are relatively rare but the consequences can be serious due to the vulnerability of the spinal cord. Instability of a vertebral injury involving the bone will accompany tearing of the posterior longitudinal ligament, thus rendering the cord vulnerable.

The spinous process of C7 may be *avulsed* due to muscular action. The condition can be very painful due largely to the muscle spasm which results, but the condition is not serious and usually requires treatment as for a muscle injury rather than a bony one.

A straight compression injury such as a fall onto the head, for example from a horse, can cause a *fracture* of a vertebral body. The intervertebral disc may be injured as well, if the force is great enough, and then disc material may be forced into the fracture site. An extension force, for example by diving into shallow water will damage the neural arch but not the posterior ligaments. This is most likely to occur at the upper two cervical levels. If the odontoid peg is fractured, the injury is of the unstable type. Extreme forced extension can fracture the vertebral body, usually posteriorly, thus endangering the cord, directly. Extension may tear the anterior longitudinal ligament without fracturing a bone. Due to the possibility of serious damage, all head injuries which are accompanied by concussion should be X-rayed for both head and neck damage the possibility of which must never be overlooked.

Neck fracture may be suggested by some unusual position of the neck. Movement of the casualty is dangerous and should not be attempted. Palpation is seldom useful as with all neck injuries there will be severe muscle spasm. A fracture cannot be palpated in this area. The athlete may complain of neurological symptoms in one or more of his limbs where it may be possible to elicit neurological signs. All suspect cases must be referred as soon as possible for further investigation. Rotational forces are usually serious as the posterior ligaments are likely to be damaged and dislocation is therefore more likely to occur. Forced flexion injuries, as can occur in rugby can also damage the posterior ligaments. Other possible causes are falls, for example from a horse or bicycle when the athlete rotates his neck as he hits the ground.

The common sites of fracture in the neck are: the neural arches of C1 or C2, the odontoid process of C2, the bodies of C3 to C7 and any of these may be accompanied by dislocation.

Once the fracture has healed, the athlete is likely to have some residual symptoms, usually from joint strains which happened at the same time as the fracture. Osteopathic treatment to these areas is essential before the athlete resumes his normal sporting activity. Any re-education of the musculature should be carried out, too.

Congenital deformities are usually of little importance but if present in the neck, may increase the chance of bony injury to the area. They are usually discovered when X-rays are taken, possibly following injury. Fusion of vertebrae, especially in the midcervical region, the presence of a spina bifida, usually in the lower cervical region, or the presence of cervical ribs should serve to dissuade the athlete from all sports where the neck is at risk from injury. Such sports as gymnastics or body contact sports will put such an athlete at too much risk and he should be cautioned as to the risk he is taking thereby.

Cervical ribs may produce their own symptom picture as they frequently pressurise the brachial plexus and/or the subclavian vessels as they pass into the arm. In fact the picture may resemble that of the scalene muscles being hypertonic. The presence of these ribs is usually suspected by the abnormal contour of the shoulder and if present, the rib(s) can be easily palpated. Pressure over the rib may reproduce the symptoms of which the athlete is complaining. Osteopathic treatment of the area is most effective; the adventitious joint may be subject to some facet locking condition, which, if treated will render the athlete symptom-free, but he may well get recurrent trouble as the rib(s) are still present. Surgical removal is not warranted but neck straining sports are contraindicated. The ribs will show on X-ray unless bony, not if they are cartilagenous. Similar symptoms may arise from unusually long transverse processes on C7. If the whole of the plexus is not affected, it is most commonly the ulnar nerve distribution which is.

14.5   **Disc injuries**

Disc injury is most likely to result from some sudden unguarded movement, a direct force to the head, or from some force upward through the arm to the neck. The former cause is probable in sports such as tennis, the second from heading the ball in football, while the last from falling or by striking the ground instead of the ball, in golf.

The patient will say that the pain came on quite suddenly, possibly following compression to the neck, a sudden movement, or a force upward from the arm. The neck will be painful and possibly held in flexion and/or side bending (away from the side of the pain). There may be symptoms of pain, tingling or paraesthesiae into the arm along the distribution of one cervical root (seldom is more than one root affected). Active extension and side bending towards the side of the pain will exacerbate it and flexion with side bending to the opposite side will relieve it. Passive movement will be limited at the level of the lesion and compression at that level will aggravate the pain. There may be a reflex change in the arm, possible loss of sensation but muscle weakness is rare in the arm. The commonest level for a cervical disc lesion is C7, followed by C6; upper cervical disc lesions are rare. Disc injury without any neurological symptoms in the arm may also occur; it is only if any protrusion or swelling of the disc is in the area of the nerve root that the athlete will complain of arm pain. It is wise to treat all cases of neck pain in which the symptoms are exacerbated by gentle compression, as disc injuries.

Treatment consists of traction with articulation as possible. Any high velocity thrust work should be avoided until the acute phase has passed. The athlete should be advised to place his head in the most comfortable position before going to sleep at night as this will enable him to get maximum rest with minimum pain. In very acute cases, a collar may be helpful and reduce the pain. The acute phase lasts about 10 to 14 days, after which corrective osteopathic treatment can be started. Full recovery, when the athlete is fit for full sporting activity may take as long as three months, but even after full recovery, he should be advised against further neck compression. Full mobility should render him safe for activities which do not risk compression; if golf was the cause, a few lessons might reduce the risk of further similar injury!

A severe cough or sneeze may also injure a cervical disc; the symptoms will be similar but the history different. Should the athlete know he is subject to attacks of 'hay fever', it may be wise to suggest he does not expose himself to pollen or whatever aggravates his mucous membranes. Tennis players may be less at risk on hard rather than grass courts.

Disc injuries predispose to degenerative changes in the apophyseal joints. Full restoration of mobility seems likely to reduce the risk, so osteopathic treatment is indicated in all cervical disc cases. Occasionally the case is of intractable pain. Other, more serious causes must be considered then, or the possibility of surgical treatment but this is comparatively rare in the neck.

14.6

Joint and ligament injuries

Injury to the *apophyseal joints* in the neck is extremely common in athletes. It is usually caused by some sudden movement when locking of the articular facets results. The history is usually clear and seldom is there any neurological involvement but there may be severe pain. There will be muscle spasm of a protective nature and loss of one or more active movements. Passive movement will be lost or limited in the same range. There will be palpable swelling over the affected apophyseal joint and often more than one joint is affected. To osteopaths, the 'feel' of such a joint is classic, and osteopathic treatment to the joint itself and to the surrounding soft tissues will render the athlete symptom-free.

Facet locking of the *upper cervical joints* is often accompanied by head pain, usually worse first thing in the morning. Relief results from normalising the mechanics of the area. All such conditions may be accompanied by abnormalities in the upper thoracic area, which should always be examined and treated as well as the neck. The athlete can resume full activity when the mechanics are normal again and a full range of movement is restored. This type of case is very often seen in active people; it seems unlikely that anyone is immune, but restriction of movement may not be noticed in an inactive person.

Spondylosis in the cervical area will render the joints more easily strained, but it does not contraindicate treatment if facet locking has occurred. These athletes, who are somewhat older, will benefit from daily exercises to keep the area as flexible as possible and the soft tissues well stretched. Degeneration of the lower cervical apophyseal joints occurs prematurely in athletes who have an increased cervical curve. This is usually secondary to an increased thoracic kyphosis. In these cases it is obviously imperative to increase the thoracic mobility and attempt to reduce the kyphosis in order to reduce the cervical curve and the strain on the cervical joints.

Forced extension of the neck can damage the *anterior longitudinal ligament*, the sort of injury which can result from the collapse of the scrum in rugby. However it is comparatively rare as usually one or more joints and/or discs take the brunt of the force. Repeated extension injury, especially of the lower cervical area can render a joint hypermobile. This is in extension, and can be palpated or demonstrated on mobility films. It is difficult to treat and the best approach is to prescribe exercises to strengthen the anterior muscles. Any other hypermobile joint should be treated to take as much stress off the hypermobile one as possible. Some hypermobile joints require a few weeks in a collar to reduce movement.

Dislocation occurs occasionally in the neck and can be very serious. It can only occur if either the posterior or the anterior longitudinal ligament is torn. This will occur in forced flexion or forced extension. Following such an injury it must be assumed that a dislocation has occurred until such time as the possibility has been eliminated by X-ray examination. Plates will be taken in full flexion and full extension when the dislocation will show, if present. These cases require specialist treatment but once the dislocation is reduced and stabilised, osteopathic treatment to the affected area and the surrounding areas is most helpful and will relieve any residual symptoms.

14.7   **Blood vessel injury**

The subclavian vessels can be pressurised by the presence of a cervical rib or extra long transverse processes of C7, or by a hypertonic condition of the scalene muscles. In either case there will probably be associated symptoms of pressure on the brachial plexus. Pressure on the vessels may give rise to some degree of ischaemia in the arm, or even paraesthesiae. There may be some congestive swelling of the limb, blueness and coldness of the fingers. The athlete is likely to be a lady in her early thirties, and her symptoms will be made worse by any sporting activity. Osteopathic treatment to the offending rib and/or costovertebral area will invariably relieve the symptoms. Sport which involves strong use of the arm above the head may well cause recurrence.

Injury to the neck is considered to possibly implicate the vertebral artery blood flow. Compression of the artery can occur in forced extension of the neck. However it seems unlikely that the cerebral circulation would be severely impaired as the majority of flow is via the cartoid arteries. Nevertheless, all cervical techniques should avoid extension especially accompanied by rotation, as such a risk must never be taken. It is a controversial point.

14.8   **Nerve injury**

Nerves of the neck can be pressurised by disc lesions, cervical ribs, or long transverse processes of C7. All these conditions have already been discussed and the treatment outlined.

With *disc lesions*, the neck movements are limited and pain is usually felt along the distribution of one nerve root.

With a *cervical rib*, the adventitious bone (or cartilage) is palpable and may show on X-ray. Usually the whole of the brachial plexus is involved and there may be signs of pressure on the subclavian vessels. Frequently there is wasting of the thenar muscles and weakness. There may be sensory changes especially in the distribution of C7 and T1.

In addition, occasionally the phrenic nerve is irritated, resulting in *intractable hiccoughs*. This nerve can be inhibited by pressure as it passes over the first rib. It arises chiefly from the C4 nerve so such a problem should lead the examining osteopath to that level of the neck where any mechanical abnormality should be corrected.

Headache is often associated with upper cervical problems. The exact mechanism is unsure but treatment of the upper cervical region will often relieve symptoms. In all cases of head pain, the lower cervical and upper thoracic areas should also receive treatment if necessary. Athletes will complain of head pain after head injury or possibly following neck injury in some cases.

Foraminal encroachment usually occurs in older athletes, especially those who have been subjected to head or neck injury earlier in life. The pain is felt more when the neck is extended and side bent to the side of pain. X-rays will show some degree of degeneration. Osteopathic treatment to increase the foraminae and increase the general mobility of the neck is very effective. Extension should be avoided as much as possible by the athlete so certain sports are contraindicated.

Chapter 15   The Thorax, Ribs and Diaphragm

15.1

Anatomical review

Twelve thoracic vertebrae comprise the *thoracic spine*, which increase gradually in size from above downwards (see Fig. 15.1). The distinguishing feature of the thoracic vertebrae is the presence of 'half articular facets' on the sides of the bodies which articulate with the heads of the ribs, and articular facets on the transverse processes which articulate with the tubercles of the ribs. The exceptions are the first rib which has a complete facet on the superior border of the body as well as the usual half articular facet on the inferior border of the body; the ninth which may not articulate with the head of the tenth rib, in which case the lower facet on the body will be absent; the tenth which may not have a facet for articulation with the tubercle of the tenth rib; the eleventh and twelfth ribs which articulate with the heads of the corresponding ribs only and are 'free' anteriorly − i.e. do not articulate with the sternum nor are they attached to the ribs above them.

The spinous processes of the thoracic vertebrae overlap each other as they are directed downwards and posteriorly, so the tips of the spinous processes of the middle vertebrae lie one to one and a half vertebrae below their corresponding bodies. This angulation reduces in the lower thoracic vertebrae as they become more like lumbar vertebrae.

The supporting ligaments are described in section 14.1. In addition there are ligaments of the costovertebral and costotransverse joints.

The joints of the heads of the *ribs* are plane joints; these form joints with the articular facets on the adjacent margins of the vertebral bodies and the intervening intervertebral discs, the costovertebral joints (see Figs. 15.2 and 15.3). Apart from the first, eleventh and twelfth ribs, these joints are dual; each rib articulates with the facet on two vertebrae and there is a ligament, the intra-articular costal ligament which runs from the head of the rib to the intervertebral disc of that costovertebral joint dividing the joint. The capsule is attached to the margins of the articular facets and is strengthened by the superficial radiate ligaments which are attached to the anterior part of the head of each rib and to the sides of the adjacent vertebral bodies and intervening disc.

The costotransverse joints are between the tubercles of the ribs and the transverse processes of the vertebrae. The capsule of each joint is fine and is supported by the costotransverse ligaments

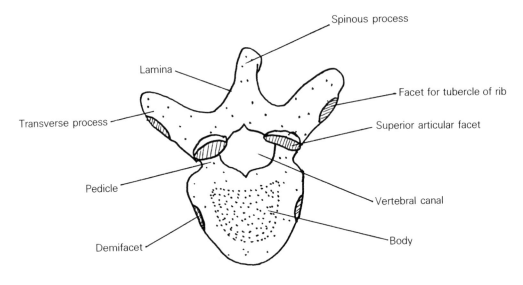

(a)

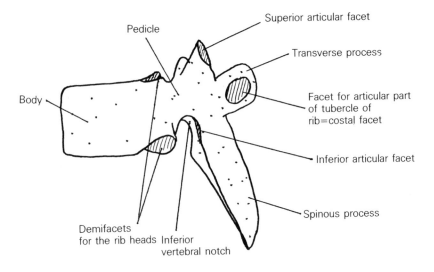

(b)

Fig. 15.1   A typical dorsal vertebra. (a) Superior aspect; (b) lateral aspect.

which run from the neck of the rib to the adjacent transverse processes both above and below the joints. The first rib has no costotransverse ligament above. The twelfth rib is connected to the transverse process of the first lumbar vertebra by the lumbocostal ligament.

The *sternum* is a flat bone forming the central portion of the anterior chest wall. It consists of the manubrium, the body and the

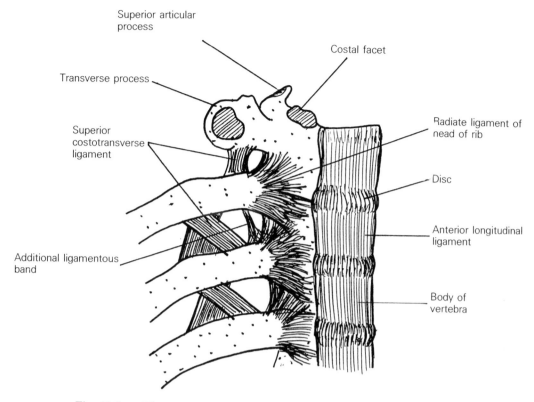

Fig. 15.2   The costovertebral joints, right anterolateral aspect.

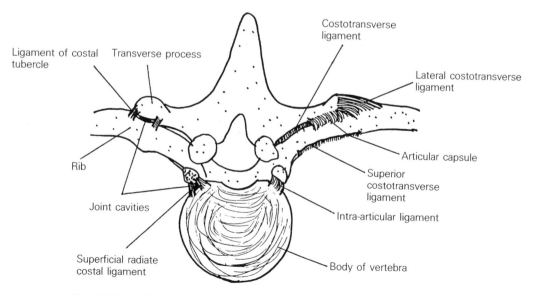

Fig. 15.3   The costovertebral joints, superior aspect.

xiphoid process and this process may ossify in later life or it may remain partly cartilagenous. The sternum articulates with the clavicles forming the sternoclavicular joints and with the first to seventh ribs inclusive (see Fig. 15.4). Some movement also occurs between the three parts of the sternum. There are sex differences in the sternum; the body is longer in men than in women and is narrower in men.

Each rib consists of a bony and a cartilagenous part. Each bony part has a head, a body and a neck joining the other two parts. The tubercle lies at the junction of the neck and the body of the rib. Articular facets are present on the head and the tubercle, for articulation with the vertebrae. The ribs are curved, the obliquity increases downwards to a maximum at the ninth rib and decreases below that level.

Movement of the ribs in relation to the vertebrae and sternum varies according to the plane of the articular facets. The upper ribs, in inspiration, tend to increase the anteroposterior diameter

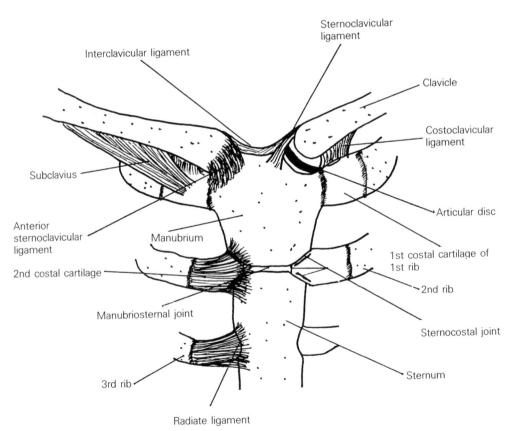

Fig. 15.4   The sternoclavicular, manubriosternal and sternocostal joints, anterior aspect.

of the chest, while movement of the lower ribs tends to increase the lateral or transverse diameter in inspiration. During inspiration the sternum moves upward and forwards and the relative position of rib and sternum is maintained by the elasticity of the costal cartilages which form the bond between the ribs and the sternum. The sixth, seventh, eighth and ninth costal cartilages articulate with each other; the capsule of each joint is strengthened laterally and medially by the interchondral ligaments which pass from one cartilage to the next.

The *diaphragm* is a dome-shaped musculofibrous structure, convex superiorly, which forms the lower border of the thoracic cavity (see Fig. 15.5). It is the principal muscle of inspiration. The sternal part of the diaphragm arises from the inner surface of the xiphoid process. The costal part arises from the inner surface of the seventh to twelfth ribs inclusive, the slips of origin alternating with the slips of origin of the transverse abdominal muscle. The lumbar part is composed of two parts, namely the medial crus which arises from the anterior surfaces of the upper four lumbar vertebrae and intervening discs on the right, and from the upper three on the left; and the lateral crus which arises from the medial arcuate ligament which is an arch of tendinous material where the

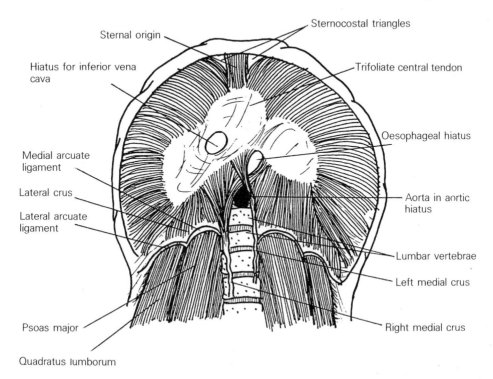

Fig. 15.5   The diaphragm, inferior aspect.

crura meet, and lies in front of the aorta. The fibres of origin converge to be inserted into the central tendon of the diaphragm which is a thin but strong aponeurosis of interwoven fibres. Above the diaphragm lie the lungs enclosed in the pleura, and the heart enclosed in the pericardium, and below is the peritoneum, the liver, the kidneys and suprarenal glands and on the left, the fundus of the stomach. The nerve supply consists of the phrenic nerve from C4 and the lower six intercostal nerves which supply the periphery.

In sport there is need for full inspiration and expiration and training can increase the volume of air taken in and expelled by as much as 30%. During inspiration, the ribs are elevated mainly by the action of the intercostal and levator costarum muscles (see Fig. 15.6), while the scalene muscles assist elevation of the upper two ribs. Sternomastoid assists indirectly by acting on the clavicle. At the same time the diaphragm contracts, thus lowering the central tendon and increasing the vertical diameter of the thorax and reducing the thoracic pressure. This pressurises the abdominal viscera and causes the abdominal wall muscles to contract and expiration follows. The muscles of the abdominal wall are assisted

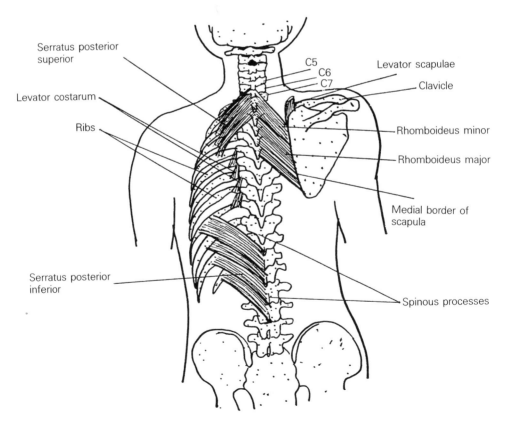

Fig. 15.6   The serratus posterior muscles, the rhomboids and levator costarum.

by the passive recoil of the thorax, due to it's elasticity. In addition muscular assistance is given by the internal intercostals, the subcostals, the transverse thoracis, the lower fibres of iliocostalis, the longissimus thoracis, serratus posterior inferior (see Fig. 15.6) and quadratus lumborum. The antagonistic action of the abdominal muscles on the diaphragm is essential for the full efficiency of respiration. The range of movement of the diaphragm will be affected adversely in cases of abdominal distention or enlargement of the abdominal viscera, for example following a heavy meal.

There are a number of openings in the diaphragm which allow the passage of structures between the thorax and abdomen, namely the aorta, oesophagus and vena cava and there are lesser apertures on each crus for the greater and lesser splanchnic nerves. The oesophageal opening is the commonest site for a *diaphragmatic hernia*, which may be congenital, and will interfere with the efficiency of diaphragmatic function.

The *intercostal muscles* are necessary for movement of the chest wall (see Fig. 15.7). The *external intercostals* are eleven in number on each side of the chest. They arise from the tubercles behind, almost as far and as the cartilages of the ribs forward. The fibres pass downwards and forwards to become attached to the upper border of the rib below. The fibres therefore are directed laterally on the back of the thorax and medially on the front. The nerve supply consists of the intercostal nerves 1−11. They act as inspiratory muscles in full respiration. The *internal intercostal* muscles are also eleven in number on each side. Each muscle arises from the sternum, between the attachment of the costal cartilages, from the floor of the costal groove and the corresponding costal cartilage and inserts into the upper border of the rib below. The direction of the fibres is oblique, and at right angles to the external intercostal muscles. The nerve supply consist of the intercostal nerves 1−11. These muscles act as expiratory muscles in full respiration. See Fig. 15.7.

The *subcostal muscles* lie in the region of the costal angles. They are fibres of the internal intercostal muscles which pass to the second or third rib below. They are well developed in the lower part of the thorax only and also act as muscles of expiration.

The *transverse thoracis muscle* arises from the deep surface of the xiphoid process and the body of the sternum and the fibres pass upward and laterally to become attached to the lower border of the second to sixth costal cartilages. Its nerve supply consists of the intercostal nerves, 2−6. This is a muscle of expiration. These muscles form strong elastic supports between the ribs.

The *sternocostalis muscle* is situated on the inner surface of the front wall of the chest; it arises from the posterior surface of the xiphoid process and the adjacent surfaces of the costal cartilages and becomes inserted into the inner surface of the second to sixth

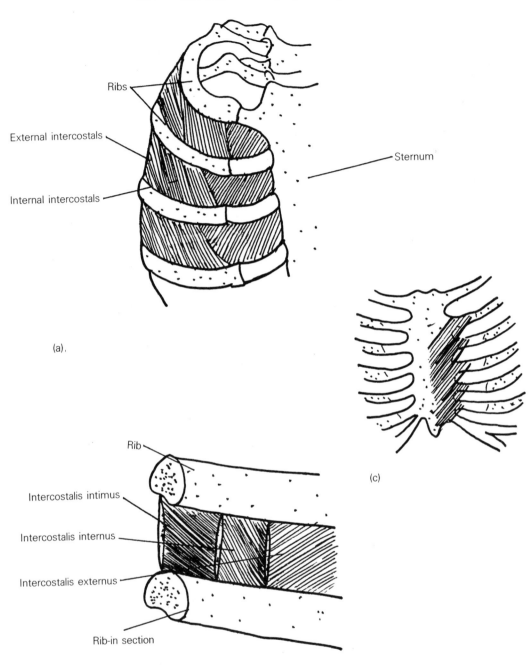

Fig. 15.7   The intercostal muscles. (a) Anterior aspect; (b) section through intercostal muscles; (c) sternocostalis, retrosternal.

costal cartilages. The nerve supply consists of the intercostal nerves 2−6.

The *levatores costarum* are twelve in number on each side. They arise from the transverse process of C7 to T11 and each muscle passes obliquely downwards and laterally to become inserted into the rib below, between the tubercle and the angle. The nerve supply consists of the intercostal nerves. These act to side bend and rotate the thoracic spine and help to stabilise the ribs, posteriorly. See Fig. 15.6.

The *serratus posterior superior* arises from the spinous processes of C7 to T2 and from the ligamentum nuchae in that area. The fibres pass downwards and laterally to become inserted into the second to fifth ribs, close to the angles. The nerve supply consists of the intercostal nerves, 2−5. See Fig. 15.6.

The *serratus posterior inferior* arises from the spines of the lower two thoracic and upper two lumbar vertebrae and passes upwards to become inserted into the lower four ribs close to their angles. The nerve supply consists of the anterior primary rami of T9 to T12. Both the serratus posterior muscles assist inspiration in full respiration.

The *scalene muscles* are described in section 14.2.

The deep muscles of the thoracic spine have been described in section 14.2 as their anatomy is similar to those of the cervical area. However, the rotatores are well defined in the thoracic area and are able to assist in rotation of the thoracic spine.

The *sacrospinalis muscle* lies in a groove on the side of the vertebral column throughout it's length. It can be divided into three columns and is continuous from the sacrum to the occiput. In the thoracic area, the lateral part is called the iliocostalis and is inserted into the angles of the lower six ribs. The intermediate part is the longissimus thoracis and is inserted into the tips of the transverse processes of T1 to T12 and into the angles of the lower nine ribs. The medial part is known as the spinalis thoracis and actually arises in the thoracic region, from the transverse processes of T6 to T10 and the fibres pass upward to become inserted into the spinous processes of C6 to T4. The nerve supply consists of the posterior primary rami of lower cervical, thoracic and lumbar nerves in the related areas. These muscles are responsible for extension, side bending and rotation of the thoracic spine. See Fig. 14.16.

Superficially lie the rhomboids, trapezius (see sections 6.7 and 14.2) and latissimus dorsi, all of which are muscles of the shoulder.

On the anterior aspect of the thorax, three muscles attach the thorax to the shoulder girdle, subclavius and the pectoral muscles, major and minor (see Fig. 15.8). *Subclavius* arises from the junction of the first rib and it's costal cartilage and is inserted into a groove on the intermediate one-third of the clavicle. Its nerve supply

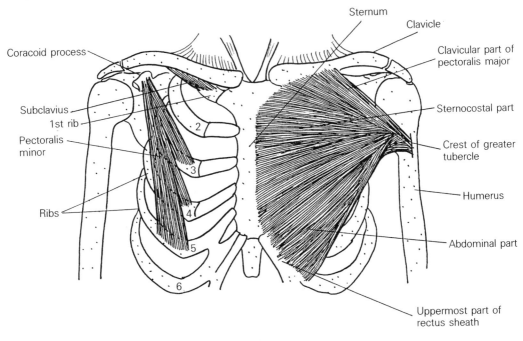

Fig. 15.8   The pectoral and subclavius muscles.

consists of C5 and C6. This muscle stabilises the clavicle during shoulder movements. See section 6.7.

Pectoralis major arises from the medial half of the clavicle, the anterior surface of the sternum as far down as the seventh rib and from the upper seven costal cartilages. It is inserted by means of a tendon into the lateral lip of the bicipital groove. Its nerve supply consists of, for the clavicular portion, C5 and C6; sternocostal portion, C7, C8 and T1. This muscle adducts the arm and medially rotates it. With the arm in abduction, the muscle anteverts the arm, a movement used in swimming. It also acts as an accessory muscle of respiration; that is why an exhausted athlete will prop up his arms on his trunk, to increase the thoracic movement.

Pectoralis minor arises from the anterior part of the third, fourth and fifth ribs and is inserted into the coracoid process of the scapula. It stabilises the scapula by lowering it and can also act as an accessory muscle of respiration. Its nerve supply consists of C6, C7 and C8.

Serratus anterior arises by fleshy slips from the outer surface of the upper nine ribs (see Fig. 15.9). It passes around the chest wall and is inserted into the costal surface of the medial border of the scapula and into the angle of the scapula. Its nerve supply consists of the long thoracic nerve, C5, C6 and C7. It is the principal muscle involved in pushing and punching. It stabilises the scapula

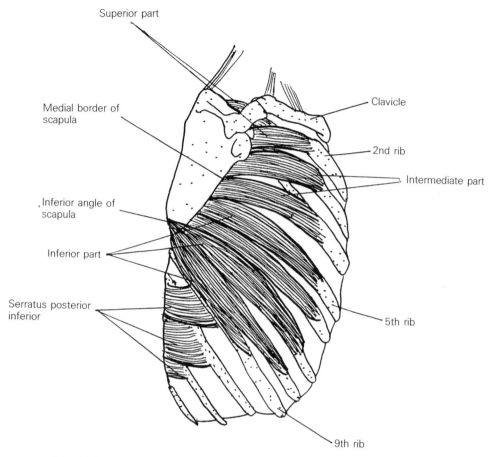

Fig. 15.9   Serratus anterior, right lateral aspect.

in the initial stage of abduction of the arm. When weights are carried in front of the body, serratus anterior prevents backward rotation of the scapula. It can also act as an accessory muscle of inspiration.

The *rhomboid muscles* are antagonists of serratus anterior. *Rhomboideus major* arises from the spinous processes of T2 to T5 and is inserted into the medial margin of the scapula. *Rhomboideus minor* arises from the spinous processes of C6 and C7 and is inserted into margin of the scapula immediately above the rhomboideus major. The two muscle are sometimes fused. Its nerve supply consists of C4 and C5. The two rhomboids act together and retract the scapula, thus bracing it in movements of the arm. They are synergistic to serratus anterior.

The *latissimus dorsi* is the largest muscle in the body (see Fig. 15.10). It arises from the spinous processes of the lower six thoracic vertebrae, from the spinous processes of the lumbar and sacral vertebrae via the lumbar fascia, from the posterior one-third of the

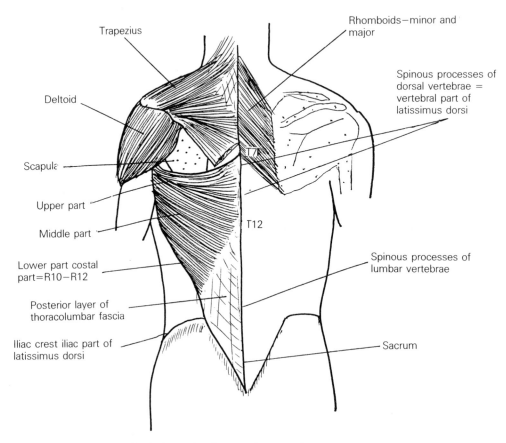

Fig. 15.10   Latissimus dorsi, posterior aspect.

iliac crest, from the lowest three ribs and usually from the inferior angle of the scapula, where there may be an interposing bursa. The fibres converge to be inserted into the crest of the lesser tubercle of the humerus. The nerve supply consists of C6, C7 and C8. Acting together the two muscles pull the shoulders backwards and downwards (as in weight training). The elevated arm is pulled down and adducted and when adducted the muscle rotates the arm medially through a wide range of movement. Together the muscles act as muscles of forced expiration, as in coughing.

The movements of flexion, extension, side bending to either side and rotation to either side are necessarily limited by the presence of the rib cage and sternum. Extension is checked by the spinous processes approximating one another and although the plane of the facets would permit side bending, this is limited by resistance from the ribs and sternum. Rotation is comparatively free but even this movement is limited by the ribs and sternum. In the young the elasticity of the thorax permits more movement than in the older athlete where the ossification of the costal cartilages reduces the

Table 15.1 Muscles supplied by the thoracic nerves

	Anterior primary rami	Posterior primary rami
T1	Small muscles of the hand	Deep muscles of the back
T2	2nd intercostal 2nd levator costae Serratus posterior superior	Deep muscles of the back
T3	3rd intercostal 3rd levator costae Serratus posterior superior Sternocostalis	Deep muscles of the back
T4	4th intercostal 4th levator costae Serratus posterior superior Sternocostalis	Deep muscles of the back
T5	5th intercostal 5th levator costae Sternocostalis	Deep muscles of the back
T6	6th intercostal 6th levator costae Rectus abdominis	Deep muscles of the back
T7	7th intercostal 7th levator costae Subcostal External oblique Internal oblique Transversus abdominis Rectus abdominis	Deep muscles of the back
T8	8th intercostal 8th levator costae Subcostal External oblique Internal oblique Transversus abdominis Rectus abdominis	Deep muscles of the back
T9	9th intercostal 9th levator costae Subcostal External oblique Internal oblique Transversus abdominis Rectus abdominis Serratus posterior inferior	Deep muscles of the back
T10	10th intercostal 10th levator costae Subcostal External oblique Internal oblique	Deep muscles of the back

Table 15.1 continued

Anterior primary rami		Posterior primary rami
	Transversus abdominis	
	Rectus abdominis	
	Serratus posterior inferior	
T11	11th intercostal	Deep muscles of the back
	11th levator costae	
	Subcostal	
	External oblique	
	Internal oblique	
	Transversus abdominis	
	Rectus abdominis	
	Serratus posterior inferior	
T12	12th levator costae	Deep muscles of the back
	External oblique	
	Internal oblique	
	Transversus abdominis	
	Rectus abdominis	
	Pyramidalis	

chondrocostal elasticity, progressively with age. This limitation of thoracic spinal movements renders the intervertebral discs free from torsional strains, so problems with the discs are seldom seen. The only way they can be injured is either by compression injuries along the axis of the spine or from injuries which damage the bone structure and so the intervening disc as well.

15.2   Spinal curves

The thoracic spine retains the *primary kyphotic curve*, but in some athletes this may be reversed or reduced. Such a condition seems to be associated frequently with excess extension in the growing stage, but may also be hereditary.

More commonly an increase in the *thoracic curve* is seen, the commonest cause being the residual deformity left following Scheuermann's disease of adolescence. This may be localised to one or two segments or it may be generalised throughout the area. The lumbar spine can be affected, too. Such an alteration of the 'normal' thoracic curve will render extension limited and side bending and rotation will be less free. In addition the movements of the thorax required for full respiration will be limited and this can be a disadvantage to an aspiring athlete. It will be especially noticeable in sports requiring deep respiration.

If the condition is discovered during the adolescent stage of the athlete, or even earlier, osteopathic treatment to reduce the kyphosis, and exercises to do the same are extremely helpful.

Backstroke swimming is ideal as this will assist thoracic extension and stretch out the developing curve. Even in later stages, the curve can be modified somewhat by similar means, but the results will be less spectacular. Rib raising and stretching techniques are also helpful to improve mobility. Breathing exercises must be prescribed in all such cases as these will help to increase the range of movement during respiration. All these measures will improve the adverse, exaggerated kyphosis, but an athlete with a marked thoracic kyphosis is unlikely to become a top class sportsman in any of the energetic sports. This does not, however, mean that he will be unable to enjoy such activity. For scoliosis see at the end of section 15.3.

15.3   **Muscle injuries**

Direct injury may injure any of the superficial muscles in this area. A force applied to the back may bruise the thoracic part of the *sacrospinalis*. Bruising may be obvious and the history helpful. The athlete will complain of pain in the damaged area which is made worse by extending the spine; resisted extension may be painful, too. High jumpers can bruise the thoracic area by habitually falling onto the bar as they land — almost an occupational hazard!

A blow to the rib cage may damage the *intercostal muscles* without necessarily damaging the ribs. In this case the athlete will complain of localised pain and pain on full respiration.

Similarly a blow to the posterior part of the lower ribs may injure the *posterior inferior serratus muscle* which is only protected superficially by the latissimus dorsi. It can also be strained when excessive rib movement has been carried out, for example in certain throwing activities or when sneezing. Again the pain will be localised and deep breathing will be painful.

Latissimus dorsi is involved in movements of the arm especially in sports such as racket games and throwing activities and in such activities it can be strained. When the arm is fixed and raised above the head, for example in gymnastics on the overhead bar or in weight training or weight lifting, latissimus dorsi helps to stabilise the shoulder girdle and in doing so can be strained. Active movement of the shoulder will be painful and resisted extension and medial rotation of the humerus. The pain is likely to be at the site of injury.

The *pectoral muscles* are involved in any pushing activity and are fairly commonly strained. Again the athlete will complain of pain at the site of injury on active use of the muscle. Resisted movement will accentuate the pain.

All these muscular injuries respond well to deep soft tissue treatment especially if given cross-fibre. Bruising can be relieved by the application of ice packs (having oiled the skin beforehand)

and homeopathic arnica is advised. If fibrotic areas are palpable, Tiger balm is useful to help break down the nodules and congestion. Return to full athletic activity is contraindicated until complete recovery has taken place. Osteopathic examination of the surrounding joints and soft tissues is essential and any adverse conditions should be treated. The area of origin of the nerve supply to the affected muscle and the area of origin and insertion of the damage muscle must be examined and treated if necessary. This is to ensure that the muscle will be able to work normally once the local lesion has healed.

Serratus anterior is sometimes bruised at its points of origin from the ribs. Usually only one or two digitations are affected. The cause may be a direct injury or overstrain from pushing or punching; hence it is seen in boxers most frequently. Locally the area will be painful and bruising may be seen. Resisted pushing will aggravate the symptoms. This is difficult to treat locally and if it is not possible, treatment should be aimed at gentle articulation of the scapula to carefully stretch and decongest the damaged fibres of the muscle. In addition, any treatment that is necessary to the surrounding areas and to the lower cervical region from where the nerve supply arises must be given. Weakness of serratus anterior results in the so-called 'winged scapula', when the lower angle and medial border of the scapula stand out prominently from the posterior chest wall. Exercises to strengthen the muscle are required but recovery is slow.

Of all muscles in the thoracic area, the *rhomboids* are probably the most frequent source of pain. That is because they are involved in maintaining the stability of the scapula in movements of the arm, both in activity and strength sports, for example in ball games and in weight events, and especially in rowing (see section 6.8). The athlete will usually complain of pain in the interscapular region which will probably have come on insidiously over a period of time. The pain will more often be aggravated by stretching the muscles rather than by the resisted use of them, because the commonest problem is one of shortening of the fibres of the rhomboids. It is possible for an athlete to actually tear some of the fibres, in which case he will be aware of the sudden onset of pain. Palpation of the muscles is the best guide as to the problem — the fibres may feel fibrotic and shortened, or may feel acutely tender in one small area in the acute injury. Soft tissue treatment together with articulation of the scapula to gently stretch the fibres is helpful and active stretching is necessary before full sporting activity is resumed. Being fleshy, these muscles respond well to treatment. The lower cervical and upper and mid thoracic areas will have to be treated to eliminate any hypomobility which may have been a contributory factor in the original injury. These injuries are frequently seen in swimmers, weight lifters, rowers, and often unilaterally in racket players who may have developed a localised scoliosis which will predispose to rhomboid strain.

Muscular pain is often indicative of some underlying bone or joint condition, when there is a degree of muscular protection. This will involve more than one muscle and be localised to the underlying problem. Having stated that, it must be remembered that it is possible to injure more than one muscle at a time as several muscles work together in most sporting activities.

A localised *scoliosis* is often seen in the thoracic area especially in athletes who partake of one sided-sports, for example throwing events and racket sports. This inevitably leads to asymmetrical movement of the spine and ribs which in turn may predispose to muscular problems. These athletes should be encouraged to actively reduce the scoliosis by exercises and partake of symmetrical sports, for example swimming, to help stretch out the scoliosis. In all such cases it is the mobility of the area which is of most importance and this can be improved by osteopathic treatment to both joints and soft tissues.

A more serious condition arises when there is a generalised scoliosis which is contrary to the predominantly used arm – i.e. there is a developmental scoliosis where the right handed player has a right thoracic concavity; this will reduce the active movements of the right arm and may lead to muscular and joint problems. Again it is possible to improve the mobility of the area by osteopathic treatment but it is not possible to equalise the movements of the right and left.

Muscles which are well developed and well stretched are less likely to be injured in sporting activities, but the body is more efficient if the muscular development is balanced. This includes balance on the right and left and also between the muscle and it's antagonist. Such balance will reduce the risk of muscular problems.

15.4   Bone injury

Bruising of any of the bones of the thoracic area is not uncommon in sport, invariably due to some form of a blow. The fact that there may be an underlying fracture must always be considered and excluded by X-ray examination. Only then can the treatment be as for a bruise.

Rib fractures are commonly seen in athletes, usually from direct injury as in rugby, football or from a fall as from a horse. Several ribs may be fractured at any one time depending on the extent of the injury. The most serious complication of a rib fracture is the possibility of some underlying damage to the viscera and any suspicion of such must lead the osteopath to refer the athlete for further investigation immediately. Uncomplicated rib fractures do not receive treatment in hospital usually, and union takes place within about six weeks. However, the pain can be lessened by strapping the rib along the whole of its length but this should be localised to the fractured rib only and not to a wide area of the chest. Any residual pain following bony union has to be from damaged intercostal muscles which respond well to osteopathic treatment. In addition there may be some residual problem following strain of the costovertebral and/or costotransverse joints, or, if anterior, of the costochondral region and these conditions should respond well to treatment.

Diagnosis of a rib fracture from an X-ray is often difficult because of the overlying bony structures. Fortunately the athlete will point to the exact site of injury and the fracture can usually be palpated. Springing the chest wall by pressure on the rib away from the fracture produces pain as does full inspiration, thoracic extension and rotation to either side.

The *clavicle* is very often injured following a fall from a horse or bicycle and fractures of this bone are common. The history will be helpful; the athlete will complain of pain at the site of injury which will be exacerbated by any movement of the arm, except flexion; this is the position in which he will hold his arm. Palpation will reveal the fracture and the diagnosis can be ensured if the bone is sheared and crepitus is felt. The commonest complication of this fracture is residual shortening of the bone; this can be avoided if the shoulder is held backward during the initial stages of healing. The arm should not be supported in a sling which will feel comfortable but will tend to shorten the bone. In cases of a shortened clavicle, the shoulder is held forward thereafter and the anterior musculature becomes shortened, thus predisposing the area to muscular injury. There will also be some residual muscular weakness and sport can be interfered with as a result of bony shortening. Horse riding and cycling will not, however, be affected as the shoulder is flexed during these activities but throwing, ball games and even swimming can become difficult.

Both the *sternum* and the *scapula* can be injured by a direct blow in sport, but fracture of either bone is rare. However it has to be considered if there is a history of a severe blow in the area. The commonest cause is either when the athlete is thrown violently, as from a horse, or possibly in motor racing or speedway.

The *thoracic spine* may be bruised but fractures are rare as the area is well buttressed by the elastic rib cage. If fracture does occur it will be as a result of a compression with rotation strain, such as a fall striking the head, for example in horse riding or skiing. The commonest fracture is an anterior wedge type of a vertebral body which is stable and does not warrant specialised treatment and is better treated with activity. Fractures of T4 to T9 are very rare due to the protection given them by their spinous processes. The condition is painful and should not be stressed by sport until union has occurred. Residual joint and soft tissue problems will require treatment following bony union.

Scheuermann's disease occurs frequently in the thoracic spine. It is in it's active stage in adolescents when it may interfere with sport because of the pain factor. Being an inflammatory condition, the athlete should be advised to reduce stress on the spine; adequate rest is essential and any sport which risks spinal compression is contraindicated during the active phase. Osteopathic treatment to reduce the degree of spinal deformity is indicated and activities such as swimming which encourages mobility (especially extension) while non-weight bearing should be advised. The kyphosis which results from this condition can be a nuisance factor in later life (see section 15.2). The condition can be diagnosed from X-rays when the characteristic appearance of Schmorl's nodes is seen (see Fig. 15.11). The cause of this condition is unknown but it is thought by some authorities to result from overuse of the growing spine.

Osteoporosis occurs commonly in the thoracic spine in middle-aged ladies, postmenopausally. Some of these are still physically very active, for example in golf or marathon running. It seems likely that these active ladies are less liable to suffer from severe osteoporosis but the possibility must always be borne in mind. The far-reaching consequence of osteoporosis can be collapse of the

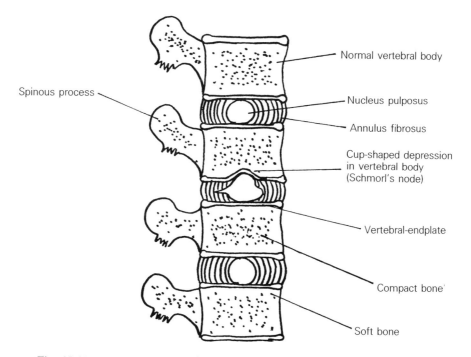

Fig. 15.11   A Schmorl's node.

vertebral body. X-rays must be taken to confirm the diagnosis and osteopathic treatment together with orthodox medical advice and a regime of non-weight bearing exercise will benefit the patient. It is also wise to increase the calcium and vitamin intake of these people. Once the inflammatory stage is over, this condition does not often handicap the athlete who is not likely to partake of sports which require excessive flexibility of the spine, but full mobility of the area should be maintained osteopathically if necessary.

Joint and ligament injury

15.5

There are a great many joints in the thoracic area, any one or more of which may be subjected to strain. *Flexion strains* are comparatively rare but extension and rotation in particular, can strain thoracic joints. The long ligaments of the spine are not easily traumatised in this region as this usually occurs with a flexion strain and the area is protected by the rib cage. The commonest joints to become strained are those between the vertebrae and ribs. The athlete will complain of pain and may give a history of the pain starting after some activity which involved rotation. The pain will be aggravated by deep breathing as the intercostal muscles will be protecting the injury. Passive examination reveals some intercostal hypertonia but the movements of the joints are not usually restricted; in fact they may, on occasion, be excessive. Rest from physical activity will relieve the pain.

Costochondral strain is often seen. There may be visible deformity but the condition does not cause great pain in most cases. It is probably the deformity which leads the athlete to seek advice. If there are no symptoms, the condition is best left alone. If there is pain, the best treatment is an injection either of a corticosteroid or a sclerosing fluid. Occasionally surgical treatment is needed to stabilise the joint. If the symptoms originate from the intercostal muscles, osteopathic treatment is indicated − see section 15.3.

Heavy lifting can cause injury to the sternal joints, but this is not often seen in athletes. The pain will be aggravated by deep breathing unlike pain in the same area, of cardiac origin. The condition responds to rest. The xiphoid process can be depressed by direct injury; this will require surgical treatment if it is handicapping the athlete.

Facet locking

15.6

This can occur at the apophyseal joints, the costovertebral joints or the costotransverse joints, or, more often, at more than one site at any one time. A group lesion is commonly seen in this region. The athlete will complain of pain, the onset usually being related to some sudden or awkward movement. Active movement in at least one direction will cause pain and passively there will be restriction in the same direction. Movement in the opposite direction may be free. There will be peri-articular muscular guarding which is palpable and may be visible as well, and there may be palpable swelling around the joint(s). There may be irritation of one or more intercostal nerves, referring pain posteriorly at first and then possibly anteriorly later. The joint(s) will have the classic 'feel' which is so well known to all osteopaths. Correction, followed by stretching and corrective articulation will relieve the athlete's pain. It is often necessary to treat a wide area as there may be contributory factors in other parts of the spine or thoracic cage.

15.7   **Mobility injury**

Hypermobility of the *sternoclavicular joint* results from a fall onto the point of the shoulder, common in horse riders and cyclists. The medial end of the clavicle is forced upward and forward. If the force is sufficiently great, the joint will dislocate, resulting in a prominence at the medial end of the clavicle which is tender (see Fig. 15.12). Shoulder movements will be painful due to the soft tissue injury which accompanied the joint strain and the ligamentous damage. The soft tissues will repair with rest, but the dislocation is difficult to treat. Some stabilise with a corrective pad and strapping but most do not. In time, which is usually several months, full pain-free shoulder movements return but the bony prominence remains.

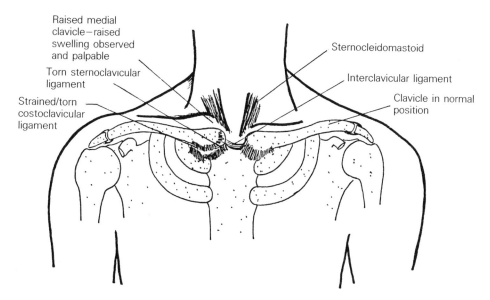

Fig. 15.12   Dislocation of the right sternoclavicular joint.

More commonly the *acromioclavicular joint* becomes hypermobile or even dislocates with a similar fall onto the shoulder (see Fig. 15.13). The lateral end of the clavicle is displaced superiorly and shows as a lump over the joint. Again there will be pain initially but once the soft tissue damage has repaired, the residual instability does not appreciably impair shoulder movements. Occasionally surgical treatment is warranted. A fall onto the outstretched hand can also cause these problems but it is less common than a fall onto the point of the shoulder.

Stiffness of the *thoracic spine* and *ribs* may follow some unaccustomed activity and is caused by hypertonic musculature. The athlete will soon recover and the pain is lessened by heat. Osteopathic soft tissue treatment and articulation together with gentle exercises will accelerate recovery.

Stiffness which the athlete reports is progressive is more serious. The patient is likely to be a young man under the age of thirty. He will say that he is more comfortable in a position of semi-flexion and can relieve his pain by adopting that position. The pain will be an ache rather than a sharp pain. Ankylosing spondylitis gives rise to just this symptom picture and X-rays may show the condition, but these should be taken of the sacro-iliac joints as well, as the condition starts in these joints. The lumbar spine may not be affected but this is unusual. Treatment is aimed at reducing the kyphosis so that once ankylosis has occurred the patient will be upright and not held in fixed spinal flexion. Pain originates from

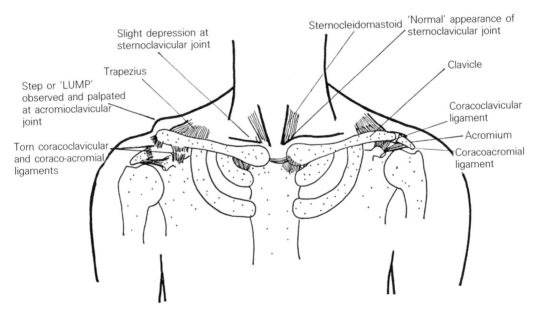

Fig. 15.13   Dislocation of the right acromioclavicular joint.

the spinal ligaments and osteopathic treatment can improve the symptom picture but not halt the progress of the condition. Some cases respond favourably to homeopathic treatment.

Degenerative changes occur in the thoracic area in middle life; they tend to be more marked following some previous condition such as Scheuermann's disease. The joints become progressively less mobile and the changes within the joints can be seen on X-rays. Articulation of the region helps to increase flexibility and soft tissue treatment especially to stretch the muscular fibres is helpful to the athlete. In addition he should be advised to exercise the area regularly to maintain mobility and keep the soft tissues stretched. Yoga is especially helpful.

An athlete may complain of stiffness in the *scapular region*, often accompanied by *crepitus* which is felt in the area of the scapula. The reason that crepitus occurs is uncertain but of itself it is of little importance. Any loss of mobility of the scapula is far more important as it will restrict athletic agility. Articulation to the scapula is particularly helpful and the crepitus often disappears as the mobility is improved.

15.8   **Nerve injury**

Nerve root irritation is rare in the thoracic area as the typical disc lesion of the cervical or lumbar areas is rarely seen. However, nerve root irritation can result from strains of the spinal and rib joints. In such a case there will be the symptoms of joint strain and pain felt along one or possibly more than one intercostal space. Treatment is aimed at the underlying joint condition. Pain from a cervical disc or joint condition can refer to the thoracic region, typically from the levels of C5 or C6 to the interscapular area and from C7 to the angle of one scapula.

Herpes zoster is commonest in the thoracic area. The athlete may have been in contact with chickenpox. He will complain of severe intercostal pain which is not affected by any movement. Small vesicles appear three or four days later and the diagnosis is clear. The pain can be relieved somewhat by medical means. Sometimes there is a residual post-herpetic neuralgia which is resistant to osteopathic treatment and may warrant further medical attention. This condition can affect athletes of any age group but is seldom seen in adolescents.

Neuralgic amyotrophy is sometimes seen in athletes. It is a viral infection usually of several nerve roots; there is often a history of a preceding viral infection. Severe pain is felt in the shoulder region and may extend to both arms. To the athlete the most worrying symptom is loss of power and the deltoid, infraspinatus and serratus anterior muscles are commonly affected, and wasting develops. Recovery takes about three months but the affected muscles may not recover full power and do not respond to osteopathic or other treatment.

Localised paralysis may be a complication of rib fracture if the nerve is damaged as well as the bone; recovery is usually spontaneous.

15.9   **The diaphragm**

The diaphrgam can be damaged by a severe blow on the chest but the condition is not often seen. Pain is felt only on respiration, not on any trunk movement; the pain may be referred to the tip of the shoulder. Rest from all activities which involve deep breathing is advised and recovery is usually spontaneous.

Hyperventilation is sometimes seen in an anxious athlete especially before a competitive event and is thought to be emotional rather than physiological in origin. The athlete breathes deeply and rapidly thus losing large volumes of carbon dioxide from the body and the acid base balance is altered. The initial signs are shortness of breath, faintness, dizziness and sweating, followed by tingling around the mouth and in the tips of the extremities. Muscular spasms may occur if the hyperventilation is not stopped. Following an episode of hyperventilation, the athlete may suffer from shock and need treatment for this. The attack is similar in many ways to an asthma attack and can be equally distressing.

Chapter 16   The Lumbar Area and Abdomen

The lumbar spine and abdomen

Five lumbar vertebrae comprise the lumbar spine (see Fig. 16.1). They are larger than the cervical and thoracic vertebrae; the body of each vertebra is large and wider from side to side than from front to back. There are no articular facets for articulation with ribs. The spinous process is thickened along its posterior and inferior border and is more or less quadrangular. The lamina is short and sturdy and the pedicles are thick. There is a lateral process on each side which is developmentally a rudimentary rib which has become fused to the vertebra. Behind this, on each side, is the accessory process which represents the remnant of the transverse process together with the mamillary process and the superior articulatory process. The inferior articulatory process points caudally and carries the inferior articulatory facets which face laterally; the superior articulatory facets face medially and are on the superior articulatory process. The intervertebral foraminae are large but the vertebral foramen is relatively small. The fifth lumbar vertebra differs from the others in that the body is thinner posteriorly than anteriorly and the transverse processes are very large, attached to the whole of the lateral surface of the pedicle encroaching on the body of the vertebra.

The apophyseal joints are strong; the capsule is attached to the margins of the apophyseal articular facets; the supporting ligaments have been described in section 14.1. In the lumbar region the ligamentum flavum is thicker than in other areas of the spine. It helps to limit flexion and also helps to restore the spine to the upright position by virtue of it's elasticity. In this way the ligamentum flavum guards the intervertebral discs from injury. The supraspinous and interspinous ligaments are also stronger in the lumbar region than in the spinal areas above.

The lumbar spine is lordotic; this curve can become excessive if the tone of the abdominal muscles is poor or the hamstring muscles are tight. The angle between the fifth lumbar vertebra and the base of the sacrum is known as the 'lumbosacral angle' which is normally about 140°.

The lower two lumbar vertebrae are joined directly to the ilium by the iliolumbar ligaments (see Fig. 16.2). The superior iliolumbar ligament is attached to the tip of the transverse process of L4 and runs downwards and backwards to become attached to the iliac

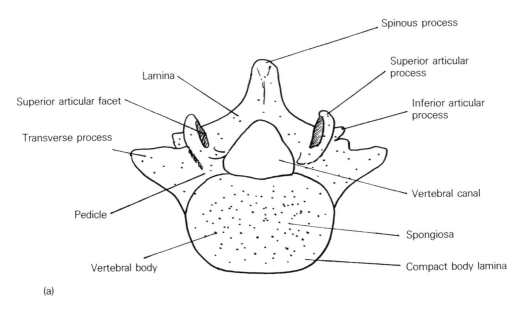

(a)

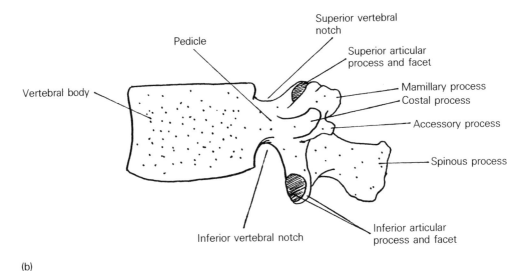

(b)

Fig. 16.1   A typical lumbar vertebra. (a) Superior aspect; (b) lateral aspect.

crest. The inferior iliolumbar ligament arises from the tip of the transverse process of L5 and passes downward to the iliac crest to become attached to it immediately anteromedially to the superior ligament (see Fig. 16.2). These ligaments are extremely strong and become stretched during movements of the lumbosacral joint and hence help to limit movements at that joint. Their strength is extremely important to athletes.

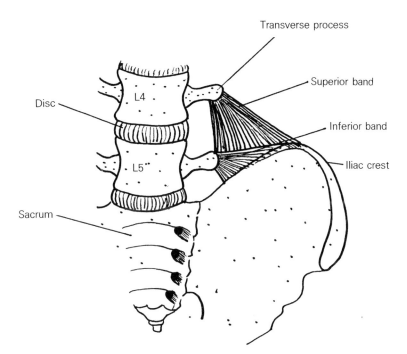

Fig. 16.2 Iliolumbar ligaments.

The movements of the lumbar region are flexion, extension, side bending to right and left and rotation to right and left. Flexion is brought about by the anterior muscles, namely psoas and the abdominal muscles and is limited by tension in the posterior ligaments of the spine. Extension is brought about by the action of the posterior spinal muscles and is limited by apposition of the spinous processes and tension in the anterior longitudinal ligament. Side-bending is brought about by the action of quadratus lumborum and the lateral abdominal muscles and is limited largely by tension in the ligamentum flavum (and the lateral muscles on the stretched side). Rotation is a very limited movement in the lumbar area due to the plane of the articular facets. It depends on the rotatores and the range is about 2° between any two vertebrae. Forced rotation beyond that range will damage the joint. Should a scoliosis be present, this movement will be unequal on each side leading to the increased possibility of joint strain.

The abdominal muscles are divisable into three groups. The superficial lateral muscles are the external and internal oblique muscles and the transversus abdominis (see Figs. 16.3 and 16.4). The medial muscles are the rectus abdominis and pyramidalis and the deep muscles are the psoas and the quadratus lumborum.

The *external abdominal oblique* is the largest and most superficial muscle of its group (see Fig. 16.3). It arises by fleshy slips from the outer surface of ribs five to twelve, interdigitating with the origin of serratus anterior between the fifth to ninth ribs and of

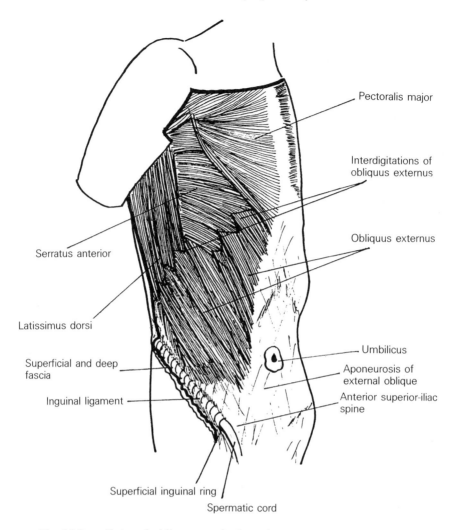

Fig. 16.3   External oblique muscle, lateral aspect.

latissimus dorsi between the tenth to twelfth ribs. The lowest
fibres, from the lowest three ribs run almost vertically downwards
and are inserted into the anterior half of the iliac crest, on the
outer lip, and into the anterior superior iliac spine. The remaining
fibres pass downward and forward and end in an aponeurosis, the
lowest fibres of which form the inguinal ligament which stretches
from the anterior superior iliac crest to the pubic tubercle. This is a
thick band of fibres folded back upon itself. The remainder of the
insertion is in the median plane where the right and left aponeuroses
interdigitate, together with those of the other lateral abdominal
muscles to form the linea alba. This tendinous raphe stretches
from the xiphoid process to the symphysis pubis. The nerve supply

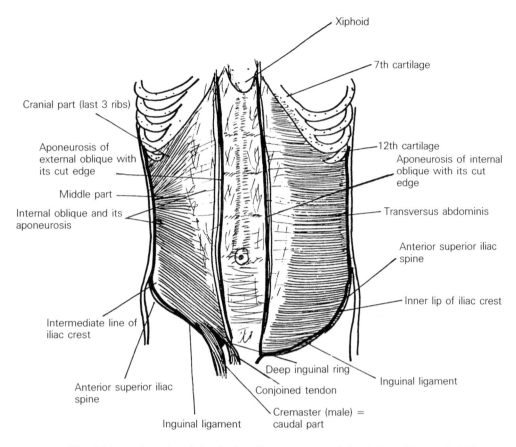

Xiphoid

7th cartilage

Cranial part (last 3 ribs)

Aponeurosis of
external oblique with
its cut edge

Middle part

Internal oblique and its
aponeurosis

12th cartilage
Aponeurosis of internal
oblique with its cut
edge

Transversus abdominis

Anterior superior iliac
spine

Inner lip of iliac crest

Intermediate line of
iliac crest

Deep inguinal ring

Conjoined tendon

Inguinal ligament

Anterior superior iliac
spine

Inguinal ligament

Cremaster (male) =
caudal part

Fig. 16.4   Anterior abdominal wall, transversus abdominis and internal oblique muscles.

consists of the anterior primary rami of the lower six thoracic nerves.

The superficial inguinal ring is a slit like opening in the aponeurosis of the external oblique muscle, forming part of the inguinal canal. It is bounded by bundles of fibre of the aponeurosis which strengthen the aperture.

The *internal abdominal oblique* lies under the external oblique and is thinner and less bulky (see Fig. 16.4). It arises by fleshy fibres from the lateral two-thirds of the inguinal ligament, the anterior two-thirds of the iliac crest and from the lumbar fascia. The posterior fibres ascend almost vertically to be inserted into the lowest three ribs and are continuous with the internal intercostal muscles. The fibres which take their origin from the inguinal ligament, arch downwards across the spermatic cord in the male, or the round ligament of the uterus in the female, and are inserted together with part of the aponeurosis of the transversus abdominis into the crest and pectineal line of the pubis. The middle fibres of the muscle pass medially into the aponeurosis which splits to encase the rectus abdominis muscle and then reunites at the linea alba. The nerve supply consists of the anterior primary rami of the lower three thoracic nerves and that of L1.

The *cremaster* muscle is composed of a few fibres of the internal oblique which pass along the lateral side of the spermatic cord in the male, forming a series of loops around the cord and testis and is finally inserted into the pubic tubercle and crest. Its nerve supply consists of the femoral nerve, L1 and L2. The muscle is principally not under voluntary control but it helps to support the testis.

The *transversus abdominis* is the deepest of the flat muscles of the abdominal wall, lying deep to the internal oblique (see Fig. 16.4). It arises from the inner surfaces of the cartilages of the lowest six ribs, where it interdigitates with the diaphragm, from the lateral one-third of the inguinal ligament, the anterior two-thirds of the iliac crest and the anterior superior iliac spine and also from the lumbar fascia. The fibres pass medially and end in an aponeurosis, the lowest fibres of which are inserted with some of those of the internal oblique into the pectineal line and crest of the pubis. The remaining fibres pass horizontally to become inserted into the linea alba, the upper threequarters behind the rectus abdominis and the lower one-quarter in front of that muscle. Its nerve supply consists of the anterior primary rami of T6 to T12 and L1.

The *rectus abdominis* is a medial muscle of the abdominal wall (see Fig. 16.5). It arises from the xiphoid process and by three slips from the outer surface of the fifth, sixth and seventh costal cartilages as well as from the intervening ligaments. The fibres pass downward and become inserted into the crest of the pubis and into the symphysis pubis. The muscle lies within the rectus sheath which is formed by the aponeuroses of the three lateral abdominal muscles passing in front of and behind the rectus before merging together to form the linea alba. Three fibrous bands pass transversely across the muscle and are adherent to the anterior part of the muscle sheath. The first is usually at the level of the xiphoid process, the second midway between that process and the umbilicus and the third at the level of the umbilicus. Its nerve supply consists of the anterior primary rami of T6 to T12.

The *pyramidalis* is a small muscle which arises from the front of the symphysis pubis and the adjacent part of the pubis (see Fig. 16.5). It is inserted into the linea alba between the umbilicus and the pubis. It acts to tense the linea alba. Its nerve supply consists of T12.

The inguinal canal transmits the spermatic cord or the round ligament of the uterus (see Fig. 16.6). The inner or deep inguinal ring lies immediately below the arched fibres of the transverse abdominis muscle between the fibrous attachment to the iliac crest

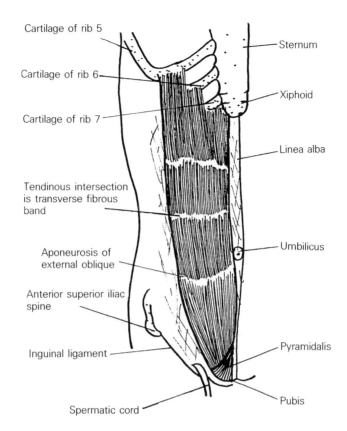

Cartilage of rib 5

Sternum

Cartilage of rib 6

Xiphoid

Cartilage of rib 7

Linea alba

Tendinous intersection is transverse fibrous band

Umbilicus

Aponeurosis of external oblique

Anterior superior iliac spine

Pyramidalis

Inguinal ligament

Pubis

Fig. 16.5 The right rectus abdominis and pyramidalis, anterior aspect.

Spermatic cord

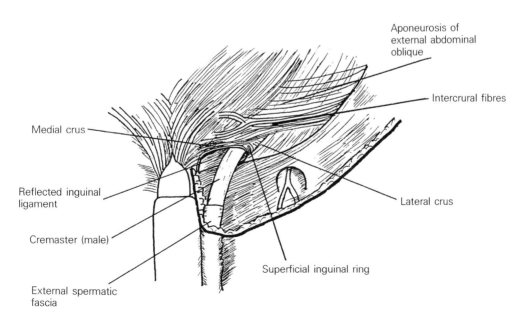

Aponeurosis of external abdominal oblique

Intercrural fibres

Medial crus

Reflected inguinal ligament

Lateral crus

Cremaster (male)

External spermatic fascia

Superficial inguinal ring

Fig. 16.6   The inguinal canal and the superficial inguinal ring.

and the pubis and forms the medial opening for the start of the inguinal canal. Anteriorly the canal is covered by the aponeurosis of the external oblique muscle and the canal ends at the superficial inguinal ring in the external oblique muscle (see Fig. 16.6).

There are sites of weakness in the abdominal wall (see Fig. 16.7), one of which is the superficial inguinal ring, where herniation is likely to occur. Other weak sites are the umbilicus, the linea alba and surgical scars. In addition the femoral canal presents a weak site but this lies below the inguinal ligament. Herniation is more likely to occur inguinally in men and femorally in women who are particularly prone to femoral herniation following multiple pregnancies which weaken the abdominal wall. See also section 17.1.

Psoas has already been described in section 9.1.

Quadratus lumborum arises from the iliolumbar ligament and the adjacent part of the iliac crest. The fibres pass upwards to be inserted into the medial half of the twelfth rib and into the tip of the transverse processes of L1 to L4 inclusive. This is a powerful muscle and acts to side bend the lumbar spine, an action which is much used in athletic activity. Its nerve supply consists of the

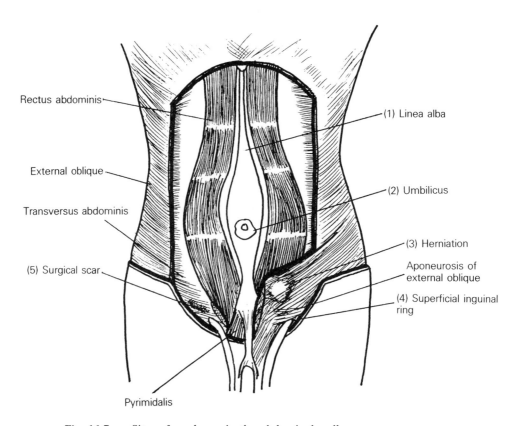

Fig. 16.7   Sites of weakness in the abdominal wall.

anterior primary rami of T12 to L4. Both muscles acting together can extend the lumbar area of the spine.

Muscle injuries

The abdominal wall is injured either by some direct force or by stretching activities especially when the arm is used above the head (see also section 17.1). Tennis players, volleyball players and netball players are likely candidates for this injury, tennis players usually causing the problem by overstretching on the service action. The athlete will complain of pain at the site of injury which may be anywhere, not necessarily at its attachment to bone. The pain is made worse on forced contraction of the abdominal wall and possibly on deep expiration. It is not an easy muscle injury to treat. Soft tissue techniques are difficult to use on these muscles but can be performed preferably with the athlete in the kneeling position. Ultrasound is very helpful. There is usually a residual area of fibrous scar tissue which tends to tear later around the periphery. To minimise the amount of scar tissue the athlete should be encouraged to carry out gentle stretching to the area while healing is taking place, such as gentle swimming. Ultrasound helps to reduce the scar tissue fibrosis. All stretching activities must be avoided until the lesioned area has completely repaired or there is a great risk of further damage.

Other damage to the abdominal wall includes *herniation* which is usually caused by heavy lifting. Some athletes have a congenital weakness in the inguinal or femoral regions and are more prone to possible herniation. In these cases herniation of one side is often followed some time later by herniation on the other side. The athlete will complain of pain: there is a palpable swelling which becomes larger on coughing. Surgical repair is advisable.

Injury to psoas is described in section 9.2.

Quadratus lumborum is often injured as a result of violent side-bending movements such as a cricketer may carry out, especially in the slips or behind the wicket (see Fig. 16.8). It is also seen in other sports such as racket sports where this movement is suddenly performed. The athlete will complain of pain in the region of the injured muscle which is made worse on active side bending. Resisted movement will exacerbate the pain. Palpation will reveal acute tenderness in the damaged muscle which may be in a state of spasm. Treatment is aimed at gently stretching out the contracted fibres and heat also helps. Rubbing the area with Tiger balm is useful. As in all muscular injuries, the athlete must not return to active sport until the condition has healed, to avoid the probability of recurrence.

Injury to the lumbar erector spinae usually accompanies a joint

Table 16.1 Muscles supplied by the lumbar nerves

	Anterior primary rami	Posterior primary rami
L1	Quadratus lumborum Internal oblique Transversus abdominis Cremaster	Deep muscles of the back
L2	Psoas major Pectineus Sartorius Adductors longus and brevis	Deep muscles of the back
L3	Psoas major Obturator externus Adductors Iliacus Pectineus Sartorius Quadriceps	Deep muscle of the back

L4	Obturator externus
	Adductor magnus
	Gracilis
	Rectus femoris
	Vasti lateralis and
	  intermedius
	Gluteus medius and
	  minimus
	Tensor fascia lata
	Quadratus femoris
	Semimembranosus
	Tibialis anterior and
	  posterior
		Deep muscles of the back

L5	Gluteus maximus Gluteus medius Gluteus minimus Tensor fascia lata Quadratus femoris Obturator internus Semimembranosus Semitendinosus Biceps, short head only All muscles of leg except gastrocnemius Extensor digitorum brevis Abductor hallucis Flexor hallucis brevis Flexor digitorum brevis	Deep muscles of the back

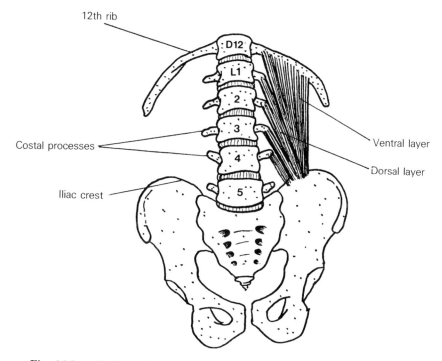

12th rib

D12

L1

2

3

4

5

Costal processes

Iliac crest

Ventral layer

Dorsal layer

Fig. 16.8   Left quadratus lumborum.

strain (see section 16.6), a disc injury (see section 16.5), or a bone injury (see section 16.4).

16.3   Tendon injuries

Tendon injury in this region is unusual, but the tendon of psoas, or more often the musculotendinous junction can be injured. The condition is described in section 9.4.

16.4   Bone injuries

The lumbar region is not likely to be injured as it is well protected both in front and behind. However, it is possible if there is a fall against a hard or sharp object such as a goal post, in which case there could be damage to a spinous process. The athlete would complain of severe pain due largely to the involvement of the posterior ligaments, especially the supraspinous ligament and inter-spinous ligaments, both of which are strong in the lumbar region. The athlete would be most likely to adopt a posture of lumbar extension to relieve the pain. Active flexion would be painful. X-rays would reveal the bone damage but as the long ligaments would not be damaged, the fracture is of the stable type and responds best to activity, gentle at first. Full activity can be resumed, only after bony repair.

An *avulsion* of a transverse process is possible due to violent muscular action usually of psoas, such as in a violent kick. It can also result from violent use of quadratus lumborum in violent side bending of the lumbar spine, for example in hockey or cricket. The athlete will complain of pain in the area of the avulsion which will be aggravated by use of either psoas or quadratus lumborum, or both muscles. As this too is a stable fracture, it is best treated by activity, gentle at first. Sometimes union is fibrous, but this does not affect the athlete in the long-term as it seems to be sufficiently strong for active use.

Compression injury such as a fall from a height can occasionally fracture a vertebral body. The history will help. If the longitudinal ligaments are not damaged, this fracture can be overlooked as the pain will be minimal. It is best treated by a corset which should be worn for about six weeks, or until healing has occurred. If the longitudinal ligaments are damaged, there will be considerable pain. Treatment is still by use of a corset. Following bony union, osteopathic treatment to the surrounding areas is indicated to make sure there are no residual joint or soft tissue problems before full sporting activity is resumed. If there are abnormal neurological signs the athlete should be referred for further investigation.

Extension strains of the lumbar spine, if severe, can fracture the pars interarticularis, usually of L5 or L4. The iliolumbar ligament is also damaged in this case. If there is an associated shift forward of the upper part of the spine the condition is known as spondylo-listhesis. The fracture can be bilateral or unilateral. This condition is often familial, which implies that there may be some congenital weakness in the pars. (If the vertebral slip is backwards above the fracture, the condition is known as retrolisthesis.) Mild cases respond well to osteopathic treatment, aimed at mobilising the surrounding joints. Sacral springing is also useful and can be marginally correc-tive. The degree of instability of spondylolisthesis can be demonstrated on mobility plates. If the condition is unstable, surgical treatment may be necessary. One orthopaedic surgeon tests the stability of an athlete by asking him to perform on a trampoline for ten minutes in addition to all the other tests; if the condition is made considerably worse, the surgeon may consider surgically fixing the vertebrae. Where surgical treatment is not needed, strengthening of the ab-dominal muscles is useful as these help to prevent hyperextension. Should the athlete's sport involve lumbar extension, surgery may be advisable, but if the sport does not, for example cycling, surgery may be unnecessary. Clinical examination will reveal hyperextension at the level of the fracture and there may be a palpable shelf. Extra care should be taken if the injury is at the level of L5 as this bone may have a short spinous process which is difficult to palpate and may have slipped so far anteriorly as to be impossible to palpate. The spinous process which appears to be that of L5 may in reality be that of L4. X-rays are diagnostic; oblique plates will show the well known 'scotty dog collar' defect. Oblique X-rays must always be taken in cases of suspected pars injury. Pain is often referred to the anterior aspect of both thighs, aggravated by lumbar extension. Low back ache is also present.

All *fractures* of the lumbar spine must cause some damage to the associated intervertebral disc. This may be evident at the time of the initial injury or may give rise to symptoms later. All fractures may cause irritation of the lumbar nerves, or in some cases, of the cauda equina.

Occasionally there appears to be a fracture of the anterior part of a vertebral body but this is incomplete union of the bone and is of no consequence. The condition is usually discovered when routine X-rays are taken; it does not give rise to symptoms. No treatment is needed.

16.5

Disc injury

Disc injury in the lumbar region is very common in athletes, often in young people but usually after growth is complete. Damage to the adolescent disc is seen in cases of Scheuermann's disease with the development of Schmorl's nodes − see section 15.4. If this condition occurs in the lumbar spine, it is most often seen in the upper two segments. If the young growing spine is subjected to repeated compression strains, the intervertebral discs can become enlarged and biconvex; the effect is some degree of erosion of the vertebral bodies which in turn become biconcave. This results in weakening the adult spine so that injuries are more likely to be seen. This used to be seen all too often in youngsters who played a great deal of rugby football but a change in the rules has decreased the incidence of such injury.

Disc injury in adults is usually a result of a lifting or twisting strain. The exact symptom picture will vary according to which tissues are damaged. Nerve root pressure will result from a posterolateral protrusion of nuclear material which can cause pressure on the nerve root (see Fig. 16.9). Low back pain is present as the posterior longitudinal ligament is also damaged. The ligamentum flavum may be involved as well and in the lower two segments, the iliolumbar ligaments may be damaged too. Nerve root irritation is nearly always unilateral and can only be bilateral if the disc protrusion is large and posterior so that both the segmental nerves can be pressurised by it. If the protrusion is anterior, the symptom picture will be one of low back pain without nerve root irritation. In these cases the anterior longitudinal ligament will be damaged

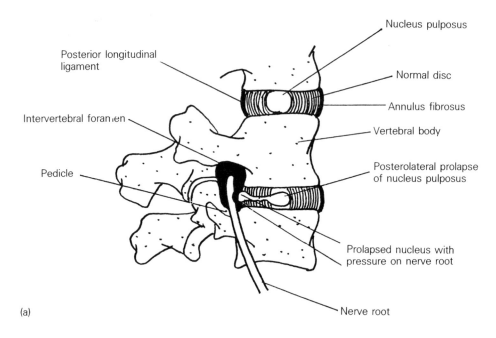

(a)

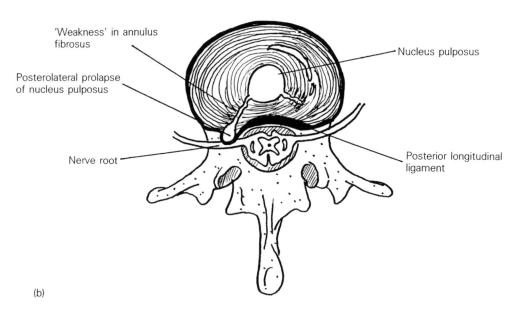

(b)

Fig. 16.9   Disc protrusion resulting in nerve root pressure. (a) Lateral aspect; (b) superior aspect.

and will give rise to low back pain. The usual symptom picture is of low back pain, the onset frequently is within the first hour of the day and may follow some unusual physical activity the previous day; often, however, the onset is for no apparent reason. There may be pain in the distribution of one nerve root, most often the fifth lumbar root. Somewhat less often the first sacral root or the third lumbar root is irritated. Upper lumbar root involvement is not often seen. The pain is accentuated by active extension with side bending to the side of the pain and is relieved by flexion and side bending away from the pain. Coughing and sneezing make the pain worse. When the athlete is asked to flex, actively, he may well side bend away from the pain as he flexes. Compression tests are usually positive. There is limitation of movement, muscular guarding, positive straight leg raising, weakness of dorsiflexion, possible numbness in an area of the foot, a reflex change, (usually a diminution is found,) and possibly an area of sensory loss. All these symptoms are unlikely to occur together in any one athlete, but the list should be a guide to the possibility of some disc injury having occurred.

Most cases respond well to osteopathic treatment which is aimed at relieving the pressure. The first line of approach is to try to increase the size of the foramen through which the irritated nerve has to pass, by foraminal gapping, and possibly by traction in flexion. Sacral springing will have a similar effect at the level of L5. Articulation in any range which relieves the pain is indicated and improving the mechanics at the surrounding joint levels to take some of the mechanical pressure off the damaged segment. Only once there is evidence of the disc being less inflamed and the associated ligaments undergoing repair is any treatment directed at the level of disc protrusion. It is an accepted fact that joint and disc injury is less likely to occur if the surrounding musculature is strong, so some re-education of the surrounding muscles is necessary before athletic activity is resumed.

In older athletes there will be a reduction of the disc due to advancing age. This, if it is severe, can lead to nerve root irritation from progressive foraminal encroachment. These athletes respond well to osteopathic treatment, aimed at improving the spinal mechanics. Exercises for these athletes should be aimed at increasing flexibility rather than muscular strength, but this may be important if the muscles are of poor tone. Yoga and swimming are particularly helpful for these athletes.

Some cases of disc injury present with intractable pain — i.e. the pain cannot be relieved by any means while the athlete is on the treatment table. These cases are probably those where there is a true herniation of the disc with some strangulation of the protrusion. In some cases, the pain gets slowly better if all weight bearing is avoided, that is, the athlete must have complete bed rest. The pain can be controlled by analgesics. Should this approach not improve the athlete's condition by the end of two weeks, surgery has to be considered. In all cases where there is any sign of spinal cord involvement or of progressive muscular weakness, an orthopaedic opinion should be sought as soon as possible, as surgery may well be the treatment of choice, but only if conventional treatment has proved ineffective.

It seems probable that many disc injuries follow some time after joint strains in the area, especially if these have been recurrent. A careful history of any previous low back problems can be a helpful guide to the possibility of disc injury in an athlete.

16.6   **Joint and ligament injury**

Simple joint strains are extremely commonly seen in athletes. The picture is similar to the typical sprained ankle. The history is of some unusual movement and the pain may come on at the time of such movement or shortly afterwards. Clinically there is ligamentous damage which may be to the capsule of an apophyseal joint or to one or more of the surrounding ligaments. The exact symptom picture will vary according to which ligament(s) is traumatised and how. Strain of an apophyseal joint will lead to pain at the site of the strain and there will be surrounding muscle spasm which is also painful. All active movement will be limited and possibly painful due to the associated muscular condition, but the pain may not be equally severe on all active movements. Examination of the range of passive movement may reveal no abnormality. In the early stage this type of injury responds well to rest; a supportive strapping will help to relieve the pain as the muscles can relax somewhat, around the injury. After about four days, osteopathic treatment to any surrounding abnormal mechanics and soft tissue treatment to the surrounding muscles accelerates full recovery. Sport can usually be resumed in about two weeks.

Hypermobility is not rare in the lumbar spine, where it is usually found to be affecting one spinal segment only. The commonest sites are L4 and L3 apophyseal joints. This condition is caused by repeated strains of the joint concerned, either from some activity or possibly from some repeated postural problem, for example the athlete may have an angular lordosis so that the joint at the apex of the curve is repeatedly overstretched on extension. In this case, the anterior ligaments become progressively stretched and the posterior ligaments remain relatively normal or marginally shortened. Passive examination in such a case will show excessive extension at that level when the range of movement is compared with that at the joints above and below. The athlete will complain of low back pain which is worse following physical activity, especially if that activity involves flexion. This is not an easy condition to treat. The hypermobile joint should be immobilised to allow the ligaments to tighten and any inflammation to subside. This may take up to a month. Following that, active osteopathic treatment to the joints above and below to reduce the strain on the joint which was hypermobile is indicated but no additional move-ment should be put through the hypermobile joint. Exercises to strengthen the muscles at the previously hypermobile joint level should be prescribed and any postural re-education given. This condition is often associated with poor abdominal tone and/or tight hamstring muscles where treatment will be needed.

Injury to any of the ligaments of the spine in the lumbar region is associated with damage to some other tissue, for example a fracture of bone or a disc injury or a joint strain. Hypermobility in extension of a lumbar joint is different from a spondylolisthesis; in the former there will be no palpable shelf, no X-ray change is likely and there will probably be no referred pain.

16.7

Facet locking

Facet locking in the lumbar region is very commonly seen in athletes; it can occur at one joint or may affect more than one at any one time. The athlete will complain of pain in the region of the injury which he may report came on after some unusual activity. There will be muscle spasm around the injured joint. Active move-ment in at least one direction will cause pain and he may adopt a particular posture to reduce his discomfort. Passive movement will be restricted in the same movement as caused maximal pain actively, but the other movements may be free. It is possible for this condition to give rise to nerve root pressure (the apophyseal joint lies in close proximity to the intervertebral foramen), but this is by no means commonly seen. X-rays, if taken, will be normal. Cor-rection of the locking will relieve the symptoms. Treatment should be given to other areas of the spine and pelvis if any mechanical fault is found as this could have been a contributory factor in the original injury.

16.8

Anomalies

Congenital anomalies occur most frequently in the lumbo-sacral area of the spine. In general, an anomaly will interfere with the normal mechanics of the area and predispose to the probability of injury, especially in activities such as weight lifting or throwing events. Reduced flexibility will interfere with activities such as gymnastics which may be contraindicated in these people.

Atypical facets at the lumbo-sacral level are very commonly seen. The facets may be of the thoracic type so the normal range of movement (which depends on the plane of the facets) will be altered. This condition may be bilateral or unilateral; in the latter case, the mechanics will be dissimilar on the right and left, a condition which predisposes to severe joint strains in some athletes. It is difficult to treat successfully as it is impossible to rearrange the facets. The best treatment is often to limit movement by the use of sclerosing fluids or a supporting belt, as at least this will reduce the risk of strain.

The fifth lumbar vertebra may be *sacralised* − i.e. have a bony bond with the sacrum. This may be bilateral or unilateral. If it is bilateral, effectively the athlete will have only four mobile lumbar segments so each will have to take additional strain during athletic activity. This condition could contraindicate any activity therefore, which requires great flexibility. If the condition is unilateral, it is also asymmetrical so the strains are unevenly placed on the segment. The result of this is usually strain of the normal side where movement can occur. Again the approach is usually to reduce movement at the level of the lumbosacral joint and thus reduce the risk of strain.

The first sacral segment may be *lumbarised* − i.e. incompletely fused to the remaining segments of the sacrum and permitting some degree of movement. This gives rise to strain of the S1 segment and stretching of the ligaments there, which causes pain on certain movements. A spina bifida occulta may be present at the first sacral level when the supraspinous and inter-spinous ligaments may be stretched with activity, and cause pain. Both these conditions are best treated by immobilising them, thus reducing the strain which movement places on them, and the flexible type sports are contraindicated.

There may be a hemivertebra, usually at the level of L5, which will result in abnormal mechanics at that level. Again, immobilisation is the most effective approach.

Occasionally an *adventitious joint* is seen, usually between the transverse process of L5 and the crest of the ilium. In this case the transverse process is obviously far larger than normal. This condition is seldom bilateral. The adventitious joint will become strained in side bending away from it and compressed in side bending towards it and give rise to pain of a ligamentous type. Any side bending should be avoided and sports which involve this movement are contraindicated.

Congenital fusion is occasionally seen in this region but is less common than in the thoracic area. It results in a degree of inflexibility.

Some athletes have an *extra vertebra* − i.e. six lumbar vertebrae. At times this may only become apparent because there may be an absence of the twelfth pair of ribs. It does not usually give rise to problems as the condition is symmetrical.

Ribs are sometimes seen articulating with the first lumbar vertebra. Pain can result from them if they are compressed, which is likely to happen on side bending movements so such movements may have to be avoided. Lumbar ribs can also irritate the kidney due to their anatomical proximity.

The sensible approach to all anomalies is to analyse the mechanical problem which the anomaly causes and relate it to the particular sporting activity of the athlete concerned.

Surgical fusion of vertebrae in the lumbar region will lead to some loss of flexibility which can cause additional strain on the remaining, flexible joints. A laminectomy sometimes leaves the athlete hypermobile in extension when support by means of a belt may be necessary for sporting activities.

16.9 Stiffness

This usually follows some unaccustomed activity and is caused by increased tone in the lumbar erector spinae muscles. It can be very distressing to an athlete, and painful. The athlete will adopt a position of lumbar extension, to reduce the pull on the affected muscles. Stretching them will cause pain. Rest from all physical activity, deep soft tissue treatment and the application of heat will relieve the condition swiftly. Degenerative changes are seen in older athletes and give rise to progressive stiffness. Osteopathic treatment can improve the mobility in these people.

16.10 Nerve injury

The lumbar nerves are invariably injured as a result of trauma to bone, a joint (rarely) or to an intervertebral disc (commonly). The exact symptom picture will depend on which nerve root is involved. The symptoms will be pain along the line of the nerve, possible muscle weakness and numbness or paraesthesia.

Herpes zoster may affect a lumbar nerve, see section 15.8. Pain can be referred to the low back from the abdominal or pelvic viscera, in which case examination of the lumbar spine will reveal no abnormality. Palpation of the abdominal region may cause the osteopath to be suspicious and the athlete should be referred for the necessary further investigation.

The nerve roots may be irritated due to *foraminal encroachment*. This usually accompanies degenerative changes in the lumbar spine, which will show on X-ray examination. If a lateral plate is taken in extension, a degree of stenosis may be seen to be present. The condition responds well to osteopathic treatment especially in the early stages. Anterior osteophytosis is frequently present and does not contraindicate osteopathic treatment, but in cases where there is considerable posterior osteophytosis, the patient does not respond well to treatment in my experience.

16.11 Visceral injury

In cases of abdominal injury there is a possibility of visceral damage, slight though this is. However, it must always be remembered in cases of direct violent injury. The kidneys and bladder (especially if full), the liver, spleen, pancreas and gastro-intestinal tract are at risk and these athletes should be kept under careful observation and referred at once if their condition deteriorates.

Chapter 17   The Pelvis, Sacrum and Coccyx

General

The bony pelvis consists of the two innominate bones, the sacrum and the coccyx.

The *innominate* consists of three parts, the pubis, ilium and ischium; they fuse together in the walls of the acetabulum (the pelvic articular surface of the hip joint) (see Fig. 17.1). The two pubic bones meet anteriorly in the midline forming the pubic symphysis (see Fig. 17.2). Posteriorly the ilium articulates with the sacrum forming the sacro-iliac joint on each side. The coccyx is the most inferior part of the vertebral column and articulates superiorly with the sacrum at the sacrococcygeal joint. Below and in front of the acetabulum is a large or oval gap, the obturator foramen.

The *ilium* is the superior part of the innominate. The upper part of the ilium forms the iliac crest; the anterior superior iliac spine projects at it's anterior part while there is a smaller spine below – the anterior inferior iliac spine which is not so easily palpable. There are two posterior iliac spines at the posterior end of the crest, the superior being more easily palpated than the inferior. The large posterior surface of the ilium is the gluteal surface, while the corresponding anterior surface is the iliac fossa. The gluteal surface has two gluteal lines, the anterior and the posterior on it. The upper part, or ala of the ilium, is separated from the lower part, or body, by the arcuate line. On the internal surface is a roughened area which is the articular surface which forms the iliac part of the sacro-iliac joint.

The *ischium* is divided into a body and the ramus of the ischium. This ramus forms the inferior border of the obturator foramen together with the inferior ramus of the pubis. The ischial spine projects downwards and medially, giving attachment to the sacrospinous ligament which divides the two sciatic notches. The ischial tuberosity is a roughened area on the lower part of the postero-inferior aspect of the ischium and is the area on which the weight should be transmitted while sitting. The ramus springs from the lower part of the body and passes forward, upward and medially to join with the inferior ramus of the pubis.

The *pubis* is the anterior component of the innominate. It consists of a body and two rami. The superior ramus borders the obturator foramen anteriorly while the inferior ramus joins the ramus of the ischium to border the obturator foramen inferiorly. The rounded

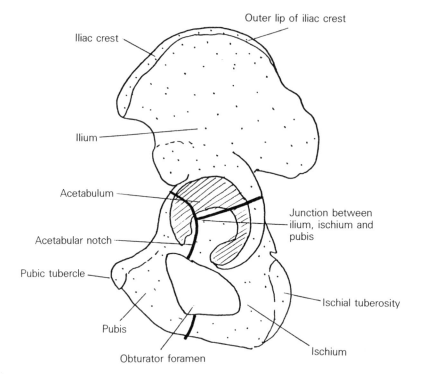

(a)

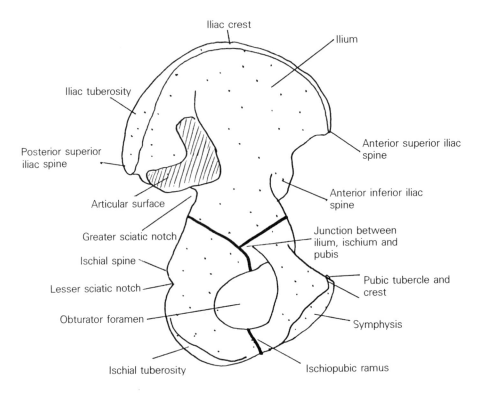

(b)

Fig. 17.1   The left innominate. (a) Lateral aspect; (b) medial aspect.

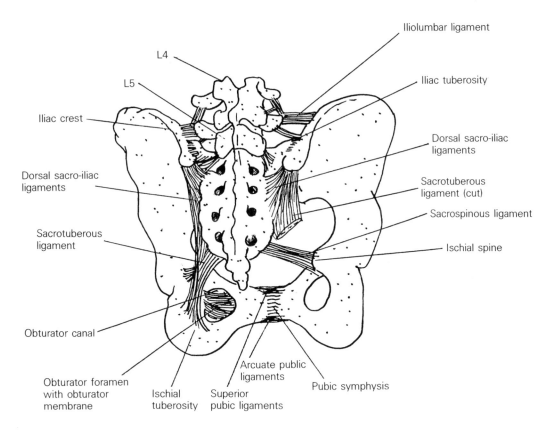

Fig. 17.2   Sacro-iliac joints, pubic symphisis and pelvic ligaments, dorsal aspect.

upper border of the body is the pubic crest which has a rounded projection medially, the pubic tubercle. The pectineal line runs laterally from the crest towards the arcuate line of the ilium. The obturator groove lies below the tubercle and has a small tubercle on it's internal surface, the obturator tubercle.

The *symphysis pubis* is formed by the two pubic bones where they meet anteriorly. It has a fibrocartilagenous disc. The superior pubic ligament connects the bones superiorly and is attached to the pubic tubercles. The inferior pubic ligament reinforces the symphysis below and is attached to the inferior rami of the pubes.

The *sacrum* consists of five fused vertebrae and their intervertebral discs. On the anterior surface there are four foraminae for the transmission of the spinal nerves. It is concave anteriorly. The posterior surface is convex. The spinous processes have fused in the midline to form the median sacral crest. Immediately lateral to this is the intermediate sacral crest which is formed by the fused remnants of the articular processes. Lateral to this crest lie the four foraminae while more lateral still is the lateral sacral crest which is formed by the fused remnants of the transverse processes.

On the superior surface of the sacrum are the superior articular processes which articulate with the fifth lumbar vertebra. On the lateral surface is the roughened auricular surface which forms the sacral component of the sacro-iliac joint. Immediately posterior to this is the sacral tuberosity, another roughened area for ligamentous attachment. Inferiorly there is a small articular surface which forms the sacral component of the sacrococcygeal joint. The male sacrum is longer and narrower than the female but the female sacrum is less curved in the A–P plane. The female pelvis as a whole is broader and wider than the male pelvis. (See Fig. 2.4).

The *coccyx* is considered to be rudimentary; it is formed from three or four vertebrae which are usually fused. On the superior surface are two cornua which project laterally above the articular surface and form the coccygeal component of the sacrococcygeal joint.

The *pelvic girdle* affords protection to the contained viscera and provides attachment for muscles of the abdomen, trunk and lower limb. Far more important is it's function to transmit the weight bearing forces from the upper part of the body to the lower extremities. Enormous strength with some degree of flexibility is needed for this task. Excessive movement at the pelvic joints would lead to instability of this function, especially during sporting activities which require a great deal of flexibility elsewhere in the body.

The *sacro-iliac joint* is the articulation between the auricular surface of the sacrum and the auricular surface of the ilium (see Fig. 17.3). Each surface is covered by fibrocartilage and there is a strong taut capsule which is attached to the margins of the articular surfaces. Further strong ligaments support the joint, an anterior, an interosseous and a posterior ligament. In addition, the joint is indirectly reinforced by the iliolumbar ligaments – see section 16.1 – and by the sacrotuberous and sacrospinous ligaments.

The *sacrotuberous ligament* is attached medially to the posterior iliac spines, (where it partly blends with the posterior sacro-iliac ligament), the posterior aspect of the sacrum and the posterior aspect of the coccyx. The fibres run obliquely laterally and downwards to become attached to the ramus of the ischium. It is extremely strong.

The *sacrospinous ligament* is much thinner; it is attached to the lateral margins of the sacrum and coccyx, anterior to the sacrotuberous ligament, and the fibres converge to become attached to the spine of the ischium. These two ligaments convert the sciatic notches into foraminae.

The *sacrococcygeal joint* is a cartilagenous joint, having a fibrocartilagenous disc within. It is reinforced by an anterior, a posterior and a lateral ligament on each side. The movement which occurs is largely passive and secondary to movement of the lumbosacral and pelvic joints. This combination of movement is complex as there is

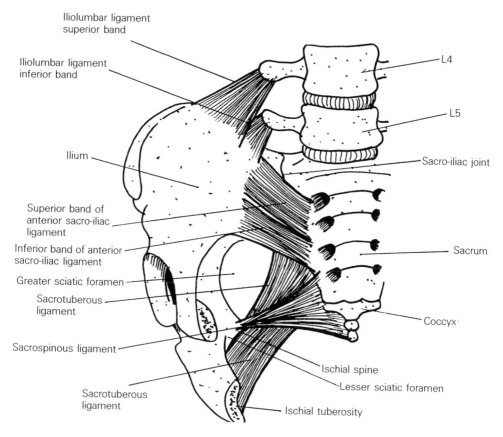

Fig. 17.3   Right sacro- iliac joint, anterior aspect.

no active movement directly on the pelvic joints, yet the movement which occurs is of critical importance in the total pelvic mechanics. Greater stresses would be placed on the lumbosacral joint and on the hip joint if the pelvic joints were not capable of movement. These joints come into use at or near the extremes of movement of the lumbosacral and hip joints. Total rigidity of the pelvis would increase the probability of bony injury there as some of the forces exerted on it are absorbed into the passively mobile pelvic joints. Logically, therefore, extreme stresses are capable of damaging these joints which do not have protective peri-articular musculature.

The movement which occurs at the symphysis pubis is of a shearing type, as the sacro-iliac joints move. In addition a small amount of separation occurs with certain hip joint movements, for example when kicking a ball. Excessive sudden movement of this type can cause a greater range of articular surface separation due to the attachment of the strong thigh muscles to the pubis.

The sacrum can flex and extend between the ilia, carrying the ilia with it. A small amount of rotation and side bending of the sacrum is also possible and the ilia will travel with the sacrum if the sacro-iliac joints are in a stable relationship to the sacrum. In addition, the ilium is capable of rotating around the sacrum, the axis of movement being through the level of the second sacral vertebra. Although this movement is not a primary one, it occurs with certain movements of the hip joint or of the lower lumbar spine due to the muscular attachments to the pelvis. These muscles act primarily on joints other than the sacro-iliac joints. The stability of the pelvic joints depends solely on the integrity of the supporting ligaments which can become damaged and stretched and less taut following childbirth. It also seems likely that they are affected by the hormonal changes which occur during the menstrual cycle – they seem to be more vulnerable just before the onset of the menstrual flow.

Muscles of the pelvis

All the muscles of the abdominal wall with the exception of the external oblique are attached to the pelvis – see section 16.1.

The muscles of the anterior aspect of the spine, namely psoas and iliacus are largely pelvic – see section 9.1.

Rectus femoris, pectineus and sartorius are also described in section 9.1. Also gluteus maximus, the hamstrings, gluteus medius, gluteus minimus, tensor fascia lata, adductor longus, adductor brevis, adductor magnus, gracilis, obturator internus, the gemelli, obturator externus, quadratus femoris and piriformis.

In addition to the above muscles, those of the pelvic floor are attached to the pelvic bones. They are divisible into the pelvic and urogenital diaphragms. Levator ani and the coccygeus muscles make up the pelvic diaphragm (see Fig. 17.4).

Levator ani arises from the body of the pubis, lateral to the symphysis, from the inner surface of the spine of the ischium and from the fascia covering the obturator muscles. The left and right muscles converge and unite in the median plane; some fibres end in the sphincter ani externus muscle and some extend into the perineum, dividing the urogenital from the anal tract. The genital hiatus is bordered posteriorly by this muscle; the vagina and urethra pass through this hiatus which is broader in the female so a second mechanism of closure is needed, the urogenital diaphragm (see Fig. 17.4).

The *coccygeus* muscle arises from the spine of the ischium and is inserted into the coccyx. Although small, this muscle is very important in the maintenance of the integrity of the pelvic diaphragm. The nerve supply of these two muscles is S4 and S5 (see Fig. 17.4).

The arrangement of the *urogenital diaphragm* differs in the male and female.

In the male: the *transversus perinei superficialis* arises from the

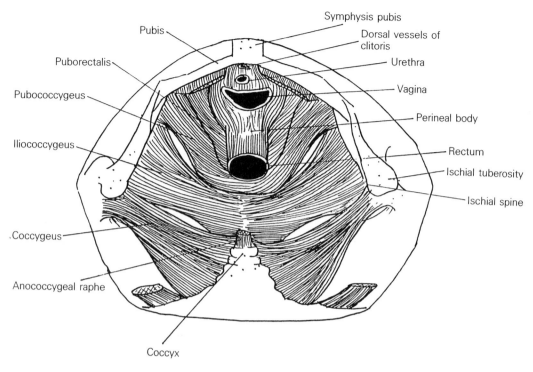

Fig. 17.4   The pelvic diaphragm (female).

ischial tuberosity and is inserted into the perineal body, which is a fibromuscular node in the midline. It is important in the maintenance of the integrity of the pelvic floor (especially in the female). This muscle helps to fix the perineal body.

The *bulbospongiosus* arises from the perineal body and is inserted into the penis. It's action assists the emptying of the urethra at the end of micturition.

The *ischiocavernosus* arises from the inner surface of the tuberosity of the ischium and is inserted into the crus of the penis. It's action maintains erection of the penis.

The *transverse perinei profundus* arises from the ramus of the ischium and is inserted into the perineal body. It also fixes the perineal body.

The *sphincter urethra* surrounds the membranous part of the urethra. The two act with the bulbospongiosus at the end of micturition. All these muscles are supplied by the perineal branch of the pudendal nerve, S2, S3 and S4.

In the female: the *transversus perinei superficialis* is as in the male.

The *bulbospongiosus* inserts into the periphery of the vagina. On contraction this muscle reduces the diameter of the vagina.

The *ischiocavernosus* is inserted into the clitoris and helps to maintain erection of the clitoris.

The *transversus perinei profundus* and the *sphincter urethra* are as in the male. The nerve supply is as in the male.

The function of the pelvic floor is to support the pelvic contents especially against the force of gravity and it is capable of affecting the intra-abdominal pressure. See Fig. 17.5.

17.2

Muscle injury

Many of the muscular injuries of the pelvic muscles have already been dealt with, see section 9.2 and section 10.4.

However, many of these muscles are extremely strong in athletes and violent contraction can lead to damage to the pelvic attachment. The periosteal-tendinous region can detach from the bone. The condition can be very painful, the pain being localised to the site of the lesion and exacerbated by use of the muscle. Bone avulsion can also occur − see section 7.5. The muscles which can be thus damaged are the long muscles of the thigh, especially the adductors, the hamstrings, sartorius and rectus femoris. The adductors arise from the pubis (mainly) and can be injured by those who do a great deal of horse riding. In fact the tendon of adductor longus frequently becomes ossified and is known as the 'rider's bone'.

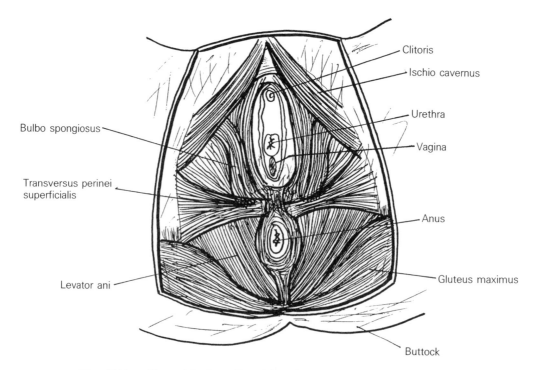

Fig. 17.5   The pelvic floor (female), pelvic and urogenital diaphragms.

During the process of ossification, the periosteal tissue is sensitive and can cause pain, especially when the muscle is contracted.

Similarly, the periosteal attachment of the rectus femoris muscle from the anterior inferior iliac spine and from the brim of the acetabulum, can detach or become inflamed, the former being the commoner site of this injury. Pain will be felt on extension of the knee, actively and resisted with the hip straight and there may be pain on hip flexion as well. Periosteal swelling and tenderness are present.

The origin of the hamstrings from the ischial tuberosity is another similar site of periosteal inflammation, caused by repetitive violent use of the hamstring muscles. The athlete will complain of pain at the site of the tuberosity which is aggravated by active and resisted contraction of the hamstring muscles – i.e. on knee flexion. There will be localised swelling and tenderness over the tuberosity, difficult to differentiate from a bursitis (see section 17.9).

The balance of strength, tone and flexibility of the hamstrings and the quadriceps is vitally important. Many athletes spend a great deal of time developing their quadriceps and relatively ignore their hamstrings. This leads to muscular imbalance and an increased probability of damage to the weaker muscles which should have extra time invested in their training and development.

Pain in the gluteal muscles is very common in athletes, for example following prolonged running as in marathon runners or cross country running where the ground is uneven. This is dealt with in section 9.2.

The pelvic floor can be damaged, especially in water sports where the athlete hits the water at speed. Because of their anatomy, females are more vulnerable than males, but both can be affected. The injury will cause pain in the muscles of the pelvic floor especially when they are tightened. Rest from all physical activity is essential until the fibres have completely healed as there is a risk of damage to the pelvic viscera. This is an example of an injury which is entirely preventable by wearing suitable protection during competition and training. Similarly the external genitalia of the male should always be suitably protected from the possibility of direct injury. Should there be any haematuria, this must be investigated at once and the athlete referred immediately.

17.3	**Tendon injuries**

These result from violent use of the muscles and have been mentioned in the section above. The common sites are the adductor origins from the pubis, the quadriceps rectus femoris component, sartorius and the hamstring origin from the ischial tuberosity. To determine whether the periosteum is involved or not will depend on careful palpation. The prognosis is far better and recovery swifter if the periosteum is not involved. Treatment of the tendon injury is to give soft tissue treatment to the muscular component of the muscle concerned, thereby relieving some of the tension on the tendon fibres. Local ultrasound and ice packs to the injured tendon are also helpful, but the athlete must not resume active sport until the injury is completely healed as recurrence is common. Full recuperation can take several weeks in a severe tendon injury; during that time the athlete should be encouraged to gently stretch the muscle and use it only without weight bearing – i.e. gentle swimming can be undertaken.

In cases where the periosteum is involved, recovery takes a great deal longer. Some cases respond well to local injection which may be needed to accelerate healing. Frequently a residual exostosis remains but seldom causes problems.

<table>
<tr><td>17.4</td><td>

Musculotendinous injuries

</td></tr>
</table>

The musculotendinous junction of any muscle is a vulnerable site. In the pelvic region these injuries usually occur, yet again, in the long muscles of the thigh because of the great leverage they exert. The cause of the problem is invariably some violent muscular contraction. Iliopsoas and the gluteal muscles can also be injured at their musculotendinous junctions.

In the case of the *adductor muscles*, the athlete will complain of pain on active and resisted adduction of the thigh and possibly on passive abduction. He will probably give a history of a sudden onset of pain which increased over the next few hours and was caused by some sudden violent movement such as kicking a ball. The site of the injury will be palpable, painful and swollen. Precise palpation is essential to differentiate a musculotendinous injury from a muscular or peritoneal one.

Treatment is aimed at the muscular tissue to relieve the strain on the musculotendinous junction. Friction to the site of the injury is indicated and ultrasound is useful to promote healing. Attention must be paid to the balance of the injured part and it's antagonist; the weaker muscle is liable to become injured. Osteopathic treatment will also be needed to the surrounding joints, as should there be any deficiency in joint function, this can impose additional strain on the muscle concerned and may therefore predispose it to injury. The spinal area from which the muscle is innervated must also be treated if necessary, as any interference of the nerve supply can also predispose the muscle, it's musculotendinous junction or it's tendon to being injured.

Similarly, injury to the *hamstring* or *quadriceps* at the site of the musculotendinous junction is occasionally seen in athletes and is dealt with in section 10.4; injury to the tendon, however, is much more frequently seen.

The musculotendinous junction of the *iliopsoas* is the commonest musculotendinous injury seen around the pelvic region. It is dealt with in section 9.4.

The *gluteal muscles* may be injured at the musculotendinous junction, but are more commonly injured within the substance of the muscle or tendon itself. Exact and precise palpation will reveal the site of the injury which is important to determine, in order to give a precise prognosis to the athlete. If gluteus maximus is injured, there will be pain on active and resisted extension of the hip and this is more often seen than injury to the other gluteal muscles. If gluteus medius or gluteus minimus is involved, there will be pain on active and resisted medial rotation of the hip joint. Treatment is as described above for the adductor injury, but adapted for the glutei.

17.5   Bone injuries

Bruising of the pelvic bones can occur as a result of direct injury, the commonest sites being the iliac crest or the sacrum. There will be a history of a blow or fall; the area will be discoloured and swollen, and a skin abrasion may be present. It is very important to eliminate the possibility of a fracture. Only if there is a break in the pelvic circle as a result of a fracture will the athlete be unable to walk. One discernable break is invariably accompanied by another lesion but this may well be a strain of one or both sacro-iliac joints.

To test the integrity of the pelvic circle, pressure is placed horizontally across the pelvis by placing the hands on the iliac crests and squeezing them together. In addition, each ilium is sprung backwards and forwards by pushing against the anterior iliac spines in an A−P direction. Pain will be felt if a fracture is present. This test should be done very carefully if the athlete is able to walk, albeit painfully, and *not* if he is unable to walk. In this case he must be referred for X-rays as soon as possible. Fracture of the pelvic circle can be extremely serious as there may be visceral involvement. The above tests will cause pain in the presence of a fracture but if there is any doubt at all, the athlete must be X-rayed before it can be assumed that there is no fracture.

Should the injury be bruising only, any skin abrasion should be treated. The athlete should apply ice packs to the injured region and take homeopathic arnica to accelerate healing. There is likely to be associated muscle bruising and spasm which can be treated with gentle soft tissue treatment once this is found to be tolerable and not exacerbate the discomfort. Recovery is swift and total but the pelvic joints may have been injured in the original accident and will require osteopathic attention. The spine, too, should be treated if necessary.

Fracture of the *pelvic circle* results from violent injury only, for example in motor racing or motor bike crashes. If the circle is broken, the athlete will be unable to walk and will require expert attention. Once he has been discharged from hospital, the surrounding areas will need osteopathic treatment as there is bound to have been associated injury, most probably in the spine and in the pelvic joints, ligaments and muscles. There may well be residual pain and/or disability which should be treated before full athletic activity is resumed.

Other fractures occur in the pelvic region which do not disturb the pelvic circle and the injured athlete can therefore walk, albeit painfully. Stress fractures of the pubic rami are not rare and may occur for no apparent reason in an athlete, or there may be a history of some violent muscular action. The athlete will complain of pain in the region of the ramus which will be aggravated by activity, especially abduction of the hip. Resisted adduction may or may not be painful. Palpation will reveal an area of tenderness and swelling and gentle springing of the ramus will cause pain. The defect will show on X-ray. No special treatment is required and the fracture will heal with rest. Once this has happened, osteopathic treatment to the adductors and other surrounding muscles will be needed, in addition to treatment to the surrounding joints and ligaments. During the healing period, gentle swimming, possibly using a float between the feet, may be permitted if this does not aggravate the pain.

Avulsion fractures, due to some violent muscular action are not rare in athletes. The common sites are, the anterior superior iliac spine due to the pull of sartorius, the anterior inferior iliac spine due to the pull of rectus femoris, the ischial tuberosity due to the pull of the hamstrings, part of the pubic bone due to the pull of the adductors, or the iliac crest due to the pull of the abdominal musculature. All these avulsion fractures are more likely to be seen in young athletes but can occur at any age. Any avulsion is visible on X-ray; the appearance may be alarming but the disability may not be severe. Rest is needed for bony union to occur, after which osteopathic treatment to the muscle concerned and to the surrounding joints and ligaments is needed to ensure normal mechanical efficiency before full activity is resumed. Some cases will benefit from gentle swimming, possibly using a float between the feet, during the recuperative stage. This is only prescribed if it does not aggravate the pain factor.

Fracture of the *sacrum* is rare but can occur as a result of direct and violent injury. In this case there will be a history of severe injury and X-rays should be taken. If a fracture is present the athlete may not be able to walk without great discomfort; he requires expert attention. Following union, osteopathic treatment will be required as for cases of avulsion fracture.

The *coccyx* can be fractured by a severe fall onto it; this is more likely to occur in females as the pelvis is wider and does not afford as much protection to the coccyx as does the male pelvis. This can be very painful and the athlete will probably be unable to sit down because of the pain. The fracture will show on X-ray. Rest is needed and the athlete may have to lie prone in the early stages. Following bony union, there is likely to be some misplacement of the bone which will require osteopathic treatment; before correction, the athlete may still be suffering pain despite the fact that the fracture has healed. The pain probably emanates from the sacro-coccygeal ligament and the coccygeus muscle and both will be rendered pain-free following correction of the coccyx. Some treatment may also be needed to other pelvic and spinal structures which may have been injured at the time of the fracture or may have been disturbed later, due to the effects of the fracture. It is important to make sure that the coccyx is functioning correctly as if it is not, it can cause trouble during childbirth. Most female athletes become mothers at some later stage in their lives!

Anomalies are fairly common in the sacral region and are dealt with in section 16.8. Incomplete union of the first and second sacral segments or their spinous processes are the commonest anomalies seen in the sacral area and can give rise to a great deal of trouble in athletes, if present. Anomalies of the lumbosacral joint are also frequently seen and will disturb the normal mechanics of this joint, causing trouble at the site of the anomaly and in the surrounding tissues. Incomplete fusion of the sacrum seems to be more likely when the adolescent sacrum has been subjected to extreme stress, for example in young gymnasts, or when the sacrum has been traumatised at or about the age when fusion might have been expected to occur, for example by a severe fall onto the back at that time.

17.6 Joint and ligament injuries

Osteitis pubis is an inflammation of the pubic articular surfaces of the symphysis pubis. It can be very painful with associated pain and tenderness over the symphysis. X-rays may or may not show displacement of the articular surfaces. The condition is most frequently seen in footballers and must be differentiated from an adductor strain. In the former there will be pain felt on springing the symphysis but not in the latter, yet both conditions will cause pain on resisted adduction and on passive abduction of the hip. The ligaments of the joint have become stretched and this can become chronic. Some cases resolve with rest and some with an injection into the region but many do not respond to treatment, in which case the condition can end a football career. If associated with a true urethritis, this condition can be a manifestation of Reiter's syndrome.

The ligaments of the *sacrococcygeal joint* can become stretched and painful, usually due to some slight misplacement of the coccyx in relation to the sacrum. Careful palpation will reveal the displacement and the stretched ligament. Correction of the coccyx relieves the condition but the athlete should sit on a ring pad and not ride a bicycle for four weeks following correction to minimise the chance of recurrence.

The *iliofemoral ligament* can be injured especially in excessive extension of the hip joint for example in gymnastics or in body contact sports where the hip has been forced into extension. The athlete will complain of a deep pain in the front of the hip area which is worse with activity involving hip joint movement. Deep palpation will reveal tenderness there. The hip joint should be rested until the symptoms have subsided, after which osteopathic treatment to the flexors, extensors and other muscles of the hip will be needed. The joint mechanics should also be normalised if necessary, of the hip, the pelvis and of the spine.

The *sacrotuberous* and/or *sacrospinous ligaments* can become injured, the reason for such an injury is not certain but it is usually a secondary injury, the primary one being to the lumbosacral joint and/or one or both sacro-iliac joints. The athlete will report that he has pain in the deep gluteal region which is worse when he starts to run. There is pain after activity. There may be additional symptoms of lumbosacral and sacro-iliac origin. Even when the primary condition has been successfully treated, pain may persist in these ligaments. Deep palpation will reveal sensitivity when the ligament(s) are pressurised and passive hip flexion with adduction may cause pain as the ligament(s) are stretched. Treatment is deep inhibitory soft tissue work, to which the condition responds well, and recurrence is unusual.

The ligaments of the *sacro-iliac joints* may be injured; this is usually secondary to a facet locking condition of the joint or of the lumbosacral joint, or to hypermobility − see sections 17.7 and 17.8.

The sacro-iliac joint can become inflamed, the condition being known as *sacroilitis*. This condition usually affects young males and the early symptoms appear before the age of 30, (even as early as the late teens). The athlete will complain of low back pain which is usually relieved somewhat by adopting a posture of a few degrees of flexion. The pain is aggravated by physical activity. There will be no apparent reason for the onset. There may be a family history of ankylosing spondylitis. The condition is frequently prespondylitic or may be an early symptom of Reiter's disease. X-rays are diagnostic. The athlete should be referred for further rheumatological investigation. Any sport which requires great flexibility will be impeded by ankylosing spondylitis but Reiter's disease responds well to medical treatment.

Facet locking

The sacro-iliac joints are subject to this condition, with or without the lumbosacral joint being involved as well.

During activities such as running, the pelvis rotates around the sacrum, the axis of the rotation being the second sacral level. During running, the quadriceps and hamstrings contract and relax alternately (together with other muscles). As the quadriceps contract, they pull the pelvis forward and downward; conversely as the hamstrings contract they pull the pelvis downward and backward, so the repeated action involves pelvic rotation about it's normal axis. Although the range of rotation is small, it is nevertheless important in running, jumping, cycling etc. Should the pelvis be pulled excessively in either direction, it is possible for the sacro-iliac joint to become locked. There are, of course, other reasons for the joint to lock, but this is the common cause in athletes. Direct forces of an extrinsic nature can be responsible for facet locking, for example a fall or blow.

An *anterior rotation* of the innominate can result from excess activity of the quadriceps, for example while kicking a ball, or it may result from some rotational movement, for example while swinging a golf club, or it may be secondary to a rotational type facet lock of the lumbosacral joint. The athlete will complain of pain which usually centres lateral to the locked joint. The pain may radiate into the anterior aspect of the thigh as far as the knee. The condition is invariably unilateral, although there may be a posterior rotation of the opposite sacro-iliac joint. Active movement of the joint, such as it is, is tested by asking the athlete to flex one knee only while standing and retaining both heels on the floor. A sacro-iliac joint which is locked will not rotate as the other side will. Examination will reveal some hypertonia in the gluteus minimus muscle which can be palpated deep in the gluteal region. The mobility of the affected joint is found to be restricted and whereas the innominate (pelvic) bone may rotate anteriorly, it will not rotate posteriorly. The movement is also found to be restricted on sacral springing. On the anterior aspect of the thigh the sartorius and gracilis muscles are hypertonic and there is often some tenderness at their insertions into the tibia.

Correction of the facet lock will relieve the athlete's symptoms; it is essential to make sure that the lumbosacral joint is functioning normally; if not this too should be corrected. It is usually unnecessary to give any other treatment unless there is a short lower extremity on that side or some other predisposing factor which may require treatment.

A *posterior rotation* of the innominate is the opposite of an anterior rotation. The athlete will complain of low back pain which is centred over the posterior aspect of the joint. This may be associated with a hamstring injury or with chronic shortening of these muscles such as is seen following repeated injury. As the two conditions are so often associated with one another, it seems that there may be a chicken and egg situation. Violent rotation of the pelvis may cause the condition, or possibly a blow or fall. It can also happen with a bad fall when the body is twisted, for example from a horse or skiing.

Pain over the posterior ligament of the joint is aggravated by movement especially rotation forward of the innominate. This condition, too, may be associated with a facet locking of the lumbosacral joint. Examination reveals a loss of movement when the innominate is rotated anteriorly and on sacral springing. There may be increased tone in the gluteal muscles but this is not a small isolated area as in the anterior innominate lesion. There may be hypertonia in the hamstrings which may ache somewhat. Treatment consists of correcting the facet lock; attention to the lumbosacral joint is essential, if this joint is involved in the overall clinical picture. This rotation may also be associated with a short lower extremity but in this case the short leg will be on the opposite side from the sacro-iliac lesion.

Facet locking can also occur at the lumbosacral joint which is primarily a sacral condition, where the sacrum becomes rotated between the innominates. This may simulate an innominate condition but the sacro-iliac joints will have normal mobility. The sacrum then needs correction, not the innominate. If the innominate is erroneously 'corrected', the sacro-iliac joint may be strained and possibly become hypermobile if the procedure is repeated.

17.8   Mobility injury

Stiffness can be muscular in origin. If this is the case, in the pelvic region, the muscles most likely to be involved are the glutei, especially following some unusual physical activity. The athlete will complain of pain and stiffness which is worse when he tries to use the muscles (i.e. extend the hip) and is easier with warmth and massage. This is the treatment for choice and the condition resolves very quickly.

Stiffness without severe muscular spasm may result from a sacro-ilitis and if the stiffness persists, this condition should be suspected and X-rays should be taken.

Stiffness can also affect the pelvic area from conditions within the lumbar region, which should be carefully examined in all cases of pelvic stiffness and treated as necessary.

Hypermobility results from stretched ligaments. This condition is seen in the symphysis pubis. It may be due to minor repeated traumata to the joint or it may result from osteitis pubis once the acute phase has passed. Repair of the stretched ligaments is only partial at best, but a residual hypermobility does not necessarily give rise to symptoms. However if pain persists, it is wise to examine the sacro-iliac joints as a problem there can cause stretching of the ligaments of the symphysis. Sometimes the condition resolves following an injection of a sclerosing fluid, but the condition may be persistent and not respond to any treatment.

Hypermobility of a sacro-iliac joint is not rare. It is seen most frequently in young female athletes. The condition gives rise to pain which is worse with physical activity as this causes strain of the already stretched ligaments of the joint. The hypermobility may be caused by repeated minor traumata or can be due to repeated correction of sacro-iliac facet locking where the pre-disposing cause has been overlooked and therefore not treated. Support is needed for several weeks to assist healing of the stretched fibres and osteopathic treatment to any mechanical problem in the surrounding joints and/or ligaments as well as muscles, is necessary. Sporting activities which require a great deal of rotation of the pelvis should be avoided until there is greater stability of the sacro-iliac joint concerned. Severe cases may require an injection of a sclerosing fluid, followed by a period of rest from sports which stress the joint. This condition can result from childbirth but what-ever the cause, the treatment remains the same.

17.9	**Bursitis**

There are many bursae in the pelvic region. In general they lie under tendons, separating the tendon from a bony prominence.

The common sites of bursitis are between the ischial tuberosity and the tendon of origin of the hamstring muscles, between the tendon of insertion of gluteus maximus and the greater trochanter of the femur, between the tendon of insertion of piriformis and the upper border of the greater trochanter into which it inserts, between the tendon of gluteus medius and it's point of insertion on the lateral surface of the greater trochanter, and between the tendon of iliopsoas and the pubis and front of the hip joint. Should any of these be inflamed the athlete will complain of pain at the site of the bursa which is worse following activity and worse on active and resisted movement of the muscle concerned. The bursa may be palpable and swollen and tender to pressure.

Treatment is designed to reduce the pressure on the bursa, so rest from use of the muscle is essential. Ice packs may help to reduce the inflammation and an injection may be needed. Return to full sporting activity too soon, i.e. before the inflammation has subsided will cause further inflammation and recurrence of the condition.

Table 17.1 Muscles
supplied by the sacral
nerves

	Anterior primary rami	Posterior primary rami
S1	Gluteus maximus Tensor fascia lata Piriformis Obturator internus Quadratus femoris Gemelli Semitendinosus Biceps All muscles of leg and foot except tibialis anterior and posterior	Deep muscles of the back
S2	Gluteus maximus Piriformis Obturator internus Gemellus superior Biceps − long head Gastrocnemius Soleus Flexor hallucis longus Flexor digitorum brevis Abductor digiti minimi Flexor digiti minimi Interossei 3rd and 4th lumbricals	Deep muscles of the back
S3	Biceps − long head Ischiocavernosus Transversus perinei Bulbospongiosus Sphincter urethra	Deep muscles of the back
S4	All muscles of pelvic floor	Deep muscles of the back
S5	Levator ani Coccygeus	Deep muscles of the back

17.10

Nerve involvement

The *sciatic nerve* is closely related to the piriformis muscle and the
superior gemellus in the region of the buttock where the former
muscle is frequently pierced by the lateral popliteal nerve. Hypertonic conditions of these muscles can cause pressure on the related
nerves and symptoms peripherally.

The *sacral plexus* lies in front of the piriformis muscle on the
posterior wall of the pelvic cavity and can also be irritated by
piriformis spasm.

The *femoral nerve* passes through the fibres of psoas and passes
downward between it and iliacus, above the inguinal ligament, so
it can be affected by muscular conditions of either of these muscles.

Pain can refer to the pelvic region from the lumbar spine. Pain can refer to the lower lumbar and sacral regions from the pelvic viscera.

These points should be borne in mind when there is some unusual clinical picture; the fact that pelvic pain need not necessarily arise from the musculoskeletal components of the area must always be remembered and further examination carried out if indicated.

Chapter 18   Various Sports and their Commonly Related Injuries

Some sports are more commonly undertaken than others. Some carry a higher risk of injury than others. To understand fully the injury with which the athlete is presenting, it is essential to have some knowledge of the sport itself, preferably from personal experience, or at least from spending time watching the sport. Television coverage is useful, but much more is learned by actually attending the sporting event when the body stresses can be more fully studied.

As an osteopath who is interested in the treatment of sporting injuries, it is a wise investment of time to actually go and watch the various sports in action, not only at the top (professional) level but also at the grass roots level. The injuries which occur among the keen amateurs are frequently different from those which occur among the professional athletes, who are experts at their sport, understand the techniques involved, and above all are careful not to endanger their own or their colleagues' professional careers. The keen amateur has the added disadvantage of a lack of time to invest in physical fitness and general body training; he may have to do his training after a day's work when he is mentally and physically tired. Try as he will, therefore, he is unable to benefit from training as much as the professional.

A fuller understanding of the parts of the body which are particularly stressed in any particular sport will arm the osteopath with background information and make the diagnosis of any athletic injury easier and hopefully accurate.

Athletes are always anxious to talk about their particular sport and if asked will give invaluable information, for example at adult classes, or during the treatment session. My advice to my colleagues is to glean as much information as possible; the time will come during your own career when it will come in useful!

American football

This is a sport which has increased in popularity enormously during the past few years and is likely to increase still further. It is widely played in USA and has an enormous following there.

Basically the game can be divided into two parts, the running aspect and the physical contact aspect which can be bordering on the violent at times.

The average player is of a heavy build so the injury which one player can inflict on another can be severe.

The protection which is worn is great, from a protective helmet to shin pads, including shoulder padding, hip or thigh guards, knee pads, a box, elbow guards and some players also use gum shields. The vulnerable areas, therefore, are the hands and feet but injuries often occur despite the protective clothing.

The majority of injuries fall into the extrinsic group, including: head and neck injury, shoulder and arm injury, rib and thoracic injury, hand injury possibly including the wrist, and foot and ankle injury. Knee and elbow injuries do occur despite the protection worn.

Spinal strains and strains are commonly seen, especially of the lumbar region and pelvis.

Angling

This is a widely practiced sport, involving enthusiasts of all ages, most of whom are males.

Sea angling exposes the participant to the dangers of the ocean, which include sea sickness, hypothermia and navigational problems. They commonly suffer from the effects of cold, i.e. muscular pain and spasm, especially of the glutei and shoulder girdle muscles.

Bites from the caught fish are common. Shoulder and elbow strains result from repeated casting. Hooks can be embedded in the skin − they must never be pulled out against the barb, but should be pushed through. The line can be caught around a finger causing damage if tightened by a fish resisting being landed.

In addition, many anglers spend a full day by a river or lake. They habitually sit on a stone surface or at best on a folding stool which has no insulation. The result is pain in the gluteal muscles which are especially sensitive to exposure to cold.

Sea anglers may suffer from cervical problems as they spend a great deal of their time watching their lines, i.e. in a position of cervical extension, when fishing from the beach.

Low back problems arise from digging for bait, a pastime of most anglers.

Archery

Although this is an Olympic sport, it does not have a great many participants. It is probably the oldest of all sports dating back 25,000 years when it was used for killing. At one time a bowman could shoot faster with a bow than with a pistol! There is no age limit and archery can be used for the Duke of Edinburgh award. It is always an individual sport.

Good posture is essential, with sound abdominal tone. The arrow flies at 100 mph as it leaves the bow and the draw force line extends from the fingers to the shoulder girdles. Females pull about 26 lb, while males may pull up to 47 lb, and during competitions they may shoot all day.

The female archers, in olden times, used to have the left breast amputated as it would obstruct shooting!

The injuries seen include, assuming the archer is right-handed: the posterior muscles of the right shoulder girdle, the muscles of the right upper extremity, the right elbow joint, the right pectoral muscles (only if the bow is too long), and extension strain of the cervical spine from recoil.

Protective wear includes a bracer on the left forearm to avoid bruising, a tab on the second and third fingers and a left breast protector for female archers.

It is said that the derogatory 'V' sign originated during the Battle of Agincourt, when if an English archer was captured, his second and third digits were amputated by the French. If, however, he escaped, he would raise these to his enemy, presumably as he ran off.

Baseball

This is a very popular sport in North America and is gaining popularity in this country. It involves four distinct activities: pitching, hitting, running and catching.

Pitching causes several problems to the shoulder girdle and elbow, namely: injury to the conjoint tendon, subacromial bursitis, degenerative changes in the acromioclavicular joint, hypermobility in the sternoclavicular joint, subglenoid exostosis at the origin of the long head of triceps, bicipital tendinitis, little league shoulder — in adolescents, and inflammation of the bicipital aponeurosis when supination is used to curve the ball.

Hitting can strain the muscles and joints of the arm from the shoulder girdle to the wrist inclusive. This, and pitching can cause a stress fracture of the olecranon, exostosis on the inner edge of the trochlea, or thickening of the medial ligament of the elbow which can affect the ulnar nerve.

Running can injure the muscles of the leg and joints of the leg, pelvis and spine — see running. In addition, sliding causes particular injuries in baseball, mostly to the thigh, hip and gluteal region. Spiking injuries occur. Ankle injuries are common, frequently resulting from a spike catching in the grass as a player slides towards a base.

Catching injuries are to the hands. Fracture of the finger or thumb with or without dislocation is not rare.

Basketball

This is another sport which is increasing in popularity.

The commonest injuries are to the hands, from catching the ball. Other injuries result from jumping, landing, falling and to a lesser degree from running.

Catching the ball can cause a fracture and/or dislocation of finger or thumb, or strain of a joint (especially the metacarpo-phalangeal) from forced hyperextension of the joint. In addition, in defensive rebounding, the ball is caught and brought forcibly down in a protective position when it can be inadvertently rammed into an opponent's finger.

Jumping and landing frequently injures the ankle – a sprained ankle being the commonest basketball injury of all. The incidence of this injury is increased by the soles of the shoes withstanding slipping, to enable quick turns and stops to be made. Periostitis of the lateral aspect of the ankle is seen in some cass. Violent twisting and turning movements can injure the knee, especially the collateral, coronary and cruciate ligaments and possibly the meniscus (medial).

Falling to the floor is common and can result in contusions to the elbow, wrist, hand and knee; some players wear protective pads to the knees. A fall onto the outstretched hand can cause injury to the shoulder, clavicle and clavicular joints.

Play close to the basket involves vigorously contested exchanges between opponents. Elbows are often raised to protect the ball and numerous injuries can occur from intentional or accidental use of the elbow. These may be to the head, including the eye and nose as well as the mouth, or to the ribs.

Abdominal wall injuries result from overstretching upward for the ball.

Running can injure the muscles and joints of the leg, pelvis and spine – see running.

Bowls

Bowling has a popular image of being a tranquil sport partaken in the open air, involving little physical strain but a good deal of concentration, an image which is only partly true.

During a game of 21 ends of pairs, each athlete will bend 160 times and will walk approximately one mile. Imperfect body balance at the time of delivery of the wood can cause strain on the body, especially the left leg (assuming the athlete is right-handed) as this takes most of the weight of delivery. It is flexed and the anterior muscles of the thigh and iliopsoas can fatigue if the technique is incorrect.

Lower extremity muscles which can be injured are the iliopsoas and the quadriceps. The knee joint may be strained as flexion is maintained. The flexor muscles of the right hand may be strained especially in cold weather. The muscles of the shoulder girdle may be strained.

The lumbar spine may be injured, especially if flexion in that region is already limited (many bowlers are elderly).

Ten pin bowling

This also stresses the hip and thigh as above and injury to the quadriceps and to iliopsoas is commonly seen.

In addition, the grasp of the ball is different, the thumb and first two fingers being inserted into holes in the ball. The actual technique of delivery results in the thumb being released last, whereby strain is placed on the thenar muscles which become sore and painful. Repeated use of these muscles commonly leads to tenosynovitis and to strain of the joints at either end of the first metacarpal bone.

The action by which the ball is gripped predisposes to this type of injury as it is a heavy ball, whereas a wood is held and carefully balanced in a more natural way, prior to delivery.

Boxing

The commonest injuries in boxing occur to the head and are caused by being punched, rather than by punching.

Head injuries include: nose bleed with possible deflection of the nasal septum, abrasion and/or laceration to the face especially the eyebrow, haematoma of the eye – the 'black eye', concussion, strain or dislocation of the temperomandibular joint, and fractures.

Injury to the hand results from punching rather than being punched.

Hand injuries include: a bursa which may develop on the dorsum of a metacarpal head, most frequently the second, and become inflamed producing a bursitis there; the intermetacarpal ligament may become strained leading to a classic deformity of the hand – this is caused by the strapping applied to the metacarpal bases with the fingers in extension, before fighting; a Bennett's fracture of the thumb, with or without dislocation; a possible chip fracture at the base of the thumb.

The ribs may be bruised. There may be a dislocation of a sternocostal joint. Serratus anterior may be strained.

Worst but not uncommonly, the boxer may suffer from the condition known as 'punch drunk' when he will display mental and emotional changes. Some degree of this condition is thought to occur in over half of the boxers who have been in the ring regularly for a period of five years or more.

Canoeing

This sport is carried out in either flat or rough water; in the latter there is the additional problem of balance of the craft.

The athlete is exposed to possible cold weather with resultant muscular problems and his body may chill as he becomes wet.

In both events there is enormous strain on the muscles of the wrist and hand and the forearm muscles often suffer from cramp. Tenosynovitis of the wrist extensors is common.

There is no support to the back in sprint racing; the paddler sits on a raised seat with his legs out in front of him, thus straining the low back. Lumbar spine problems occur. (Fig. 18.1(a).)

In Canadian canoeing, the athlete kneels on one knee with the other leg out in front of him, producing an asymmetrical vertebral strain, and the possibility of a pre- or infrapatellar bursitis developing. (Fig. 18.1(b).)

In rough water canoeing, the shoulder girdles are placed under additional strain. Turning manoeuvres are executed with the arms extended away from the body. With unexpected incidents, for example striking a rock under the water, the sudden movement of the athlete can result in strain of the shoulder girdle and even possible dislocation of the glenohumeral joint.

To provide as much stability as possible, the paddler gets as low as possible in the kayak or canoe. In Canadian canoes, the paddler kneels on both knees which can injure the knee joint especially if sudden movements of the body occur. There is a possibility of a bilateral bursitis developing anteriorly in the knee. (Fig. 18.1(c).)

Cricket

This is a complex sport involving numerous different activities. These are running, catching, bowling, throwing, batting, wicket keeping and exposure to the elements over a long period of time.

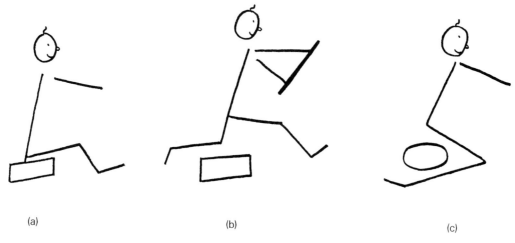

(a)   (b)   (c)

Fig. 18.1   Canoeing positions. (a) Sitting; (b) kneeling on one knee; (c) kneeling on both knees.

Running injuries include those to the muscles and joints of the leg, pelvis and spine — see running.

Catching frequently injures the fingers; hyperextension strains of the finger or thumb joints are common as is a Mallet finger and a Bennett's fracture dislocation of the thumb.

Bowling lays stress on the shoulder girdle and injury to the conjoint tendon and the subacromial bursa can follow. Spin bowling can injure the flexor tendon and synovial sheath of the spinning finger, usually the second or third digit. Fast bowling produces its own problems; first, the bowler sprints, thus putting his hamstrings at risk; then he side bends suddenly, possibly straining his quadratus lumborum muscle; thirdly that same sudden side bending combined with extension of the lower lumbar spine risks an injury to the pars interarticularis of the fifth lumbar vertebra. A spondylolisthesis is extremely common in fast bowlers.

Throwing stresses the shoulder girdle, elbow, wrist, pelvis and spine where injuries are commonly seen — see throwing.

The batsman has his own problems. His action is essentially one-sided and he strains one leg repeatedly. Injuries to the hip, knee and ankle are common, the hip injuries being mainly to muscles and the knee and ankle injuries to ligaments. Repeated batting over a period of years predisposes the batsman to osteoarthritic changes in the hip (most frequently) knee and ankle joints.

The wicket keeper lays a great deal of stress on his knee joints. He remains in a position of flexion for several minutes at a time and repeats this continuously. Strain to the ligaments of his knee are often seen or possibly to the quadriceps expansion which is put on stretch by his crouching position. Many injuries occur to the hands of the wicket keeper, the long-term result of which is a predisposition to osteoarthritic changes in the joints of his hands. Fielding in the slips and wicket keeping involve a great many sudden movements which can result in strain to the legs, pelvis and spine and these are often seen. Sudden stretching to catch a ball may injure the shoulder girdle.

In conclusion, injuries from cricket can occur anywhere in the body, but the site will depend largely on the position played.

All cricketers are subject to possible sunburn or chilling, depending on the weather conditions.

All cricketers are also at risk from direct injury by being struck by the ball which can travel fast and is very hard. The chance of this type of injury increases as the pitch wears, so is more likely in three or five day matches. Although they wear protection to the head, legs, hands (wicket keeper and batsman wear gloves) and genitals, direct injury often occurs. The bones of the forearm may be bruised or even fractured by a fast rising ball, the ribs may be hit and bruised or fractured and the ankles and feet may also be bruised or fractured.

Cycling

This is an extremely popular sport, at all levels and is engaged in by athletes of all ages. It is a well balanced sport, is self-limiting and convenient, hence its enormous popularity. The injuries which occur are invariably as a result of falling off, or of a machine which is not correctly balanced for the cyclist.

It is easier to consider the problems with which cyclists present on a regional basis throughout the body.

Feet

Pain under the long arch, usually due to the plantar fascia, probably caused by ill-fitting shoes. The shoe should have a sole which bends easily having no steel plate. Otherwise the condition may be due to the foot being too far forward on the pedal; the ball of the foot should be just over the axle of the pedal. The alignment of the shoe and the shoe plate should be parallel.

Pain in the tendo Achilles is usually caused by shoes which have the back too high and therefore rub, or the shoe may be too far back, thus exaggerating the motion of the ankle. Using gears which are too high can also cause this, and may have to be altered.

Ankle

Pain on the lateral aspect is usually as a result of falling off. There may be evidence of this elsewhere in the body.

Pain medially is usually caused by hitting the ankle on the crank. It may be secondary to a foot problem or shoe problem.

Knee

Pain in the patellar tendon is usually due to sitting too far forward on the saddle or using too high a gear, so the saddle or gearing may need altering.

Pain over the medial collateral ligament is usually due to abduction strain. The pedal or crank may be twisted from a fall or propping the machine against the curb. The shoe plates may not be straight.

Pain on the lateral aspect of the knee may be due to strain of the superior tibiofibular joint either from the biceps or possibly secondary to a short leg on that side, stretching the area. This usually resolves if the saddle is marginally lowered.

Pain in the popliteal region is due to strain of the popliteus muscle and may be because the cyclist is not doing enough cycling frequently enough, or the gears may be too high. It usually resolves if the gearing is lowered.

Pain in the patellar region is often chondromalacia patellae and is an overuse condition. The gears may be lowered to reduce the stress and a free wheel is advisable.

Hip

Pain in the adductors may result from a fall or from some imbalance, either of the body or the machine, for example a short leg or a twisted saddle.

Pain in the region of the ischial tuberosity is due to increased weight being put upon it while cycling. This is probably due to the saddle being too far back or twisted and uneven.

Low back pain

This may be because the spine is not flexible enough for the correct position while cycling. The position may be incorrect if the cyclist is too far back, so the saddle may need adjusting.

Cervicodorsal pain

This is probably caused by too much weight being placed on the arms. The saddle may be too far forward or tilted. Pain in the low back or cervicodorsal areas of the spine may be secondary to injury from falling off, or the handle bars may be too low.

Neck

Pain in this area is often caused by sitting too high with the handle bars too low, so that the cyclist has to extend his neck to see where he is going. Cold weather and cold winds can also cause pain here as perspiration evaporates, chilling the region. A scarf worn in cold weather will prevent this problem.

Shoulder girdle

Injury to this area is very common and usually results from a fall off the machine. Skin damage may occur and possible bruising. There may be damage to the glenohumeral joint but the commonest injury is to the clavicle and/or the clavicular joints. Fracture of the clavicle is almost an occupational hazard of serious cyclists! Falls are almost inevitable when a tyre bursts or when the riding surface is slippery and skidding occurs.

Elbow

Pain around the elbow is usually caused by too much weight being placed on them or to holding the handle bars in the 'twisted wrist' position. The elbow can often be injured by a fall off the cycle.

Wrist

Falls, jolts and repeated pressure can cause injury to the flexor retinaculum giving rise to a carpal tunnel syndrome. This is very often seen in cyclists.

To measure the position of the cyclist

With cyclist standing, feet six inches apart, in socks but no shoes, measure inside leg length. Height 'A' should be nine-tenths of this (see Fig. 18.2).

The average cyclist should be at least one inch 'behind the bracket', long femurs can go to as much as 3″. This is length 'B'. It will also be governed by the length of the foot, as the ball of the foot should be vertically under the knee joint when the pedal is going down and the cyclist sitting correctly and working.

With the elbow on the front of the saddle, the fingertips should just clear the handlebars. This is length 'C'.

Finally the frame, measured from the middle of the joint to the middle of the joint on the frame should be two-thirds of the crutch height, see length 'D'.

This may all sound very complicated, but it is important to understand the relationship between the cyclist and his machine as incorrections can lead to problems in his body.

Equestrian sports

This is unique in that it involves a partnership between two totally different beings, emphasised especially in rodeo events and by occupations such as the mounted police.

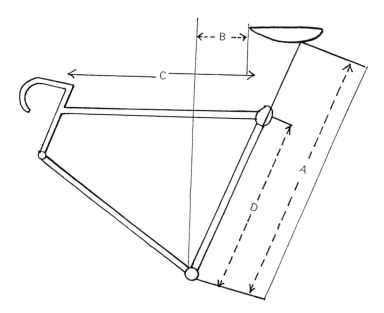

Fig. 18.2 Measuring the position of a cyclist.

The riding position requires the centre of gravity line of the rider to be immediately above that of the horse – see Fig. 18.3.

The jumping position allows the rider to follow the movements of the horse using his thigh, knee and ankle as shock absorbers, while the back is kept straight; the stirrups are shortened so the riding angles are narrowed thus putting more weight on the thighs and stirrups, the extreme of this is seen in the flat-race jockey. See Fig. 18.4.

The most serious injuries result from falls, with the added risk of being kicked or trodden on by the horse. They are: head injuries including concussion and fractures; neck injuries – whiplash injury is common; shoulder injuries including subluxation or dislocation of the clavicular joints, fracture of the clavicle and dislocation of the shoulder; spinal injuries especially to the lumbar discs; rib

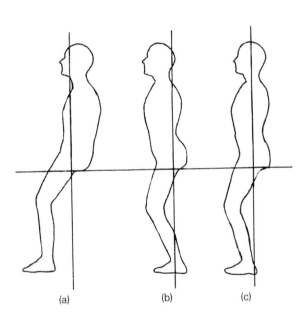

Fig. 18.3 Riding position. (a) Rounded back; (b) hollow back; correct position.
From *Fit for Riding* by Richard Meade (1984); reproduced by permission of the publishers B.T. Batsford Ltd, London.

(a)   (b)   (c)

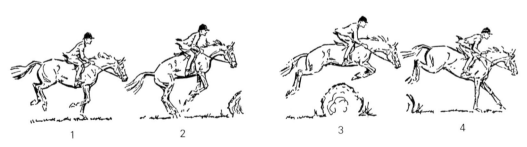

1   2   3   4

Fig. 18.4   Jumping position.
From *The Manual of Horsemanship of the British Horse Society and The Pony Club* (1966).

injuries; pelvic fracture or damage to the coccyx (especially in females); hip joint injury from the foot being caught in a stirrup and; knee and ankle from the foot being caught in the stirrup. Occupational strain of the adductor muscles causes development of the so-called 'riders bone'; low back pain is often a result of poor posture while in the saddle, leading to muscular and ligamentous strain and may be cumulative.

Some protection is given by the use of a riding hat which has decreased the incidence of major head injury. See Fig. 18.5.

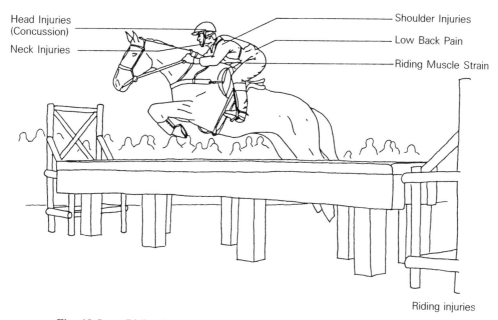

Riding injuries

Fig. 18.5   Riding injuries.
From *Fit for Riding* by Richard Meade (1984); reproduced by permission of the publishers B.T. Batsford Ltd, London.

Fencing

This is a sport increasingly practiced throughout the world, yet it is an art of the greatest antiquity. Figures 18.6–18.9 show some of the positions employed and the stresses which are placed on the fencer's body. The effects of the sport are shown in Fig. 18.10.

The injuries which occur can be divided into traumatic and overuse.

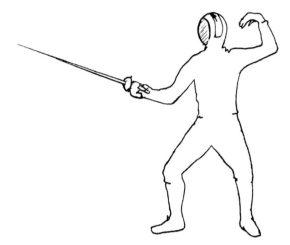

Fig. 18.6 The on guard position.

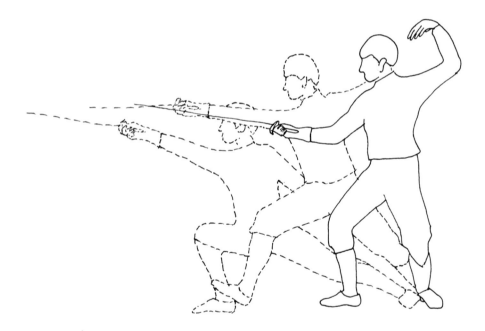

Fig. 18.7 The lunge.

Traumatic

Inversion sprain of the ankle, due to the fast footwork involved; there is instability during the take off in the fleche attack which is not overcome by fencing shoes which have no ankle support.

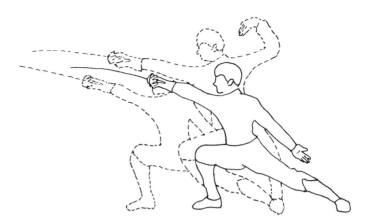

Fig. 18.8 The reprise.

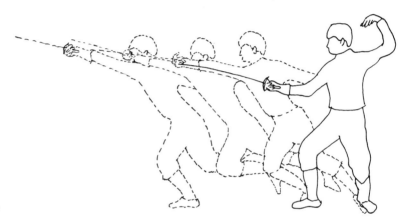

Fig. 18.9 The flèche.

Hamstring tears commonly occur during lunging which is an explosive action requiring forced flexion of the hip of the leading leg under great load. Slippery floors can cause this with possible avulsion fracture of the ischial tuberosity especially in young fencers. Poor hip mechanics and lumbar extension predispose to this.

Erector spinae tears occur when the fencer employs the 'reposte around the back' which requires a lot of spinal rotation. This is limited in the thoracic spine so the movement comes from the dorsolumbar region, predisposing to hypermobility there.

Upper thoracic rotatores tears result from the above movement and are predisposed to by the fact that most fencers have a flattened upper thoracic area encouraged by the 'on guard' position, with the associated shortened muscles and ligaments.

Dislocation of the shoulder has become less frequent since the rules have been altered, prohibiting bodily contact between contestants during a bout.

Damage to the olecranon is common in fencers who do not wear an elbow guard. In sabre, the arm is part of the target and the

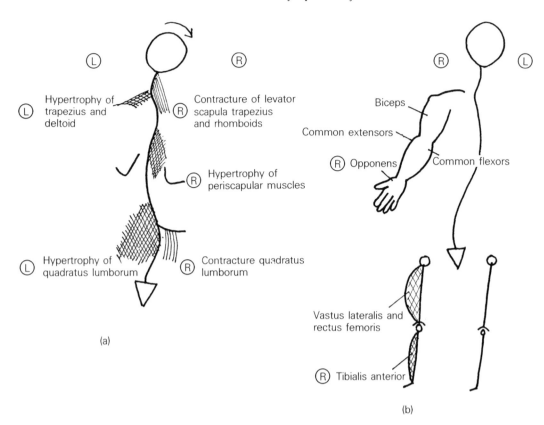

Fig. 18.10   The effects of fencing. (a) Posterior view; (b) anterior view.

fencer can use the blade with a cutting action to score a point. Blisters occur on the second and third digits of the sword hand and on the first metatarsal head of the rear foot if this is turned.

Overuse

Osgood-Schlatters disease is common in young fencers on intensive training schedules who overlunge on the front knee, see Fig. 18.11.

Chondromalacia patellae occurs commonly, especially in female fencers as the female pelvis predisposes to this condition, while fencing develops the vastus lateralis leaving the vastus medialis relatively weak. This imbalance causes poor tracking of the patella in the femoral groove.

Dysfunction of the right hip and sacro-iliac joint results from the fact that the right hip is held in medial rotation in the 'on guard' position, putting abnormal stress on the knee and ankle especially when lunging, see Fig. 18.12.

Pain in the extensors of the rear knee results from strain, see Fig. 18.13. Pain over the lateral epicondyle of the humerus caused by gripping the weapon too tightly is common in beginners.

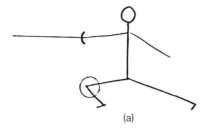

(a)

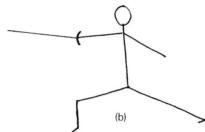

Fig. 18.11 Overlunge on the front knee.
(a) incorrect.
(b) correct.

(b)

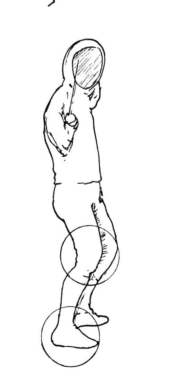

Fig. 18.12
Dysfunction results from abnormal stress on the knee and ankle.

Stiffness in the shoulder can lead to thoracic outlet problems, tension head pain and shoulder girdle muscle pain. See Fig. 18.14.

Anterior compartment pain is often due to the constant dorsiflexion of the front foot. The tibialis muscle can hypertrophy causing damage to the deep peroneal nerve.

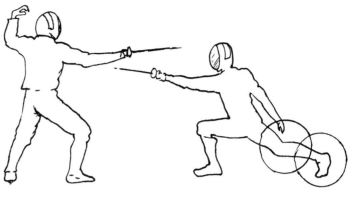

Fig. 18.13 The attacker's rear knee is strained as the rear heel comes off the floor.

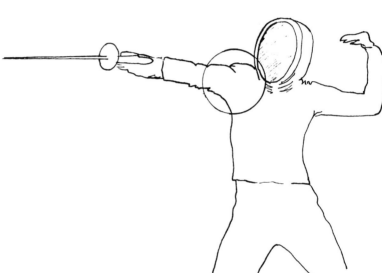

Fig. 18.14 Stiff and lifted shoulder.

Sprains of the inferior radio-ulnar joint occur as a result of the complex hand movements especially if these are practiced with too much vigour.

Football/Soccer

More males probably play football than any other game, and females are now starting to play in some areas. Hence injuries from the game are commonly seen.

Injuries from running are frequent. They involve the lower extremity and seem to account for over 50% of the total; sprains are the commonest. The ankle is the most frequent joint injured, closely followed by the knee.

According to a paper published in the *British Journal of Sports Medicine* in September 1984, by S. Maehlum MD, and O.A. Daljord MD, the following injuries were sustained:

Injury	Number
Sprain	545
Contusion	311
Laceration	103
Fracture	254
Dislocation	27
Rupture of tendon, ligament or muscle	44
Other	45
Total	1329

Most frequent localisation of sprains and fractures:

Location	Sprains	Fractures
Ankle	312	24
Knee	71	—
2–5 fingers	41	23
Wrist	40	45
Thumb	32	—
Rib	—	33
Toes	—	27
Total	496	132

It is interesting to note that 86% of the ruptures of tendon, ligament and muscle occurred in players over 20 years of age.

Muscle injuries can be extrinsic or intrinsic. Extrinsic injury is most frequently seen in the quadriceps muscle following being kicked by another player.

Intrinsic injury may occur in iliopsoas, adductor longus, gastrocnemius, the gastrocnemius/soleus junction, sartorius, the hamstrings, and most often in the quadriceps, overcontraction of which can cause injury within the belly, at the quadriceps expansion or even fracture of the patella. Powerful contraction of the adductors can lead to an avulsion fracture of the pubis, and osteitis pubis is a common sequel.

The tendo Achilles may be injured at the musculotendinous junction, within its tendinous substance or at the insertion into the calcaneum. This may occur with an associated bursitis.

The ligaments of the ankle, especially the lateral ligament and the anterior aspect of the capsule, frequently become injured. The latter results in osteophytic development if repeated often enough.

Chondromalacia patellae results from quadriceps overuse and possibly from disturbed patella tracking. Bursitis is common around the knee joint often as a result of extrinsic injury or from a fall.

The shoulder joint is particularly vulnerable in goalkeepers who reach up repeatedly and often fall onto the shoulder with low dives. The areas most often injured are the clavicle and the clavicular joints while the humerus may be fractured, either from a fall onto the elbow or onto the hand. Chronic injury to the conjoint tendon is common, possibly with an associated bursitis and chronic tendinitis of the biceps is often seen too.

Trochanteric bursitis may result from falling. Shin soreness from repeated running is not rare in footballers.

The ligaments of the knee are vulnerable in football due to repeated kicking of the ball, especially the medial ligament, the coronary ligaments and the cruciates as well as the medial meniscus.

Problems in the low back are often seen and frequently become chronic due to repeated overstrain. The lumbar discs may be injured.

Neck injury results from heading the ball and from repeated falls when the neck is probably forced into extension.

Golf

Almost every muscle in the body is used at one time or another in this sport, from the intrinsic muscles of the foot to the muscles of the neck. The vast majority of injuries seen, result from a faulty swing which should be corrected in cases of recurrent trouble. The hip joints and the low back are the most vulnerable areas.

Trochanteric bursitis results from repeated contraction of the gluteus medius and gluteus minimus muscles while the hips are abducted and the spine is suddenly rotated; this happens if the feet are firmly planted on the ground − the correct action is for the force to be dissipated to the ground via a swing through the legs. This action can also give rise to a bursitis under the iliopsoas tendon, anterior to the hip joint.

Strain of the low back results from excessive rotation there. Again that rotation should be taken through the legs to the ground.

Tension in the shoulder girdle and neck at address of shot gives rise to pain in the muscles of that region and can also cause facet locking of the joints of the neck.

The knee joint may be damaged if the joint is not kept flexed. This is most likely to occur at the medial collateral ligament which will be forced to take the strain of abduction.

'Golfer's elbow' is a strain of the common flexor origin at the elbow and can occur if the wrist is flexed while striking the ball. Injury to the wrist can occur when making a shot out of a bad rough lie.

Striking the ground instead of the ball can cause injury to the cervical and upper thoracic spine and a disc injury may result. Flying sand can enter the eye if the ball is being struck in a sand bunker.

Golf injuries do not happen easily and are rare in professionals.

Gymnastics

The majority of gymnastic injuries are as a result of overuse. The sport requires a high degree of flexibility which has to be counteracted by muscular strength. Many gymnasts are young and therefore not fully developed physically, which can lead to overuse problems of growing bone.

Falls account for the smaller group of injuries, the result of which will depend on the exact forces imposed on the body while falling. Fractures and dislocations are therefore not rare.

The ankle is the most frequently injured area, a sprain being the commonest injury of all. The tendo Achilles may be damaged or a sesamoiditis may occur, especially as most of the events are undertaken barefoot. Stress fractures of the metatarsals occur frequently, especially in females.

The knee joint is subjected to extreme strain in certain events and damage to the ligaments is common, especially to the medial and cruciate ligaments, giving rise to pain and instability.

Low back injuries result from overuse mainly, especially from hyperextension. Hypermobility or a spondylolisthesis may result, the former most often in the dorsolumbar, lumbar or sacro-iliac joints and the latter at the level of L5. Trampolinists are especially vulnerable. Adolescents may suffer from an epiphysitis of the bones of the hand or wrist due to overuse. A pulled or pushed radius may occur.

Wrist problems are often seen in those who use the pommel horse, and they may suffer from 'wrist splints', a condition of the forearm muscles akin to shin splints in runners.

Strains of the shoulder and especially of the conjoint tendon are common in gymnasts who are ring specialists, possibly with an associated bursitis and damage to the clavicular joints.

Muscular injuries occur most often in the erector spinae, latissimus dorsi and in the groin muscles and are often recurrent.

Hockey

This sport has experienced a revival since England won a medal at the Los Angeles Olympics. The injuries which occur can be divided into those resulting from running, especially suddenly in various different directions and those which result from the ball or from being struck by an opponent or his stick.

The running injuries may be exacerbated by the fact that the game is usually played in cold weather conditions when injury to muscles is more likely. The muscles of the leg and low back may be damaged and the joints of the legs and low back are vulnerable too. Knee and ankle injuries occur most frequently and the shins are often injured by being struck by a stick.

Ice hockey is a much more dangerous sport, yet it is very popular in North America and it is gaining popularity in the north of England. Facial injuries are the most common, followed by sprains, strains and avulsion injuries, but the incidence of facial injury is reduced by wearing a helmet.

Injury to the knee, ankle, wrist, elbow and hand are most often seen, including laceration, bruising, fracture and dislocation, the majority of injuries being caused by high sticking rather than from the puck. Rib injury is comparatively common, usually caused by the stick. Damage to the clavicular joints and to the clavicle itself are frequently seen and concussion may occur, even when wearing a helmet. Other sources of injury are the skates and goal posts which can cause extrinsic type injuries. These risks do not occur in hockey played on grass where the majority of injuries are from the stick or are intrinsic in origin.

Repeatedly striking the ball or puck can result in progressive instability in the glenohumeral joint which is a common complaint of hockey players. It can also give rise to epiphysitis at the elbow in adolescents or less commonly at the wrist.

Fractures of the proximal phalanges of the hand result from direct injury from a stick, ball or most often from the puck in ice hockey.

Judo

This is a sport which commands great courtesy and the rules of safety are carefully upheld by the officials during competition. Otherwise the number of injuries would undoubtedly be greater than it is.

However, injuries do occur either as a result of falling or as a result of some leverage imposed on the judoka by an opponent, or by throwing. Falls account for several injuries and are most often seen in the shoulder region. There may be muscular damage especially to the muscles of the shoulder girdle or to the neck or back or to muscles of the arm. Similarly joints of the shoulder girdle, neck, back and upper extremity can be injured by a fall. The clavicle and the clavicular joints are particularly vulnerable and dislocation of the sternoclavicular and/or acromioclavicular joints is not infrequent. Fracture of the clavicle may result from a bad fall with resultant involvement of the clavicular joints.

A fall onto the outstretched arm does not often happen, but if it does the wrist, hand and elbow may be injured.

Leverages used in the sport may injure the opponent's joints and the elbow is the joint most at risk where damage to the joint and/or the surrounding ligaments and muscles is frequently seen. An increase in the normal carrying angle is one of the commonest injuries, but the olecranon may be fractured or severely strained.

The shoulder girdle can also be injured this way where the muscles are particularly vulnerable.

Throwing techniques can injure the competitor and result in back injuries or shoulder and arm injury. The low back is often damaged this way and hypermobility of a joint due to repeated insults is common, where the technique may need modifying to prevent recurrence.

Injury to the foot is often seen as the sport is undertaken barefoot, so there is no protection to the foot. Stubbing of the first toe is a common injury and may result in the development of hallux rigidus later in life. Dislocation of a toe is not uncommonly seen.

The hand can be damaged in two ways, either directly, or more often as a result of losing the hold on the opponents garments when the tendons at the wrist may be injured or the wrist ligaments strained. Tenosynovitis is a common injury in the wrist in judo.

Jumping – hurdling, high and long jump

Hurdling is often termed 'rhythm sprinting' as it essentially involves sprinting with ten hurdles carefully placed in each lane so that very precise rhythm is required to clear them.

High hurdles (3 ft 6 in) over a distance of 110 m and low hurdles (3 ft) over a distance of 400 m both require a fairly tall physique with long legs to comfortably produce the necessary stride pattern for the sport. Basic speed is of paramount importance while the clearance style is of secondary importance only.

The approach to the first hurdle is eight fast accelerating strides. Crossing the hurdle produces a flight stride of about 11 ft; the leading leg is kicked up fast, high and bent at the knee, then driven across the hurdle so that it becomes straight. There has to be associated trunk lean, and compensating movement of the opposite arm to keep the trunk square. The trailing leg is at 90° assuring a good stride for landing. Timing between the hurdles is vital requiring three running strides. After the last hurdle is crossed speed is essential and there are six strides to the finish. (See Fig. 18.15).

The common injuries are: Medial collateral ligament of the trailing leg from repeated lateral gapping of the knee joint. Strain of the hip joint muscles due to inadequate stretching and possible muscular imbalance. The hamstring muscles are the most frequently injured and the injury can be within the muscle belly or at the ischial tuberosity where a bursitis may develop or a tendinitis or periostitis may occur. An avulsion fracture is not uncommon here. Osteitis pubis is not rare. Injuries around the patella include quadriceps pull, tear of the quadriceps expansion, chondromalacia patellae, injury to the patella ligament and possibly Osgood-Schlatters disease

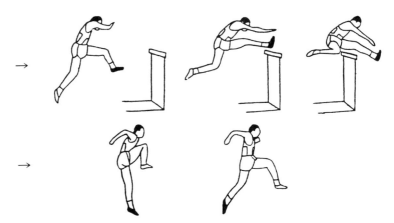

Fig. 18.15 Hurdling. From *Track and Field Athletics* by Wilf Paish.

in adolescents. Shin splints and anterior compartment syndrome may occur. The ankle may be damaged by bad landing or the tendo Achilles may be traumatised by repeated pounding.

Sacro-iliac strains are not uncommon due to the unequal strain placed on these joints during this sport.

In high jump the aim is to project the body as high as possible in a vertical direction which is achieved by extension of the take off leg, aided by the free limbs. The straddle jump depends largely on pelvic rotation (see Fig. 18.16(a)). The Fosbury flop has revolutionised high jump and depends largely on spinal extension followed by flexion for landing with some rotation while crossing the bar (see Fig. 18.16(b)).

The common injuries which occur are: the ankle and foot are subjected to great force during landing in the straddle high jump. Impaction or facet locking of the tibiotaloid joint may result. Injury to the tendo Achilles is common and sesamoiditis under the first metatarsal-phalangeal joint is seen. Periostitis on the lateral aspect of the ankle joint is an injury unique to those who jump and is particularly common as a result of the Fosbury flop. Overstrain of the pushoff leg at the knee or in the calf muscles is usually due to inadequate stretching. The muscles around the hip joint of the push off leg need to be extremely strong to withstand the strain of this action; any weakness or imbalance can result in injury to these muscles. The fact that high jumpers wear spikes on one foot only can increase the take off imbalance.

Long jump requires a fast controlled approach run, an explosive take off, a controlled flight and a sound landing (see Fig. 18.17).

The common injuries which occur are: strain of the hamstring muscles which is the commonest injury of all as is the case in sprinting. The lumbar spine is extended in midflight and jack-knifed forward for landing, leading to strain on this region of the spine and on the psoas muscle. Facet locking of the lumbar joints may occur or hyper-mobility due to repeated insult, with associated

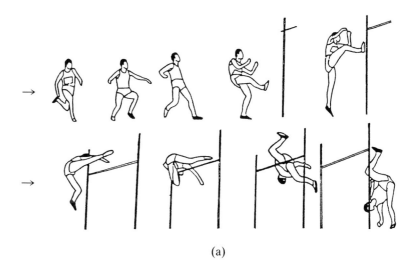

(a)

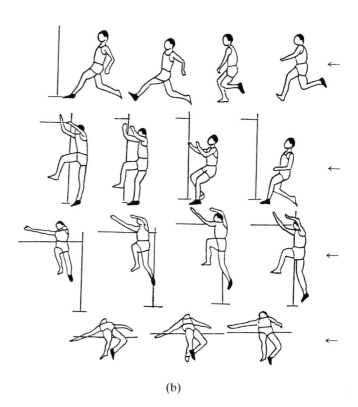

Fig. 18.16 High jump. (a) The straddle; (b) the Fosbury Flop. From *Track and Field Athletics* by Wilf Paish.

(b)

ligamentous strain, muscular guarding and pain. Morton's metatarsalgia can result in the push off leg from ill-fitting footwear, 'slapping' the foot on the board, or from possible intrinsic foot imbalance. Neck injury is seen less often but can result from bad landing in any of these three jumping events.

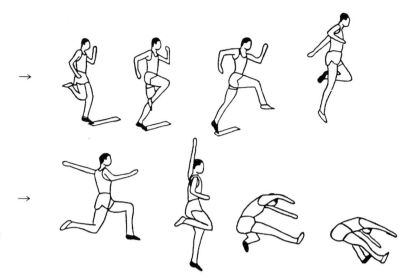

Fig. 18.17 Long jump. From *Track and Field Athletics* by Wilf Paish.

Karate

This sport principally involves the use of the hands and feet to deliver a variety of strikes to the opponent's body. Kicking is particularly aimed at the upper body and head so hip joint mobility is of paramount importance.

The front kick rapidly stretches the hamstring muscles as does the axe kick when the heel of the kicking leg is brought down to strike the opponent on the top of his head. Hamstring injuries, tears, bursitis, periosteal injuries and possible avulsions of the ischial tuberosity are likely to occur. Hyperextension strain of the knee joint may accompany this kick.

The side kick will stretch the adductor muscles resulting in possible tears, musculotendinous junction tears or even pubic avulsion. Osteitis pubis may result from repeated strain of the joint.

The back kick will stretch the rectus femoris and abdominal muscles as the athlete kicks his leg directly backwards while facing forward. The quadriceps and abdominal muscles can be injured by this kick. In addition, there is a risk of an extension strain of the low back. As the technique requires that the upper torso remains as straight as possible, strain is placed on the sacro-iliac joints which may be hurt.

Much of the training involves punching at an imaginary opponent, i.e. into thin air. This can force the elbow into hyperextension with resultant injury to the olecranon which is often locked as a result. There may also be a distraction type injury to the shoulder joint with possible damage to the conjoint tendon.

Sparring is often undertaken without protection to the hands; there is risk of the thumb being abducted and injured, the scaphoid, trapezium, and first metacarpophalangeal joints being damaged.

Some enthusiasts strike at a straw-covered post repeatedly and form scar tissue on the dorsal aspect of the third and fourth metacarpophalangeal joints in particular, which can result in the extensor tendons becoming thickened and damaged.

The common sites of muscular damage in the thigh and pelvis are: iliopsoas where the bursa between the tendon and the hip joint may become inflamed, or an avulsion fracture of a lumbar transverse process may occur as a result of violent kicking, or the muscle may be injured within its fleshy part; the quadriceps, especially at its insertion or expansion or this may involve injury to the patellar tendon. The cruciate ligaments of the knee joint may be stretched by the violent kicking action involved in the sport, leading to instability of the knee joint and resultant pain.

Motor bike scrambling

Participants of this sport make up for their comparatively low numbers by their enthusiasm. The injuries which occur are due to falling off the machine or to the jolting and jarring of the body during riding.

Falls are usually onto the side of the athlete, so injury to the shoulder, clavicle and clavicular joints are the most commonly seen. There may be damage to the skin as well as to the underlying structures. Fracture of the clavicle is the commonest bony injury but the bones of the arm may be injured in this way, depending on the way the athlete falls. Injury to the neck or back may also occur thus and the possibility of fracture must always be remembered.

Actually riding the machine over rough ground results in enormous compression forces being sustained by the spine and shoulder girdles as well as the arms. The commonest injury is to the lumbar spine which is repeatedly subjected to compression forces. These are somewhat reduced by wearing a support belt which is usual these days. The muscles of the lumbar region may become hypertonic, in an effort to reduce the compression factor on the underlying ligaments and joints. The ligaments may become stretched and the joints are frequently subject to facet locking. Repeated insults to the intervertebral discs may render them liable to premature prolapse.

The ischial tuberosities often become inflamed from sitting on them and subjecting them to repeated jolting. The shoulder joint is also subjected to jolting and the tendons and surrounding muscles may become inflamed as a result. Inflammation of the elbow and wrist also occur, and tenosynovitis of the wrist extensors is common.

Netball

This is principally played by females and most schools include netball in the curriculum, so there is a large number of participants, albeit most of them young. For this reason, epiphysitis is commonly seen particularly in the weight bearing bones of the leg. Overuse giving rise to pulling osteochondritis of the tibial tubercle is also frequently seen in young netball players.

Among adult players, injury to the ankle is more often seen than any other problem. This seems to be at least partially due to the footwork rule which permits one foot only to be moved on landing with the ball. The effect of this is that the fixed foot is subjected to a compression injury from which it cannot escape by its normal method of moving with the momentum of the body. Awkward landing may sprain the ankle and/or foot which is made more likely as the game is played on a hard surface.

The knee may be injured by a bad landing, or by a twisting movement such as is needed when marking or dodging; knee injuries come second to ankle injuries.

Hand and finger injuries are due to the digits being hit by the ball usually, or because of faulty catching when one or more joints may be stressed. The joints of the fingers may be forced into extension.

Back injury is due to bad landing, when the spine is jarred. It may be stretched by jumping up to reach the ball, causing muscular, ligamentous or joint injury.

Injury to the shoulder girdle results from throwing the ball. The surrounding muscles or tendons can be damaged this way especially if the throw has to be awkward due to an opponent marking closely. The neck may be strained in a similar manner.

Injuries seem to be most frequent amongst those players in the positions of goal defence and wing attack, possibly as those players tend to cover a greater area of the court. Muscular injuries are more likely to occur in cold weather conditions and usually affect the shoulder region and the legs and back.

Racket sports

All racket sports involve running, twisting, turning, jumping and holding the racket. Tennis players run a greater distance than other racket players, so are more prone to leg problems. These are chiefly of the calf muscles – indeed a tear of the midcalf is so common that it is termed 'tennis leg'. Injury to the thigh muscles is also seen. Fatigue may well play a part in these injuries as tennis players often play for long periods of time during drawn out matches.

Twisting and turning lay stress on the joints of the legs and on the pelvis and spine. Knee strains are common as are spinal problems. Analysis of the injuries has revealed that low back problems account for just over 50% of the total (my figures).

Jumping stresses the ankle joint in particular; sprains and compression injuries account for the second most frequently seen injury. The knee joint is often damaged this way.

Holding the racket produces problems. Squash and badminton rackets have a smaller handle than tennis rackets which increases the chance of elbow trouble, especially 'tennis elbow'. This is not so often seen in tennis players with the exception of inexperienced players who tend to strike the ball late, thus using the arm rather than the shoulder and body as a whole.

Wrist injuries occur frequently in squash, badminton and table tennis players because the action of the game involves flicking of the wrist. In enclosed courts, squash and real (or court) tennis, there are wrist injuries resulting from colliding with the wall. This can also lead to head and shoulder injuries.

Shoulder strains usually involve tendons around the joint, the conjoint tendon being the most vulnerable, but the biceps tendon may be damaged. This is more often seen in real tennis and lawn tennis because of the power which is generated from the shoulder during a stroke. Bursitis is a frequent complication.

Tennis elbow occurs in lawn tennis players who put a great deal of top spin on the backhand and is then associated with hypermobility of the inferior radio-ulnar joint.

The shoulder musculature of racket players is usually overdeveloped; this results in a thoracic scoliosis which can predispose to thoracic spine and rib strains. The acromioclavicular joint usually shows premature signs of degenerative change and there are many players who have developed chronic changes in the conjoint tendon.

The neck is subjected to strain especially in the service action of lawn tennis and in badminton where cervical extension is repeated. Squash and real tennis players as well as table tennis players do not stress the neck so much.

Overstretching can injure the abdominal wall; this is most often seen in lawn tennis and badminton players. The upper ribs can become strained due to excess elevation of the racket arm, common in squash, badminton and lawn tennis.

The low back and pelvis are often injured from the twisting which these sports demand. Players who have short legs seem to be more prone to these strains, especially those involving the sacro-iliac joints. Latissimus dorsi and the erector spinae muscles are often seen in a state of hypertonia.

The knee joint is subjected to twisting strains. The resultant injuries include damage to the medial collateral ligament, the medial meniscus, the quadriceps expansion, the patellar ligament and bursitis and chondromalacia occur frequently.

Shin splints occur in lawn tennis and real tennis players. The former are more prone to the problem when they play on the hard surfaces such as 'Plexipave', but all real tennis courts have floors which are not resilient, thus increasing the risk of this. Squash and badminton players are unlikely to suffer from shin splints.

The ankle joint is very often sprained; many professional lawn tennis players routinely strap their ankles to prevent this injury. The tendo Achilles is injured in racket players due to the excessive strain placed upon it. This condition now occurs more frequently due to the tabs on the back of the heel on many shoes, which can cause friction to the tendon.

Stress fractures of the metatarsals occur especially in female lawn tennis players. 'Tennis toe' is very often seen in lawn tennis players due to the friction of the shoe on the first toenail.

Injury from the ball is most often seen in real tennis and in squash. Injury from the racket of the opponent occurs in squash, especially when the players are inexperienced. A broken string can also cause injury and is more likely in squash as the players are not separated.

In conclusion, it is obvious that racket sports can cause injury to all parts of the body, but the ankle and low back seem to be the most frequently injured areas.

Rowing

See also canoeing.

Skin abrasions and blisters are a common complaint due to the friction of the oars.

Rowing differs from canoeing in that the oarsman sits. He stabilises his position by using the extensor digitorum brevis muscle which is usually overdeveloped and may be strained, especially in rough water conditions. In addition the stabilising muscles of the shoulder girdle are frequently strained, the rhomboids in particular and the levator scapulae, scalenes and posterior muscles of the shoulder. Trapezius and latissimus dorsi may be injured as well.

On occasion the muscles of the thigh become traumatised, namely the quadriceps and the hamstrings. This is probably more likely to occur in cold weather conditions. In hot weather conditions, the oarsman may be subject to excess sunshine, and perspiration may render him liable to dehydration.

As in canoeing, the muscles of the wrist are particularly subject to injury; tenosynovitis is frequently seen at the wrist and strains of the wrist joint are not infrequent.

Rugby

This game involves body contact as well as running and is played in cold and wet weather conditions, thus increasing the probability of injury.

The Rugby Football Union now publishes an annual report on

injuries sustained in the game. According to the report published in September 1987, 1,247 injuries were reported during the previous season by 126 clubs, which averages out as one injury per 4.5 seasons, contrary to what one might expect. Most of the injuries reported were of a relatively minor nature, 592 players returning to the same game. The highest number of injuries resulted from tackling or being tackled, 47% of the total. Open play accounted for 22% and the scrum for a mere 7%.

Injury was most frequently reported during the second half and in particular in the final quarter of the game, probably due to fatigue. Ground conditions lead to variation; head and shoulder injuries increased in numbers on hard ground while knee and ankle injuries occurred most often on soft ground.

Contrary to many assumptions the 'front five' appear to be least likely to sustain an injury, the wing forward being the most vulnerable.

Back injury accounted for almost one-third of the total. These would include muscular, ligamentous and joint conditions, lower lumbar joint strains being the most common of all. Head injury occurs most often as a result of falling on hard ground. Neck injury is still too frequent for comfort, but the majority are muscular or ligamentous. However, the long-term effect of such injuries is commonly seen in osteopathic practice, the athlete complaining of neck pain and stiffness, and the clinical findings suggest compression injury in the past, often with premature degenerative changes.

Injury to the ankle usually results from an inversion strain particularly sustained on wet ground. Fracture of the fibula is not rare. The knee joint is also more likely to become injured on wet ground. The medial ligament, coronary ligaments, cruciate ligaments and the medial meniscus may be damaged. Quadriceps and hamstring injury also occurs.

Shoulder injuries are often seen, either tendon damage or dislocation, often recurrent. The elbow may also be damaged and even dislocated. Injury to the clavicle and it's joints remains a common rugby injury. The ribs may be injured either from a fall or tackle.

Bruising probably remains the commonest injury of all in this sport.

Running

Running is involved in most sports. It may be associated with torsional strains of the body, as in the various ball games, or it may be relatively predictable as in track events or road running.

Sprinting is an explosive type of activity, and many ball games involve this type of action. Middle distance running requires more endurance and even more is needed for long distance running.

However, the vulnerable areas of the body are similar in all these activities.

The hamstring muscles are the most frequently injured group. This is because there is forceful extension of a fully flexed hip with the knee extending to more than 90° at the same time, so there is some degree of stretch on the contracting muscle. This injury is often associated with muscular imbalance, either there are strong knee extensors with relatively weak flexors or there is a tone/length imbalance between the extensor and flexor compartments.

Quadriceps strains are the second most often seen, especially of the rectus femoris as this muscle acts on two joints. Adductor muscle strains are usually a result of hurdling and jumping during training. Calf muscle strains are very common − tears, tendinitis, possible bursitis or tears of the tendo Achilles; they are most often a result of hill running.

Low back and sacro-iliac strains are common. They are frequently associated with muscular imbalance of the thigh muscles and possibly caused or at least aggravated by bend running.

Shin splints includes anterior and posterior tibial compartment syndromes, anterior tibial tenosynovitis and stress fractures of the tibia, all often associated with running on hard surfaces.

Chondromalacia patellae is very commonly seen; it is usually associated with imperfect patella tracking or a patella alta. The occurrence is increased when the left foot is forced into excessive lateral rotation on bends.

Foot injuries occur. Plantar fasciitis may result from bend running or from ill-fitting shoes, commonly. Spikes typically have little arch support and poor heel padding, so wear may exaggerate the inversion/eversion at the heel, causing subtalar problems. If the heel of the shoe is too wide, the movements at the ankle may be increased as the first contact with the ground is on the outer border. Bruising of the calcaneum is seen; stress fractures may occur in the foot (especially the metatarsal bones in females), or in the tibia or fibula.

Ankle sprains are most often seen as a result of running on uneven surfaces such as rough grass, but can result from bend running. Starting from blocks can produce excessive strains as there is a greater range of movement required at the hip, knee and ankle. If the lumbar spine is not sufficiently flexed (i.e. relaxed) the stresses are greatly exaggerated. See Fig. 18.18.

Decelerating causes a possible tendency to overstride when the tendo Achilles, low back and sacro-iliac joints become additionally stressed.

Bend running requires a sudden adaptation to the curve of the track. As all track races are run anticlockwise, the spine has to sidebend as if for a short right lower extremity. The inner knee has to flex more than the outer and there are considerable gapping

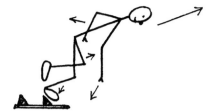

Fig. 18.18 Stresses when using starting blocks.

forces applied to the knees. Many hamstring pulls occur on the bends or on the attempt to accelerate out of the bend. The bends are sharper on indoor tracks and the slope is inadequate to prevent hamstring strains. See Fig. 18.19.

Long distance running presents different problems. This is a feat of endurance when muscular exhaustion may result in conditions such as cramp.

Dehydration is the other common problem encountered and the athlete must make sure that he has a sufficient fluid intake, particularly in hot weather conditions. Blisters of the foot are very commonly seen in long distance runners.

Sailing

Apart from the occupational hazards, this highly competitive sport involves risks from inclement weather conditions and possible navigational difficulties.

Recreational sailing, as a hobby, leads to muscular or ligamentous strain of the low back from inexpert launching or return to the shore, due to the general weight of the boat. Head injuries occur from neglecting to duck during the gybe.

Single-handed sailing

The boats are light, manoeuverable and speedy and handled by one sailor only who is responsible for all activity on board.

Use of the tiller rods places great strain on the wrist and elbow, leading to possible common flexor and common extensor origin

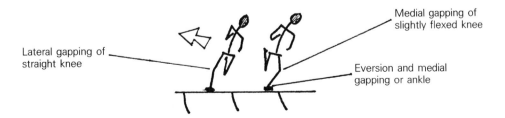

Lateral gapping of straight knee

Medial gapping of slightly flexed knee

Eversion and medial gapping or ankle

Fig. 18.19 Bend running.

problems at the elbow. This is exacerbated by holding the main-sheet against the strong pull of the wind with the arm adducted, flexed and pronated.

Much time is spent facing the bows assessing wind and boat direction, leading to rotational strain of the low back and sacro-iliac joints, together with stress on the iliolumbar ligament and the lower intervertebral discs. The speed of movement needed when tacking and more especially when gybing, accentuates the strain first on one side of the body and then on the other, for minutes at a time.

The neck is also placed under strain as the sailor keeps his body perpendicular to the length of the boat while looking forward. The lower cervical region may suffer ligamentous strain or facet locking. The upper ribs may be injured by this manoeuvre.

Balancing the boat involves leaning out, in most classes without a harness. The feet are tucked under footstraps, placing strain on the quadriceps, patellofemoral joint and patellar ligament. Chondro-malacia patellae often results from incorrect patella tracking. The traction placed through the knee joint can result in meniscal injury when a quick gybe is attempted. Great agility is needed to sail.

Crewed sailing

Here the tasks are effectively halved, but the boats are heavier and faster, laying additional strain on each sailor.

A trapeze harness is used which places strain on the junctional areas of the spine especially the lumbosacral joint leading to liga-mentous and annular injury.

Increased tension in the sheets adds extra strain on the forearm. Responsibility for the mainsheet and rudder rests with the helms-man; both place strain on his forearm increasing the possibility of tenosynovitis.

Torsion of the upper body may cause injury to the ribs. Ischial bursitis occurs as a result of sitting and moving swiftly on a hard, cold, damp surface.

The fact that two grown adults are performing agile activities in an enclosed space compromises their bodies with an increased possibility of injury.

Skating

The amateur skater is liable to be injured by falling, especially in the early stages. By so doing he may be injured by the blade of a skate, be bruised, strain a joint of even fracture a bone or dislocate a joint. The exact injury will depend on how he falls. Fracture of the arm or leg is possible. Strain of the joints of the upper or lower extremity may occur, the knee and wrist being those most often hurt this way. The female coccyx is commonly damaged by falling on ice.

The more advanced skater is unlikely to be injured this way, but by various manoeuvres he may execute. Bruising is common in pairs as one of the pair is commonly struck by the other skater's blade. Speed skaters are particularly liable to neck and shoulder strains which are frequently recurrent and due to the action of skating long distances. They also tend to suffer from low back strains of muscle, ligament and joint with facet locking being especially prevalent.

The leg muscles which are most often injured, in all classes of skater, are the hamstrings, calf muscles and the anterior tibial muscles, probably partially induced by low temperatures on ice. They are less commonly injured if they are strong and supple.

Groin strains occur as a result of the strain placed on them during certain movements.

The ankle joint is comparatively well protected by the boot, but this results in an extra strain being placed on the knee joint, which is very commonly damaged. The injuries are most often to the medial ligament, the coronary ligaments, the medial meniscus and sometimes to the cruciate ligaments. The knee joint is subjected to enormous rotational strain during take off for most jumps and during landing which is on a flat blade rather than the usual heel toe action, added to which is the lack of resilience of ice. For example, in the double axel (which is 2½ rotations in the air with a forward take off, landing on the opposite foot) the knee on the take off side is twisted. Repetition of this can lead to strain of the medial ligament. The landing leg can also be twisted and this is much more likely if the take off is not perfect. The salchow, toe salchow and toe loop also place great strain on the knee joint. Back strains can result from bad landings.

The tendo Achilles is frequently a problem in skating, often due to boot pressure and restriction of normal use of the calf muscles by virtue of the restriction of the boot.

The abdominal muscles are sometimes injured by the lutz, or backward jump, when they may become overstretched.

Skiing

High speed falls account for many ski injuries. Head and neck injury occurs this way; the fall is often sideways and onto a hard icy surface. Similarly shoulder dislocation results from such a fall when the outstretched hand becomes stuck in hard snow as the rest of the body is propelled forward by the fall, a traction injury. This commonly occurs in slalom racing.

Ski pole injury occurs to the hand which is outstretched and holding the ski stick. Around 10% of all skiing injuries are to the ulnar collateral ligament of the thumb, the total number is estimated at between 50 000 and 200 000 per annum. The ski pole forces the thumb into abduction and extension, straining the ligament and possibly causing a fracture dislocation of the first metacarpophalangeal joint. Prevention of this injury is discussed controversially by the use of poles without straps.

Injury to the trunk is usually as a result of collision; bruising, strains of the vertebral joints and ribs are commonly caused this way. Knee injuries occur frequently. The medial collateral ligament is the commonest injury, usually seen in poor skiers who cannot parallel correctly and who turn by checking with the edge of the downhill ski. More advanced skiers may fail to keep their skis parallel when traversing. Forward falls tend to externally rotate and medially gap the knee thus stressing the medial ligament.

The cruciate ligaments may be injured in skiing, the anterior usually by falling and the posterior by striking a fixed object with the knee flexed, so the tibia is forced posteriorly in relation to the femur.

By far the most common skiing injury is fracture of the lower leg caused by a rotational strain when the bindings fail to release. It happens more often in powdery snow and less often in icy or hard packed surfaces. Violent twisting of the foot results in a spiral fracture.

Ankle injury is almost always due to a rotational force; half these injuries are fractures, while half are ligamentous injuries.

The tendo Achilles is subjected to repeated overload in skiing; many skiers ski all day! In order to make a turn the skier must jerk his heels up and then down. Meanwhile the ski boot is such that the foot itself is virtually immobile, so the stresses of leg movement are concentrated at the ankle, the only part which can freely move being the tendon, so it takes the strain. Hence inflammation and even rupture are common skiing injuries.

Swimming

Although this is considered to be the perfect sport and is used in many rehabilitation programs, nevertheless injuries do occur, if infrequently.

Head injury can result from striking the head on the pool edge or a diving board as was the case with the World Champion, Longhanis, during the 1988 Olympics. Goggles can cause injury especially if they are too tight or are struck by another swimmer.

Neck injury is caused by repeated hyper-rotation, extension and/or side bending and can lead to joint strain especially in the midcervical and cervicodorsal regions.

The shoulder girdle can be injured. Repetitive overuse and minor traumata can strain the sternoclavicular joint, particularly in backstroke or butterfly. Similarly the acromioclavicular joint may be damaged by the repeated trauma of backstroke or freestyle swimming.

In the glenohumeral joint, rotator cuff tendinitis, fragmentation of the conjoint tendon and impingement of the subacromial bursa may result from overuse.

The thoracic region may suffer from muscle injury, especially of trapezius, latissimus dorsi and the muscles of the shoulder girdle. Hyperextension of the area may result in facet locking most often from butterfly or breaststroke.

The lumbar area may be hyperextended in diving, butterfly and in breaststroke with associated muscle overstrain and possible facet locking of the joints. The sacro-iliac joints may be involved as well.

Cramp is a common affliction of swimmers and usually affects the abdominal muscles or possibly those of the lower extremity. Muscle injuries occur in the adductors, hamstrings and calf muscles and may well be made worse in cold water conditions.

The 'screw kick' of the breast stroke causes strain on the medial side of the knee joint where damage may occur to the medial ligament or even to the medial meniscus.

The feet are prone to infection, athlete's foot and verruccae in particular.

Throwing

Ball throwing

The muscles principally used are the triceps, pectoralis major, the abdominal muscles and the intercostals. The commonest injury is to the musculotendinous junction of pectoralis major, while the external oblique on the opposite side to the throwing arm becomes stretched.

Repeated throwing may lead to instability of the shoulder joint (glenohumeral), strain of the clavicular joints and strain of the upper ribs. Elbow pain is usually posterior and is often associated with a defect of tracking of the olecranon within the fossa.

Javelin

Injury to the elbow joint is the commonest problem amongst javelin throwers. Most frequently the lateral aspect is affected, at the radiohumeral joint. Here there is bony opposition at the final stage of the throw. The elbow is held straight, and above 90° abduction as the throw begins, thus stressing the lateral aspect of the elbow. Repeated insult to the conjoint tendon causes damage there which may be exacerbated by instability in the glenohumeral joint.

The lower lumbar and sacro-iliac joints are subjected to rotation, while extension is superimposed at the final stage of the throw, so joint strains are common in this area.

Discus

During the throw, the area which is subjected to most strain is the lower lumbar spine which is rotated and somewhat extended. This repeated action will lead to facet opposition and therefore locking as well as ligamentous and annular strains. Low back pain is common in discus throwers. Comparatively speaking, there is little strain placed on the shoulder, elbow or muscles of the arm.

Shot put

This event is traditionally that of big strong men, so their muscle bulk provides certain protection to their joints. The elbow joint and ligaments take a great deal of strain in the final stage of the put. They are, therefore liable to strain from repeated insult.

Wrist joint injury is common. The final stage of the put requires a powerful push to propel the shot. At this time the wrist is in extension and slight ulnar deviation to support the shot against the neck. The flexor muscles of the hand and wrist are stretched but will contract suddenly and powerfully as the shot starts to move forward and often become strained by this action. On the posterior aspect of the wrist, usually at the base of the second metacarpal bone, an exostosis often develops as a result of bony impingement while the wrist is in extension (Lister's tubercle). If large, this may become inflamed with repeated bony impingement.

Hammer

During the final stage of delivery, the right foot is driven down onto the ground strongly, to provide an upward accelerating force to the hammer. The lumbar spine is rotating to the left (righthanded thrower), slightly side bent to the right and extended. This causes strong contraction of the quadriceps on the right which tends to rotate the right innominate anteriorly while L5 is rotating to the left. The common symptom picture, therefore, is right-sided low back pain which is only exacerbated by throwing the hammer − i.e. pain only occurs at the extreme of this peculiar movement. The right foot may suffer from a sesamoiditis.

Volleyball − see basketball

Weights

Weight training is used 'as a means to an end', either as part of a general fitness programme or to assist training to improve performance in some other sport.

Before undertaking a weight training programme a beginner should consider the aim of the programme. This falls into the following categories:

(1) Muscular endurance. The number of repetitions a muscle or group of muscles can perform in any movement.
(2) Strength. The ability of a muscle or group of muscles to exert a force against resistance.
(3) Fitness. Muscular endurance coupled with an increase in aerobic activity.

Weight training can achieve these aims in the following ways:

(1) Muscular endurance. Light weights with high repetitions.
(2) Strength. Heavy weights with low repetitions.
(3) Fitness. Light weights 'against the clock', often referred to as 'circuit training'.

Three types of training are used:

(1) Isometric. A static muscular contraction with a constant measure of tension against the muscle. Little or no movement of a joint or joints. Ideally this process involves working at about 60–70% but this is extremely difficult to measure accurately. Injury occurs when maximum effort is involved, due to muscular fatigue and possible overload.
(2) Isotonic. This is the most commonly used type of weight training and involves a dynamic contraction. It enhances the strength of the entire muscle or group of muscles, not just a part, as in isometric contraction. The disadvantage of isotonic training is that the muscular contraction varies throughout the range of movement. The maximum tension occurs at the weakest point of the lift, for example on biceps curls when the elbow is straight (in extension). As flexion of the elbow increases the effort becomes progressively easier especially as there is an increase of momentum. Injury is most likely to occur when lifting nears the performers maximum tension.
(3) Isokinetic. This type of training is relatively new in its concept. It provides maximum (unvarying) resistance throughout the range of movement. This is accomplished by using equipment which exerts variable resistance according to the percentage of muscular contraction throughout the particular movement. An additional advantage of this type of weight training is that it does not produce muscular soreness or stiffness which usually results from isotonic lifting.

The development of gymnasia both in the public and private sector has greatly increased the number of athletes using weights for training purposes. Expensive multigym type machines such as Universal and Nautilus have made weight training more popular and much safer as it is virtually impossible to be injured by weights actually falling on the athlete. However, because the athlete no longer has to learn the techniques of lifting free weights (barbell and dumbell) he may well try to lift weights near or above his maximum, resulting in possible soft tissue and joint injury.

When training for muscular endurance, the weights used are generally light so it is easier to take care and think about technique. In strength training schedules where heavy weights are used, there is a greater possibility of injury. In most cases this is soft tissue injury caused by insufficient warm up and stretching.

The common sites of injury are:

Hamstrings.   Usually when the athlete lifts with straight knee instead of slightly bent knee, or when there is too much weight on leg curls on multigym machines.

Low Back.   Often due to excess flexion, for example in rowing exercises. Possibly when the bar is held at the back of the neck and the athlete flexes at the waist while lifting; this is unsafe. Possibly when the athlete performs sit-ups with a weight held behind the head − definitely unwise! Possibly when a weight is lifted from the floor with the back already flexed and the head looking down. The athlete should have a straight back and hold his head up.

Muscle strains.   These usually occur when a muscle or group of muscles is worked in isolation and are highly stressed, for example in triceps exercises. The muscles of the shoulder girdle are also commonly injured this way.

Weight lifting

This is an entirely separate sport which emphasises flexibility as well as great strength. Because the aim is to lift as great a weight as possible, there is tremendous strain on the body. Many of the injuries which occur result from overenthusiasm, especially in young athletes who have no idea of the potential danger.

Most injuries occur to the low back and knees. The low back area is protected by a belt but nevertheless there is still great strain placed upon it. When lifting the weight above the head, there is a great tendency to extend the lumbar spine. Many weight lifters have premature degenerative changes in the lumbar region, especially at the lumbosacral level, where anterior and posterior osteophytes may be seen on X-rays.

Both the 'Olympic lifts' clean and jerk and snatch involve using the large muscles of the legs to propel the weights. The lifter starts moving the bar upwards and then 'sits in' underneath it in a deep squat position, placing tremendous strain on the knees as he proceeds to stand. Injury to the quadriceps is common and to ligaments of the knee joint, the patellar tendon and degenerative changes tend to occur prematurely in the knee joints.

Wind surfing

Beginners at this sport spend a great deal of time pulling at a heavy, unresponsive sail which, once out of the water flaps around wildly. The result is low back strains and strains of the shoulder girdle musculature especially the rhomboids and trapezius.

Once that stage has passed, the windsurfer stands, legs apart, knees locked in extension, one foot pointing towards the mast, the other at right angles to the board. The arms are apart and the torso twisted to face the mast. This position imposes strain on the sacro-iliac joints, the lower lumbar spine and the knees, especially the anterior cruciate ligament and the collateral ligaments. Strain of the clavicular joints is common, too. The use of a chest harness added strain to the low back and shoulders but this has now been replaced by a different type, the nappy harness, on which the windsurfer can effectively 'sit in', to effect maximum counter-balance. The knees are then flexed and the strain on the knee ligaments is negligible. Many windsurfers wear a belt to reduce the strain on the low back.

The elbow joints can become strained especially at the lateral side. Tenosynovitis at the wrist is common due to overuse of the muscles. The neck may become strained as a result of the windsurfer constantly looking ahead to interpret wind change and current, while the torso is relatively fixed, so facet locking or ligament strain is common.

Freestyle windsurfing and wavejumping has brought high impact injury into the sport. The ligaments of the knee and ankle become increasingly vulnerable. Compression injuries occur to the spinal joints as do whiplash injuries, often as sailors attempt 360° jumps, off the waves.

Chapter 19   Psychological Problems of Sport

It is important to understand the problems which can affect athletes, not only from a physical but also from a psychological point of view. The following experience of Jonathan Smith who is a professional tennis player may well be typical of the problems faced in competitive sport. I am grateful to him for allowing me to use this information.

> "He has all the shots, but lacks the killer instinct".
> "Tennis playing is all in the mind".
> "British tennis players are not tough enough".

These are all phrases bandied about on television and in the press and have been for many years. Indeed I have been the subject of statements of this kind, and it is worth noting that tennis players, myself included, do seek advice and help from a number of different sources, including the growing number of sports psychologists.

However, it is reasonable to suggest that one visits the chiropodist when one realises one has a foot problem, the osteopath when one realises one has a skeletal problem, generally through the onset of pain. Dentists and doctors, too, are more often consulted when one is suffering pain than for a regular check up.

So it is that the tennis player will probably seek advice for any psychological problem only when he has exhausted techniques and physical explanations as to why he keeps 'blowing' matches, and becomes aware that he has a problem inside his own head. So it was with me.

I had been playing tennis, professionally, for ten years, had a number of Grand Prix doubles titles to my credit, a World Singles ranking in the top 100, with wins against such players as Ilie Nastase, Johan Kriek, Peter Fleming, Steve Denton etc. I had represented Great Britain in the Davis Cup and Kings Cup, but had reached a stage where no matter how hard I tried, I was not playing as well as I felt I should be.

I was playing a circuit in Austria, had been involved in a number of long matches on the slow clay courts, was tired as a result of having been "on the road" for three months, and was not winning matches which I felt I should have won. Generally I was making heavy weather of those matches which I did win.

It was during a specific match against a good Swedish player when, after being 6−1, 3−1 ahead, hitting the ball sweetly, concentrating at a high level, and just playing and enjoying being part

of the drama, that things started to go horribly wrong. At this
point I became aware that the match was there for the taking. I
needed only to "keep playing the same" and "keep doing the right
things" and victory would be mine. I can remember missing shots
which I had been making; my legs and arms stiffened up, making
movement difficult and striking the ball uncomfortable, while the
harder I tried to keep playing well, the less control and power I
had. I became anxious, frustrated and finally angry with myself
and with my inability to finish off my opponent and bring the
match to an end, in my favour. These feelings were so extreme
that my technique broke down, resulting in a 6−0 final set loss and
a slanging match going on in my head.

It is hardly surprising, therefore, that I then decided to stop
playing competitive tennis until I could find some reason for what
was happening to me, making match play unenjoyable and in fact
a conscious nightmare.

So I drove home and decided to see a sports psychologist who I
had met some time earlier when he was working with a contem-
porary of mine. The psychologist has adopted the theory of *The
Inner Game* as written by Timothy Galway.

The suggestion was made that I should relive the Austrian match. I
had to identify the "voices" in my head and work out who was
talking to whom, and what sort of relationship they had, as though
they were two separate entities.

It became clear that one voice − let us call it Self 1 − seemed to
do virtually all the talking and treated me − let us call it Self 2 −
rather badly, saying that I was a lousy hopeless tennis player...
"you've missed another shot"..."give the game up"..."you've
blown another match" etc. Self 1 certainly did not trust Self 2 who
it seemed to regard as the "doer" or "striker" of the tennis ball. In
fact there was often so little trust between Self 1 and Self 2 that
Self 1 would repeat endlessly "step towards the ball, step towards
the ball" as if Self 1 thought that Self 2 had a very short memory
and was unable to do the job correctly. Then, having told the legs
to "step forwards" on account of Self 2's apparent incompetence,
Self 1 made the legs "do it right", thus tightening the leg muscles
as well as those of the arms and face! This was how Self 1 thought
it should happen. So, moving like an iron rod, the legs do not flow
freely; an off balance position is achieved forcing compensation
from the arm in the form of a stiff swing, probably a mistimed shot
and a further tirade from Self 1 as to how incompetent Self 2 is,
and so further mistrust, muscle tightness and errors result.

This vicious circle of mistrust − Self 1 trying to do Self 2's job,
creating more muscular tension and therefore more errors, brought
my career to it's knees in terms of performance and enjoyment. It
then became clear that I had to understand exactly what Self 2 did
and if Self 2 did it well enough. If so, I had to build trust between

Self 1 and Self 2, so that Self 1 would not feel the need to interfere.

Self 2 is the amazing human body. Quite apart from it's functions involved in our survival, in terms of playing tennis, it gets into position, coordinates eyes, hands and legs etc. and performs so many intricate and highly complex movements without fuss, that thousands of tennis balls are struck perfectly.

The athlete's expression of "playing out of one's mind" where there is no conscious thought, no analysis or self-consciousness, when the athlete feels an integral part of the action, where awareness is actively heightened and the athlete enjoys an addictive sense of well-being and fulfillment, accurately describes Self 2's capabilities when there is no interference from Self 1.

With such a marvellous instrument as the human body at our disposal, it seems incredible that Self 1 (our conscious, thinking, egotistic mind) could ever find fault with it, or want to take charge, yet we know that Self 1 does try to do Self 2's job and we need to understand why.

Listening to Self 1 again, one of it's favourite pastimes is to defend itself. It is constantly thinking "I am this, but not that" or "I can do this but not that", or even, "I like this but not that". It constantly identifies itself with one's performance and measures itself against others. But the problem is that Self 1's methods of building concepts and beliefs regarding one's identity, are usually distorted and debilitating.

As with my last match in Austria, I would miss a backhand and Self 1 would say "what a bad shot" and I would wonder how it had happened and if there would be others to follow. Self 1 would try to correct things, a few more would be missed and my backhand is suddenly "lousy". At this stage, two very important things have happened between the first and second thought. First, the negative thought has moved from the ball ("bad shot") to my "lousy" backhand − i.e. to one of my possessions. Already I am struggling with two distortions as there is nothing actually good or bad about a ball or a shot, even though the ball may not go where aimed. If the word "bad" is descriptive of the event, then there is no problem, but it is more often a moral judgement imposed by Self 1 and is used out of context when applied to a tennis shot.

The second distortion is that, based on past errors, the future will hold more of the same. After a few more errors, Self 1 would say "you can't hit a backhand at all". The negative judgement has now passed from a possession to the very core of my potential, so I am saying that I lack the potential to hit a backhand.

With many errors I would say "I am hopeless" and with the use of the words "*I am*" the judgement has reached my self image. "*Am*" is the most powerful word to define one's identity. Possessions can be changed, potential can be developed but "*amness*" is virtually unchangeable. Almost any word placed after "I am" limits one's potential. By this time the judgement has spread to include my whole game, so that even if I had been serving well, now that "*I am*" a lousy player, the chances are that the serve would disintegrate too!

So I had to learn to see events as they were. If, during practice, a ball I had struck landed 6″ out, that was the fact − without labelling it "good" or "bad", as judging events inevitably started the thinking/self definition process and Self 1's not-so-merry corrective interference.

But, if the tennis balls I am hitting are landing out, how hard should I try to hit then in? We are brought up with the belief that "if at first you don't succeed, try, try again". It does take effort to run for a ball and strike it back, but it does not take "trying". Trying is a word for Self 1's effort, born of self doubt, and more often than not characterised by repeated self instruction and self conscious effort to balance imagined deficiencies. We do not "try" to eat with a knife and fork, or to drive a car. These are learned skills. Yet these activities do take effort, and the body uses just enough effort to perform the action.

When I looked back at the Austrian match, I realised that I had played well, enjoyed and won the first set, so where was Self 1 at that stage?. Self 1 wasn't involved, other than seeing what was happening and encouraging me. Self 1 was happy with Self 2's progress. But as soon as the first set was over and playing in the present was supplanted by thoughts of the future − i.e. winning − and of the past − i.e. "I've hit better shots than that" − I had let go of reality and become obsessed with things over which I had no control. This leads me to the topic of concentration.

Concentration is the natural state of mind which is focused on the present, whenever the mind is not wandering into the past or future, or into a fantasy world of should or shouldn't, might or might not. When we are concentrating, we are not even aware of it; we are focused only on the object or activity in which we are absorbed. There is no conscious effort to remain in this state. Only after distraction is effort once more required to bring the attention back. So when practicing or playing a match, I worked out that as soon as I became aware that Self 1 was getting restless, forming judgements or wanting to control events, I needed and would strive to interest Self 1 in something that was happening here and now, for example the movement and properties of the tennis balls. This not only left Self 2 to do it's job without interference, but fed it with useful information as to the speed, height over the net and spin on the tennis balls for it's computer to work on.

"Watch the ball, watch the ball, watch the ball" does not tend to work, sadly. When we have seen 26,225 tennis balls coming over the net towards us, it takes a special kind of awareness to see the

26,226th ball as a new event, worth paying attention to. All things which are common, ordinary, continual, frequent and obvious, in time become barely noticed by the mind which adopts the attitude that it knows all about them. So it loses it's natural curiosity and attentiveness and therefore it's awareness.

The first thing to realise about taking one's eye off the ball is that prior to this, the mind has left. Don't blame the body. The eyes are dependent on the interest of the mind. The mind has to be sufficiently interested so that it wants to stay on the ball. When watching a gripping film or reading a thrilling book, it is quite possible that if someone offers you a cup of coffee, you may not hear them, or may answer without taking your eyes off the screen or page. During practice, therefore, when my opponent's racket face actually made contact with the ball, I would say "hit" and see, with the aid of someone watching, if my utterance was synchronised with the strike of the ball. When the ball bounced on my side of the net, I would say "bounce", again with the synchronicity of the spoken word and the bounce of the ball the main aim.

Another way of interesting the mind was to check on the way the seams of the tennis ball revolved during it's flight. Checking on the height of clearance over the net, what sort of an arc the ball traced in the air from one end of the court to the other, are useful ways of regaining concentration where Self 1 is employed as a useful gatherer of information.

So, armed with the knowledge of what had happened inside my head, and why, when I played that horrendous match in Austria, I had to work out what I wanted from tennis and how I was going to achieve it. I was set short-term goals, then longer ones and I realised that for this project to be successful these goals needed to be:

(1) Challenging
(2) Realistic
(3) Specific
(4) Measurable
(5) Time phased

The long-term goal was to become as good a player as I was capable of becoming; the short-term goal was no "spiralling down". The first three criteria were instantly seen to tally with these aims. As far as being measurable, it became fascinating to see how I became better at becoming aware of a lapse in concentration, just with practice at it. To start with, perhaps a set would go by before I noticed Self 1's antics, then perhaps four games and so on, until now, when I play, I can regain a state of concentration which I notice has disappeared during the course of the same rally.

In dealing with time phasing, we looked at the length of time it took initially for me to become aware that my attention had disappeared. If I could lessen this time by one second per week over a period of two years and the amount of time I spent on court, I would achieve my goal. This happened.

Since seeing my sports psychologist and using the course mapped out for me, I am proud to say that I have not lost or given away any match through a lack of effort of concentration. I must qualify that by saying that I have been beaten by a player striking the tennis ball too well for me on many occasions, but I can live with that. Tennis matches are once again a joy for me to play, because whoever I play, on whatever surface, in whatever country or conditions, I have the tools to get the best from myself every day. Furthermore, whether I win the match, or come off court on the wrong side of the scoreline, I know that I can beat my toughest opponent – myself. I know the meaning of "killer instinct" and being "mentally tough" and liken it to an old proverb... "one cannot control the wind, but in controlling one's reaction to it, one controls the wind".'

Chapter 20   In Attendance at a Sporting Event

Over the last few years, more and more osteopaths have become involved in the provision of an extremely effective service at various sporting events. Some do this on a regular basis, for example in American football and rugby while others attend tournaments, for example tennis and judo.

Many of the competitors may not be known to the attending osteopath and the organisation of follow up treatment is often difficult. It follows, therefore, that the task may well involve giving an 'immediate' type of treatment, rather than being able to carry out a course of treatment, which the athlete may well need.

It also follows that there will be several chronic type injuries which probably have not received the treatment they should, especially if the sport involves travelling around the world.

Acute injuries will occur sooner or later. It is therefore wise to hold a St John Ambulance First Aid at Work certificate, which has to be renewed every three years and should be kept up-to-date. Being reminded of first aid techniques is a good thing, especially the art of resuscitation, although we all hope we shall never be called upon to give it.

It is quite possible that the osteopath's attention may be needed for problems other than to the competitors, so the scope may be wider than anticipated. Officials often seem keen to receive attention, probably because it is there! They are also likely to have time readily available to attend for treatment during the course of their duties. Incidentally they can be a valuable source of patients to you or your colleagues as most will be resident in UK. They should be impressed by your professionalism.

20.1   Some helpful hints

Know your location

You will be on unfamiliar territory, quite different from the organised treatment room to which you are accustomed. You will most probably have to become an expert at compromise as the ideal set-up is unlikely to exist.

Arrive early and familiarise yourself with the geography of the event complex. You will need to know:

(a) the location of your treatment room

(b) the location of your wash room
(c) the location of the player's dressing rooms
(d) the location of the event organiser's office
(e) the location of the event schedule notice board
(f) the location of the players and their friends' relaxation area
(g) the location of the players practice/warm up area
(h) how to contact the tournament doctor
(i) what contact has been made with the local hospital
(j) the location of the dining room
(k) the location of the ice machine
(l) the availability of clean linen
(m) the location of any transport system
(n) the nearest telephone, both internal and external

Introduce yourself

Initially you will be unknown to competitors and organisers alike, a fact which is only overcome after many years attending a certain event.

Find the event organiser and the players or their representatives and make yourself known and your location for the duration of the event. Wear an easily read name badge.

Introduce yourself to players as they enter the room, even if you are extremely busy.

Case sheets

It is absolutely imperative to keep records of treatment given, even if you are really busy. Short notes on competitors – name, date and treatment given should suffice. It is extremely handy to be able to refer to the treatment you gave yesterday and so follow it logically today.

It is possible that case sheets might be needed in unlikely circumstances, for example an athlete defaulting, so be diligent here.

Organise your time

Obtain an order of play as soon as possible. This will give you some idea who is likely to attend for treatment and when. Priority must always be given to an athlete who is about to compete; one who has already done so can wait a bit, if necessary, or return later. Try to arrange your own meal time when it is unlikely that there will be great demand for your services, even though the hour may be strange for you to eat.

A different type of treatment

One of my young colleagues asked an experienced practitioner, somewhat tentatively, 'do you do anything special?'. 'No,' came the reply, 'heat before and ice after'. That sums it up in a nutshell as athletes need warming up before they compete and cooling down afterwards.

The warm up

The main object is to increase blood flow and stretch muscles and tendons. Joints should be freely mobile.

Stimulatory soft tissue is indicated. The use of a rubifacient may be necessary especially to any injured soft tissue, or to an old injury. Ultrasound may be needed. Strapping to support any injured area may be needed.

The athlete will carry out his own warm up regime and he should always be encouraged to do so diligently.

The cool down

Many athletes attend to aid their warm up, but fewer are interested in cooling down! If the event is of a knock out type, the losers are unlikely to want attention; they are often not willing to converse! Those attending at this time are likely to be suffering from an acute injury, so careful examination may be necessary. The others will be suffering from some chronic overuse injury. Both groups will need ice packs applied to the site of injury, to reduce the inflammatory changes. A good supply of freezer bags will be needed and a handy supply of ice. Reusable cold packs are available and can be used over and over again. They are particularly useful if there is no ready supply of ice. Instant cold packs are also on the market, but this is a very expensive way of providing ice treatment.

Strapping may also be needed to support an injury after competing. Relaxatory soft tissue treatment is indicated now.

The emergency bag

It is always possible that you will be called out to attend to an athlete during the course of a competition. The rules of the sport will dictate this and it is vital that you familiarise yourself with these. Some sports do not permit a competing athlete to be touched by anyone during the course of an event. Others lay down a time limit. However, it is always possible that you may have to give advice to a competing athlete or possibly supply him with some dressing or support for an injury.

An emergency bag should always be at hand for such an eventuality, containing dressings, strapping, scissors and instant ice spray and some rubifacient. You may even have to decide whether or not the athlete is fit to continue with the event. You may have to make a decision which the injured athlete does not like. You may even have to send him to a casualty unit for further investigation, but the golden rule is, if in doubt, never risk the future career of any athlete.

20.2

Contents of a sports kit

The exact contents and quantities will depend on the type of event, but this can be used as a possible guideline.

Portable treatment table and pillows (linen is usually available)
Antiseptic wipes
Airstrip plasters
Arnica − tincture of
Butterfly strapping
Callous pads
Chiropody felt
Contact lens solution
Cotton wool
Elastoplast 1″
Elastoplast 2″
Elastoplast 3″
Eye wash and an eye bath
Freezer bags and ties
Ice packs, instant
Ice packs, reusable
Instant ice spray
Kleenex tissues
Massage lotion
Massage oil
Safety pins
Scissors (take extra as they invariably walk!)
Second skin, small and large
Sporty bandage 25, 60 and 80
Surgical spirit
Tampons
Thermometer
Torch and batteries
Triangular bandages, 2
Tweezers, small

These should all be contained in a purpose made container. In addition you will need the emergency box mentioned previously.

20.3

Medication

The administration of medication is strictly speaking the job of the tournament doctor. It is unwise to give any proprietary preparation to any competitor, especially since there has been so much emphasis on the 'drugs in sport' issue.

Before the event it might be wise to check with the event organiser as to your exact position here. You may be required to carry medication for:

Pain
Sore throat
Cough
Cramp
Indigestion
Diarrhoea

If so, check with a doctor who is familiar with the drugs regulations before giving any product to a competing athlete.

Index

abdomen, 282−3, 301−20, 326
  muscle injuries, 309−10
abnormalities of musculoskeletal system, 1, 2, 6, 8, 34−45, 272, 317−19, 333
abrasions, 109, 129, 250
abscesses, 171, 214
accidents, 41, 43
  see also falling injuries
acetabulum, 35, 38, 137, 138, 166, 321, 329
ache, 63, 154, 155, 235, 313
Achilles tendon, 25, 33, 34, 54, 55, 61, 198−9, 214, 215, 217, 219, 234, 235
  injuries related to specific sports, 347, 357, 359, 362, 373, 374
acromioclavicular joint, 78, 79−80, 82, 86, 90, 94, 95−6, 97, 269, 298
acupuncture, 132, 136, 152
adenosine triphosphate (ATP), 28, 29
adhesions, 56, 57, 98, 99, 217
  see also scarring
age
  and general health, 17
  relation to injury, 24−6, 359, 366
  see also degenerative changes
alcohol, 62−3
American football, 340−1
analgesics, 315
angling, 341
ankle, 156, 181, 185, 186, 188, 195, 196, 207−220, 234
  bone injuries, 211−14
  bursitis, 219
  degenerative changes, 214
  epiphysitis and apophysitis, 214−15
  facet locking, 217−18
  injuries from individual sports, 340−79 passim
  joint and ligament injury, 215−17
  mobility injury, 218
  musculotendinous injury, 202
  skin injuries, 219−20
  snapping, 200
  sprain, 199, 203, 208, 215−17, 218, 235
  talocalcaneal joint, 209−11, 218
  tendon injury, 211

tenosynovitis, 200
  tibiotaloid joint, 207−9, 210, 216, 217−18
ankylosing spondylitis, 298−9, 334
anterior compartment syndrome, 33, 196
anti-inflammatory treatment, 56, 152, 177, 178, 204, 213, 251, 271
apophysitis, 175−6, 214−15
archery, 341−2
arm, 6, 268, 269, 272, 273, 275, 286, 287, 291
  see also elbow; hand
arnica, 46, 134, 173, 212, 292, 331
arteries, 70−2, 136, 195, 275
arthroscopic examination 98, 179, 215
articulation, 68, 117, 218, 235, 238, 273, 292, 298, 299, 315
aspiration, 109, 175, 178, 182, 216
ATP, 28, 29
avulsion
  hip tendons, 152, 154
  knee joint injury, 173, 175
  lumbar spine, 312
  neck, 271
  pelvic bones, 328
avulsion fractures, 239, 332, 353

back problems, 25, 348
  see also low back problems; spine
badminton, 367, 368
Baker's cyst, 182, 183
balance, 34, 343
  in muscular development, 293, 329, 330
  see also postural disorders
baseball, 342
basketball, 342−3
bed rest, 315
Bennett's fracture, 133, 344, 346
bleeding, 46, 48, 49, 50, 51, 68, 70−2, 243, 249
blisters, 47−8, 219, 242
blood analysis, 116
blood supply and bone tissue death, 62−4
blood tests, 8, 242
blood vessel injury, 70−2, 182, 205, 275
  see also individual areas
body temperature, 214

body type, 16−17, 26−7
bone scans, 196
bones
  abnormalities, 34−45, 272, 317−19, 333
  avascular necrosis, 62−4
  injuries to, 58−65; *see also individual areas*
bow legs, 41, 42
bowls, 343−4
boxing, 98, 133, 292, 344
brace, 178
breathing, 29−30, 54, 282−3, 286, 287, 288, 290, 291
bruising, 46, 51, 52, 109, 216, 234, 291
  of bone, 134, 173, 293, 331
bunion, 37, 241
burns, 46−7, 183
bursitis, 33, 70, 71
  see also individual areas

calcaneal exostosis, 43, 212−13
calcaneum *see* heel
calcium, 296
  deposits in muscle, 50−1
callouses, 48, 130, 226, 235, 237, 242
calorific intake, 15
canoeing, 131, 344−5
capsule injury, 68
cardiovascular system, 8, 18
carpal tunnel syndrome, 130, 136
carpometacarpal joint, 118−19
cartilages, 157, 161, 162, 178−9
case sheets, 387
catching injuries, 342, 343, 346
cauliflower ear, 250
central nervous system, 8, 244
cervical ribs, 35, 37, 130, 254, 272, 275
cervical spine, 136, 244, 253−76
  anatomy, 253−67
  blood vessel injury, 275
  disc injuries, 272−3
  injuries related to individual sports, 340−79
    passim
  joint and ligament injuries, 273−4
  muscle injury, 267−71
  nerve injury, 275−6
childbirth, 326, 333
children, 63, 117, 133, 154
  see also apophysitis; epiphysitis
chiropodist, 219, 237, 242, 243
chondromalacia patellae, 180, 354, 357, 370, 372
circuit training, 21

circulation
  improvement, 204, 205
  obstruction, 33, 99, 136, 275
claudication *see* limp
clavicle, 78, 79, 80, 82, 83, 85, 86, 87, 88, 90, 269, 282, 285−6
  injuries to, 43, 93, 96, 97, 100, 111, 294, 297−8, 365
clothing, 31, 197, 341
  see also protection
coccyx, 321, 324, 332−3, 334, 373
collar, 271, 273, 274
Colles' fracture, 133
compartment syndrome, 33, 196
complications of injuries, 33−4
compression, 178, 194
concentration, 383−5
concussion, 73−4, 249, 271
congenital abnormalities, 34−7, 272, 317−19
cooling down, 388
  see also warming up and down
corns, 242
corset, 312
corticosteroids, 62, 296
costochondral strain, 296
costosternal joint, 80−1
costotransverse joint, 80−1, 277, 278
costovertebral joint, 80−1, 277, 279
coughing, 273
cramp, 53−4, 204
cranium, 244, 250
crepitus, 57, 131, 195, 200, 234, 294, 299
cricket, 32, 152, 309, 345−6
crush injuries, 49
cuts, 129, 183
  see also lacerations
cycling, 136, 347−9
cysts, 50, 179, 180, 182, 183

Daljord, O.A., 356
Davis, Steve, 22
deficiencies, 15, 45, 296
degenerative changes
  ankle, 214
  elbow joint, 116
  foot, 238
  hip joint, 155
  knee joint, 181−2
  lumbar area, 315, 319, 378
  neck, 273, 274, 276
  thoracic area, 288, 290, 299

and weight lifting, 378
   wrist and hand, 135
   see also age
dehydration, 371
dermatomes, 10
diagnosis, 1, 7, 8
diaphragm, 281–3, 300
diet and fitness, 12, 15–16
disabled, 16
discus, 376
dislocation, 55, 57, 67
   elbow, 116
   foot, 211
   head and neck, 250–1, 274
   hip, 154–5
   shoulder, 34, 94–8
   sternoclavicular joint, 297
   wrist and hand, 134–5, 136
drugs, 13, 390
Dupuytren's contracture, 135

ear injury, 250
elbow, 88, 101–17, 133, 135
   bone injuries, 114–15
   bursitis, 109
   epiphysitis, 115
   extensors, 103–8
   flexors, 101–2, 104, 115, 130
   injuries from individual sports, 340–79 *passim*
   joint and ligament injuries, 115–17
   ligaments, 108–9
   mobility injuries, 117
   muscle and tendon injuries, 109–14
   nerve injuries, 108, 115
   skin injuries, 109
emergency bag, 388–9
emotional problems, 20
   see also psychological problems
endurance, 18, 22, 26
epiphysitis, 24, 43, 45, 60
   see also individual areas
equestrian sports, 328, 349–51
examination, 6–8, 33, 53
exercise
   effect on general health, 12, 22
   graduated muscular, 13, 18–21
   resumption after injury, 50
   see also training
exercises
   ankle, 215, 218–19
   foot, 234–5, 240, 241

hip, 155
   knee, 175, 178, 181, 182
   lower leg, 203
   spine, 290, 317
   temperomandibular joint, 251
   winged scapula, 292
exostosis, 43, 60, 134, 171, 212–13, 237, 239, 330, 376
extrinsic injuries, 13, 32, 33, 68, 150, 239, 291, 341, 346, 357, 360
eye, 250

facet locking, 69–70
   see also individual areas
falling injuries, 343, 350, 359, 360, 365, 372, 373
   ankle, 212
   elbow, 115, 117
   hip, 153
   knee, 173, 176
   neck, 271
   shoulder, 93–7 *passim*
   thoracic area, 291, 293, 294
   wrist and hand, 133, 135
fascial sheaths, 49–53
femur, 137, 138, 139, 145, 146, 148, 150, 157, 161, 164, 166, 167, 168, 170
   injuries, 153, 154, 155, 173, 174, 175, 177, 178, 181
fencing, 132, 152, 351–6
fever, 171
fibre, 15
fibula, 185–8 *passim*, 190, 192, 193, 199, 200, 203, 204, 212, 369
fingers, 127–9, 130, 132, 134
   see also Mallet finger
first aid, 386
fishing, 341
fitness, 12–14
   assessment of, 29
   see also exercise
flat feet *see* pes planus
fluid build up, 32, 33
foot, 6, 26, 34, 52–3, 59, 61, 166, 190, 195, 196, 197, 207, 210, 211
   anatomy of midfoot and forefoot, 221–33
   arches, 222–6, 227, 233, 234–8, 240
   bone injury, 238
   bursae, bursitis, 234, 237, 241
   callouses *see* callouses
   care of, 31
   degenerative changes, 238

facet locking, 238, 240
fractures, 239–40, 241
hindfoot *see* ankle
injuries from individual sports, 340–79 *passim*
metatarsal injuries, 238–40
metatarsophalangeal injuries, 240–2
muscle and tendon injuries of midfoot, 233–4
skin injuries, 242–3
football, 69, 152, 153, 333, 356–8
footwear, 31, 195, 198, 201, 213, 219, 234, 237, 239, 241, 242, 243
foraminal encroachment, 276, 315, 319
foraminal gapping, 315
forearm, 101, 121, 127, 128
forefoot *see* foot
foreign bodies, 130, 242
Fosbury flop, 362, 363
fractures, 10–11, 24–5, 58–9, 64
    accidental, 41, 43
    ankle, 212
    elbow joint, 114–15
    foot, 238, 239–40
    head and neck, 249, 250, 271
    hip and thigh, 153
    knee, 173–5, 180
    leg, 34, 195, 196, 203
    lumbar area, 312–13
    pelvis, 331–3
    rib, 293
    shoulder girdle, 93–4
    wrist and hand, 130, 133–4, 136
Freiberg's disease, 240
friction treatment, 54, 57
    ankle, 216, 217
    elbow, 111, 112
    foot, 237
    knee, 172, 177
    leg, 198
    pelvis, 330
    thumb, 133
    see also massage
frozen shoulder, 68, 98–9

Galway, Timothy, 381
ganglion, 132, 200
    cervical, 247
gastrocnemius, 34
General Council and Register of Osteopaths, 3
genu valgum, 41, 42
genu varum, 41, 42
glenohumeral joint, 77–8, 81–5, 88, 94

glenoid labrum, 98
golf, 113, 358
Golfer's elbow, 112, 113, 114, 358
gout, 57, 116, 117, 242
graduated muscular exercise, 13, 18–21
    see also weight training
grazes, 47, 48, 183, 206
greenstick fractures, 24
gripping injuries, 112, 344, 367
groin, 153, 154, 156, 171, 373
gymnastics, 218, 359

Haas, Robert, 15
haemarthrosis, 68, 178, 216
haematoma, 168, 249, 250
haematuria, 329
haemhorrages, 243
    see also bleeding
hallux *see* toes
hallux rigidus, 241
hallux valgus, 37, 241
hammer, 376
hammer toe, 242
hamstrings, 2, 34, 140, 141, 145, 146, 164, 169, 181, 317, 329, 330, 336, 378
    inflammation, 152–3, 156, 169, 171–2
hand
    anatomy, 128–9
    fall on the, 115, 117
    skin and muscle injuries, 129–30
    see also wrist and hand
Hatha yoga *see* yoga
head injuries, 248–52, 271
    from individual sports, 340–79 *passim*
    see also cervical spine; neck
head zones, 8–9, 10
headache, 274, 275
healing power of the body, 2
health, 1, 12–23
    definition, 12
Health Education Council, 21, 22
heat treatment, 51, 53
    lumbar pain, 319
    pelvic injury, 336
heel, 212–13, 214, 217, 219, 221–6 *passim*, 234, 237
    exostosis, 43, 212–13
hernia, 151, 283, 308, 309
herpes zoster, 299, 319
hiccoughs, 275
high jump, 212, 218, 291, 362

hindfoot *see* ankle
hip, 166, 183, 184, 325, 326, 331, 334, 337
    abduction, 139, 141, 143−6
    adduction, 139, 145−8
    anatomy, 137−50, 325, 326
    bone injuries, 153−4
    bursae, 139, 141, 143, 148, 150
    bursitis, 151, 155−6
    epiphysitis, 154
    extensor muscles, 139, 140−1
    flexor muscles, 139−40, 141, 142, 143
    injuries from individual sports, 340−79 *passim*
    ligament and joint injury, 154−5
    muscle injuries, 150−2
    musculotendinous injuries, 153
    neurological problems, 156
    referred pain, 156
    rotation, 139, 148−50
    tendon injuries, 152−3
hitting
    problems associated with, 342, 346, 360
hockey, 359−60
homoeopthic remedies, 220, 299
    see also arnica
hormonal changes in women, 326
horse riding, 328, 349−51
humero-ulnar joint, 101, 112
humeroradial joint, 101, 103, 105, 112
humerus, 101, 103, 105−8 *passim*, 120, 121, 291
    fracture, 93−4, 114
hurdling, 152, 361−2
hyperaemia, 239
hypermobility, 26, 34, 68, 99, 136, 270, 274,
        297−8, 316−17, 319, 336−7
hyperventilation, 204, 300

ice
    massage with, 202
    packs, 46, 47, 50, 67, 70, 151, 169, 172, 173,
        175, 176, 178, 180, 182, 194, 202, 212, 216,
        219, 251, 268, 291, 330, 331, 388
ice hockey, 360
ilium, 321−6 *passim*, 331
infection, 13, 45, 48, 50, 62
inferior radio-ulnar joint, 112, 118, 134
inferior tibiofibular joint, 185, 196, 209
infiltration, 33, 57, 68, 170, 182, 200, 201, 202,
        212
    see also injections
inflammation, 69−70, 172
    bone, 60−2

elbow, 115−16
    foot, 239, 241−2
    hamstrings, 152−3, 156, 169, 171−2
    hip and thigh, 152
    knee, 180
    shoulder, 99
    see also individual conditions
ingrowing toe nails, 243
injections, 100, 114, 131, 296, 330, 333, 337
    see also infiltration
injuries
    causes, 1, 13, 24−31
    classification of, 32−5
    related to various sports, 340−79 *see also
        individual sports*
interphalangeal joints
    foot, 231, 235
    hand, 120, 132
intertarsal joints *see* foot
intrinsic injuries, 32−3, 50, 90, 357
ischaemia, 33, 99, 136, 275

javelin, 375−6
joints, 64−5, 66
    examination, 6
    injury, 53, 67−70
    range of movement, 19−20
    restoration of mobility, 8
    sprain, 67
    see also individual joints
judo, 134, 360−1
jumping injuries, 212, 343, 361−3, 367

karate, 364−5
knee, 21, 41, 42, 65, 66, 69, 151, 154, 156,
        157−84, 203
    blood vessel injury, 182−3
    bone injuries, 173−5
    bursa, 158, 161−4, 165, 166, 182
    bursitis, 171, 172, 178, 182
    epiphysitis and apophysitis, 175−6
    extensors, 139
    facet locking, 181
    flexors, 141
    injuries from individual sports, 340−79 *passim*
    joint injuries, 178−80
    ligament injuries, 41, 65, 66, 69, 176−8
    mobility injury, 181−2
    muscle injuries, 168−70
    musculotendinus injuries, 172−3
    nerve injury, 183

patellofemoral joint, 157, 167−8, 180
referred pain, 183−4
skin injuries, 183
superior tibiofibular joint, 168, 185, 196, 209
tenderness, 165, 168, 169
tendon injuries, 170−2
knock-knees, 41, 42
Kohler's disease, 238
Korr, Irwin, 8, 247
kypholordotic curve, 38, 41
kyphosis, 43, 90, 274, 290−1, 295, 298

lacerations, 48−9
laminectomy, 319
landing injuries, 212, 217−18, 343, 366
leg, 1, 34, 234
    anatomy of lower leg, 185−94
    blood vessel injury, 205
    bone injuries, 202−3
    bursae, bursitis, 190, 201−2
    epiphysitis, 204
    fractures, 195, 196
    injuries from inidividual sports, 340−79
        passim
    mobility injuries, 204
    muscle injuries, 34, 194−8
    musculotendinous injuries, 202
    nerve injury, 196
    skin injury, 206
    tendon injury, 198−202
    see also hip; knee
lifestyle
    effect on fitness, 16
lifting, 111, 296, 309, 313
    weight *see* weight lifting
ligaments
    congenital abnormality, 34
    fitness, 30
    injuries, 21, 25, 26, 32, 65−8
    see also individual areas
limp, 63, 154, 155, 168, 205
Lister's tubercle, 376
locking of joints
    knee, 179−80
    tibiofibular, 209
    see also facet locking
long jump, 218, 362−4
loose bodies, 68−9, 116, 136, 155, 179, 180, 215
low back problems, 2, 45, 184, 313−15, 316,
    334, 335, 341, 348, 351, 358, 359, 368, 376,
    378

see also lumbar spine
lower leg *see* leg
lumbar spine, 150, 151, 156, 170, 183, 196, 214,
    244, 290, 301−20, 326
    bone injuries, 311−13
    congenital anomalies, 317−19
    disc injury, 313−17
    facet locking, 317
    injuries from individual sports, 340−79 *passim*
    joint and ligament injury, 316−17
    muscle injuries, 309−11
    nerve injury, 313−15, 317, 319
    tendon injury, 311
    stiffness, 319
lumbosacral joint, 36, 39, 40, 302, 317, 325,
    333−6 *passim*
lymph glands, 171, 214

Maehlum, S., 356
Mallet finger, 57, 58, 132, 346
manipulation, 96, 99
massage, 53, 336
    with ice, 202
    see also friction treatment
meals *see* diet
medication, 390
Medisplint, 112
meniscii *see* cartilages
mental factors in general health, 21−2
    see also psychological problems
metacarpophalangeal joints, 119, 129, 132
metatarsophalangeal joints, 231, 235, 240−2
midfoot *see* foot
mineral supplements, 15, 296
mobility
    injury, 70; *see also individual areas*
    loss, 69, 175; *see also* facet locking
    restoration, 8
Morton's metatarsalgia, 240
motor bike scrambling, 365
muscles, 28−30
    fibrotic changes, 53
    hypertonicity, 21, 92, 151, 152, 156, 180, 195,
        298
    injury, 32, 49−54, 378; *see also individual
        areas*
    spasm, 53−4, 69, 268, 270, 271, 273, 317, 331
musculoskeletal system, 1
    abnormality, 6
musculotendinous injury, 57−8
    see also individual areas

myositis ossificans, 50–1, 52, 111, 115, 169
myosynovitis, 195

neck, 133, 247, 253–76
  blood vessel injury, 275
  bone injuries, 271–2
  disc injuries, 272–3, 275
  facet locking, 272, 273, 274
  injuries related to various sports, 340–79
    passim
  joint and ligament injuries, 273–4
  muscle injuries, 6, 267–71
  nerve injuries, 269–70, 275–6
necrosis, 62–4, 133, 154
nerve injury, 72–5, 99, 100, 204
  see also individual areas
nervous system, 1, 8, 247
netball, 218, 365–6
neuralgic amyotrophy, 299–300
neuroma, 74–5, 240

oarsmen *see* rowing
observation of sports, 28, 340
occupation
  effect on fitness, 16
oedema, 8, 195
orthopaedic treatment, 63, 173, 203
  see also surgical treatment
orthotics, 217
os trigonum, 35, 61–2, 201, 217
Osgood-Schlatters disease, 24, 354, 355, 361
osteitis pubis, 333, 364
osteoarthritis, 41, 130, 155, 180, 215
osteochondritis, 24–5, 43, 45, 63–4, 238, 240
  pulling, 64, 65
  splitting, 64
osteochondritis dissecans, 179
osteoid osteoma, 173
osteomyelitis, 62, 155
osteopath
  attendance at sporting events, 386–90
  experience, 28
  observation of athletes, 28, 340
osteopathy, 1–11
  training, 3–5
osteophytosis, 319
osteoporosis, 295–6
overuse injuries, 25, 388
  ankle, 213
  arm, 269
  elbow, 115

femur, 153
hip, 151, 155
related to various sports, 354–6, 359, 366,
  374–5
wrist, 131–2
see also apophysitis; epiphysitis; shin splints;
  tendinitis

Paget's disease, 154, 214
pain
  ankle, 212–20 *passim*
  bone, 11, 60, 69
  bursitis, 70
  causes, 1, 2
  elbow, 112, 113, 115–16
  facet lock, 69
  fibrotic changes, 53
  foot, 61, 234, 237–43 *passim*
  groin, 153
  hip, 150–6 *passim*
  ischaemic, 33
  joint sprain, 67
  knee, 168–79, 182, 183–4
  leg, 1, 194–205 *passim*
  lowback and lumbar area, 45, 184, 309,
    311–20 *passim*, 334, 335, 348, 351, 376
  muscle, 50
  neck, 268–76
  on epiphyseal line, 60
  pelvis, 328–39
  referred *see* referred pain
  shoulder, 90–100 *passim*
  stress fractures, 59
  tendon, 57
  thoracic area, 291–300 *passim*
  wrist and hand, 130, 131, 133, 136
palpation, 6, 8
paraesthesia, 136, 240, 272, 275, 319
paralysis, 300
patella, 158, 166, 167, 170, 175, 181
  dislocation, 26, 34, 179–80
patello-femoral joint, 157, 167–8, 180
pathologies, 9–11, 45, 59–60, 100, 214
pelvis, 18, 19, 150, 151, 169, 170, 181, 196, 203,
  214, 321–39
  bone injuries, 331–3
  bursitis, 337
  facet locking, 335–6
  injuries related to individual sports, 340–79
    passim
  joint and ligament injuries, 333–4

mobility injury, 336−7
muscle injury, 328−9
musculotendinous injuries, 330−1
nerve involvement, 338−9
tendon injuries, 329−30
periostitis, 202, 211−12, 213, 237, 343, 362
Perthe's disease, 63, 153−4
pes cavus, 235−7, 242
pes planus, 194, 195, 234−5, 236
phlebitis, 205
physiotherapy, 237
pitching injuries, 342
plantar fasciitis, 237−8, 370
plaster, 199
poliomyelitis, 45
postural disorders, 237, 317
    see also balance
predisposition to injury, 34
pressure treatment for ganglion, 132, 200
prevention of injury, 30−1
    see also warming up and down
primary injury, 32−3
prognosis, 8, 24
protection, 329, 341, 342, 346, 351
protein, 15
psychological problems, 380−5
    of injury, 27−8
    see also emotional problems; mental factors
pulling osteochondritis, 64, 65

racket sports, 98, 99, 112, 309, 366−8
radial nerve, 130
radiocarpal joint, 118
radius, 101, 105−8 *passim*, 112, 115−18 *passim*,
    121, 122, 124, 125, 127, 133, 134
referees, 24
referred pain and symptoms, 8, 100, 154, 156,
    183−4, 214, 317, 339
Reiter's syndrome, 333, 334
relaxation, 22, 23
relaxatory treatment
    hip, 156
    shin splints, 195
respiration *see* breathing
rest, 22−3, 54, 56, 57, 59, 62, 63
    and fitness, 12
    elbow injury, 111
    epiphysitis, 60, 204
    foot injury, 238
    hip, 150, 152
    joint sprain, 67

knee joint injuries, 169−72
lower leg, 202, 203
lumbar injury, 316, 319
neck injuries, 268−70
pelvic injury, 153, 329, 332, 333
thoracic strains, 296
wrist injury, 131
retraining, 34
rheumatoid arthritis, 57, 116, 117, 135, 242
ribs, 99, 136, 263, 277−88, 291, 292, 296, 299,
    303, 304, 305
    cervical *see* cervical ribs
    injury, 89, 393−4
    lumbar, 318
rickets, 45
rider's strain, 151
rowing, 131, 135, 228, 368
rubifacients, 51, 53, 98, 169, 172, 197, 202, 268,
    292, 309
rugby, 25, 43, 368−9
running, 170, 195, 239, 240, 241, 369−71

sacralisation of lumbosacral joint, 36, 39, 318
sacro-iliac joints, 169, 183, 184, 321−6 *passim*,
    331, 334−7 *passim*
sacrococcygeal joint, 321, 324−5, 334
sacroilitis, 334, 336
sacrum, 321, 323−39
sailing, 371−2
St John Ambulance Association, 249
St John Ambulance First Aid at Work
    certificate, 386
salt deprivation, 204
scapula, 86, 101, 261, 263, 286, 287, 292
    injury, 93, 292, 294, 299
scapulohumeral rhythm, 81−9, 92, 96, 98, 99,
    100
scapulothoracic joint, 80, 82
scarring, 32, 46, 48, 50, 114, 169, 197, 309
    see also adhesions
Scheuermann's disease, 290, 295, 299, 313
Schmorl's nodes, 295
sciatic nerve, 21, 141, 150, 151, 156, 338
scoliosis, 2, 34, 35, 36, 41, 42, 43, 244, 293, 303
secondary injury, 33−4
Sever's disease, 214−15
sex
    related to injury, 26
    related to sport, 18
Sharp, Craig, 13
shin splints, 34−5, 195−6, 202−3, 367−8, 370

shingles, 299, 319
short wave diathermy, 50, 51
shot put, 376
shoulder, 76–100, 111, 133, 135, 136, 261, 269, 288, 291
  bone injury, 93–4
  bursae, bursitis, 77, 91, 100
  epiphysitis, 94
  injuries from individual sports, 340–79 *passim*
  joint and ligament injury, 34, 94–8
  joints *see individual joints*
  mobility injuries, 98–100
  muscles, 6, 53, 81–90
  musculotendinous junction injuries, 92–3
  nerve injury, 89
  referred pain, 100
  scapulohumeral rhythm, 81–9, 92, 96, 98, 99
  suprahumeral space, 78–9
  tendon injuries, 90–3, 100
skating, 372–3
skiing, 195, 373–4
skin injuries, 46–9; *see also individual areas*
sliding injuries, 342
slipped epiphysis, 60, 61
snapping ankle, 200
sneezing, 273
Spence second skin, 242
spinal curvature, 2, 37–41, 244, 290–1; *see also* kyphosis; scoliosis
spine, 1, 2, 21, 43, 99, 114, 135, 203, 244, 246, 331
  head zones, 8–9, 10
  muscle spasm, 53
  osteochondritis, 24–5
  see also cervical spine; lumbar spine; thoracic area
splinting, 57, 136
splitting osteochondritis, 64
spondylolisis, 312
spondylolisthesis, 35, 38, 312, 317, 346
spondylosis, 274
sporting events
  attendance of osteopath at, 386–90
sports
  attributes of, 13–14, 22
  injuries related to individual, 340–79 *passim*
  kit, 388–90
  rules, 24
  suitability of individual to, 13, 26–7, 34
sprains
  ankle *see under* ankle

joint, 67, 132, 134, 251
springing, 270, 312, 315, 331, 332
squash, 367, 368
stamina, 13, 18, 22, 26
stenosis, 319
sternoclavicular joint, 80, 82, 87, 94, 96, 269, 280
sternum, 278–80, 281, 283, 284, 288, 294
stiffness, 20, 51, 53, 62, 70
  ankle, 218
  elbow, 117
  knee, 181–2
  lower leg, 204
  lumbar area, 319
  pelvis, 336
  shoulder, 98–9
  thoracic area, 298
  wrist and hand, 135–6
Still, Andrew Taylor, 2
Stoddard, Alan, 43
strain
  elbow, 116
  foot, 241
  hand and wrist, 130, 134
  hip, 150–1
  knee, 170, 177–8
  ligament, 32
  lumbar spine, 312, 316
  thoracic area, 296
strapping, 56, 57, 67, 388
  ankle, 216, 219
  foot, 238, 239, 241
  knee, 176, 177, 180
  leg, 197, 199, 200, 201
  lumbar spine, 316
  rib, 294
  wrist and hand, 132, 134, 135
strength, 13, 18–19, 22, 26
stress, mental, 13, 20, 21–2
  and fitness, 13
stress, physical
  cause of intrinsic injury, 25, 32, 150
  following cartilage removal, 157
stress fractures, 18, 25, 26, 55, 59, 153, 203, 239, 359, 368, 370
stretching
  exercise to prevent injury, 20, 21, 22, 25, 30, 169, 197
  injury, 67–8, 69, 73, 116, 180, 309, 326; *see also individual areas*
  treatment of injury, 50, 53, 54, 56, 58, 135,

150, 152–3, 170, 172, 194, 199, 204, 215, 218, 235, 268, 292, 309, 330
subluxation of wrist and hand, 135, 136
Sudeck's atrophy, 218
Sunday Times, 12
superior radio-ulnar joint, 101, 105
superior tibiofibular joint, 168, 185, 196, 209
suppleness, 19–20, 22, 26 *see also* stretching
suprahumeral space, 78–9
surgical treatment, 50, 51, 52, 55, 56, 57, 58, 69
    ankle, 199, 213, 217
    foot, 240, 241
    elbow, 113
    knee, 171–82 *passim*
    lower leg, 196, 200, 201
    lumbar spine, 312, 315–16
    shoulder, 95, 99
    wrist and hand, 131, 132, 134, 135
    see also orthopaedic treatment
swelling from injuries, 52, 57, 58, 59, 62, 67, 68, 70
    ankle, 213, 214, 216, 218, 219
    arm, 275
    head and neck, 250, 273
    hip, 169, 172
    knee, 173–8 *passim*, 182
    lower leg, 194, 198–9, 202, 205
    pelvis, 332
    trigger finger, 132
    see also ganglion
swimming, 20, 214, 291, 315, 332, 374–5
    cramp, 54
sympathetic nervous system, 247
symphysis pubis, 323, 325, 333
symptoms, 6, 7, 8
synovial joints *see* joints
synovial membrane injury, 68
synovitis
    elbow, 115–16
    hip, 155
    knee, 178, 179

table tennis, 367
talocalcaneal joint, 209–11, 218
temperomandibular joint, 250–2
ten pin bowling, 344
tenderness, 53,
    ankle, 61, 213, 214, 218
    foot, 62, 237, 238, 240
    knee, 175, 176, 179, 180
    lower leg, 196, 198

    pelvis, 332
tendinitis, 32, 54–5, 90, 92, 131, 198
tendo Achilles *see* Achilles tendon
tendons, 25, 30, 34, 49–50, 54–7
    see also individual areas
tennis, 92–3, 269, 366–8
tennis elbow, 112, 113, 114, 367
tennis leg, 196–7, 366
tennis toe, 242–3, 368
tenosynovitis, 57, 131–2, 136, 200, 234, 368, 372, 379
tenseness of muscles, 21
tetanus, 49, 206
Texas College of Osteopathic Medicine, 8
thigh, 50, 51, 53, 154, 166, 184, 328, 330
    see also hip
thoracic area, 265, 269, 277–99
    bone injury, 293–6
    disc injury, 290
    facet locking, 296–7
    injuries from individual sports, 340–79 *passim*
    joint and ligament injury, 296
    mobility injury, 297
    muscle injury, 291–3
    nerve injury, 299
    spinal curves, 290–1
thrombosis, 205
throwing injuries, 98, 99, 134, 346, 361, 362, 366, 375–6
thumb, 108, 118, 124, 125, 126, 130–3 *passim*
tibia, 140, 143, 148, 157, 161, 164–8 *passim*, 184–94 *passim*, 207, 209
    injuries, 173–8 *passim*, 181, 195, 196, 202, 203, 204
tibiotaloid joint, 207–9, 210, 216, 217–18
Times, The, 13
tissues
    abnormality of, 6, 8
    fitness of, 28–31
    injuries to, 25, 46–75; *see also* individual
        areas
    palpation of, 6, 8
toes, 37, 188, 194, 195, 226, 231, 239, 241, 242
    muscles, 228–30
traction, 135, 179, 273, 315
training, osteopathic, 3–5
training, sports, 13, 23, 25, 340
    circuit, 21
    and muscles, 30
    resumption after injury, 28, 53
    weight, 377–8

see also exercise
treatment for injuries, 46–75, 388
  elbow, 109, 110–11, 112–15, 116, 117
  foot, 222, 234–43
  hand and wrist, 129–36
  hip, 150–56
  knee, 169–84
  lower leg, 194–206
  lumbar and abdominal area, 309, 311–20
  neck, 268–76
  pelvic area, 329–39
  shoulder, 89–90, 92–100 *passim*
trigger finger, 131, 132
tuberculosis, 62, 117
tumours, 173

ulna, 101, 105–8 *passim*, 112, 116, 118, 120,
    122, 127, 133
ulnar nerve, 72–3, 109, 272
ultrasound, 46, 50, 152, 169, 170, 176, 197, 309,
    330
unconsciousness, 249
uncovertebral joints, 258
upper arm muscles, 87–8, 115
urine tests, 8

varicose veins, 37, 182, 205
veins *see* blood vessels
verruca, 219–20, 242
vertebral column *see* spine
viscera, 329, 331
  pain, 100
visceral system, 1, 319–20
vitamin supplements, 15, 296
volleyball *see* basketball

Wade, Virginia, 28
warming up and down, 17, 30–1, 53, 204, 388
warmth *see* heat treatment
water sports, 329

weather conditions, 269, 341, 343, 345, 346, 366,
    368
weight distribution, 6, 203
weight lifting, 378–9
weight training, 377–8
  see also graduated muscular exercise
Wilson's sign, 179
wind surfing, 379
wobble board, 202, 215
women, 240, 275, 295–6, 326
work
  effect on fitness, 16
wrist and hand, 106, 108, 112, 113, 118–36
  anatomy, 118–29
  blood vessel injuries, 136
  bone injuries, 133–4
  epiphysitis, 134
  facet locking, 135
  injuries from individual sports, 340–79 *passim*
  joint and ligament injuries, 134–5
  mobility injury, 135–6
  musculotendinous injuries, 132–3
  nerve injuries, 136
  skin and muscle injuries, 129–30, 136
  tendon injuries, 131–2
wry neck, 263

X-rays, 8, 11, 34, 35, 51, 59, 60, 61, 62, 69
  ankle, 212, 214–17 *passim*
  elbow, 111, 113, 115
  foot, 238–41 *passim*
  head and neck, 271, 274, 276
  hip, 153, 154, 155
  knee, 171, 175, 176
  lower leg, 198, 201, 203
  lumbar area, 313
  shoulder, 90, 91, 93, 95
  thoracic area, 294, 295, 296, 298
  wrist and hand, 130, 132, 133, 135

yoga, 20, 21, 22, 299, 315

DATE DUE

DEC 0 4 2001		
DEC 0 6 2001		
DEC - 7 2005		
DEC 0 6 2005		
		Printed in USA